EMERGENCY
MEDICINE

National Medical Series for Independent Study

NMS
CLINCAL MANUALS

EMERGENCY
MEDICINE

Jonathan N. Adler, M.D.

Scott H. Plantz, M.D.

Dana A. Stearns, M.D.

William Gossman, M.D.

Joseph Stewart, M.D.

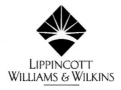

LIPPINCOTT
WILLIAMS & WILKINS

Acquisitions Editor: Elizabeth A. Nieginski
Development Editor: Melanie Cann
Senior Managing Editor: Amy G. Dinkel
Marketing Manager: Jennifer Conrad

Printed in the United States of America

First Edition, 1999

Library of Congress Cataloging-in-Publication Data

Emergency medicine / [edited by] Jonathan N. Adler . . . [et al.].
    p. cm.—(NMS clinical manuals)
  Includes index.
  ISBN 0-683-30349-X
  1. Emergency medicine—Handbooks, manuals, etc. I. Adler,
Jonathan. II. Series.
  RC86.7 .E578252 1999
  616.02'5--dc21
                                                                98-42719
                                                                    CIP

*The publishers have made every effort to trace the copyright holders for borrowed material. If they
have inadvertently overlooked any, they will be pleased to make the necessary arrangements at
the first opportunity.*

To purchase additional copies of this book, call our customer service department at **(800) 638-
0672** or fax orders to **(800) 447-8438.** For other book services, including chapter reprints and large
quantity sales, ask for the Special Sales department.

Canadian customers should call **(800) 665-1148,** or fax **(800) 665-0103.** For all other calls
originating outside of the United States, please call **(410) 528-4223** or fax us at **(410) 528-8550.**

99 00 01 02
2 3 4 5 6 7 8 9 10

EDITORS

Jonathan N. Adler, M.D., M.S., FACEP, FAAEM
Associate Program Director
Harvard Affiliated Emergency Medicine Residency
Assistant in Emergency Medicine
Massachusetts General Hospital
Instructor of Medicine
Harvard Medical School
Boston, Massachusetts

Scott H. Plantz, M.D., FAAEM
Assistant Professor of Emergency Medicine
Chicago Medical School
Department of Emergency Medicine
Mount Sinai Medical Center
Chicago, Illinois

Dana A. Stearns, M.D., FACEP
Instructor in Medicine
Harvard Medical School
Assistant Director of Undergraduate Medical Education
Department of Emergency Medicine
Massachusetts General Hospital
Boston, Massachusetts

William Gossman, M.D.
Assistant Professor of Emergency Medicine
Chicago Medical School
Project Medical Director
Mount Sinai Hospital Medical Center
Chicago, Illinois

Joseph Stewart, M.D.
Attending Physician
Department of Emergency Medicine
Augusta Regional Medical Center
Augusta, Georgia

DEDICATION

To my friend Scott—thanks for your unending dedication to this

project.

JNA

CONTENTS

1 **Cardiovascular Emergencies** 1
2 **Dermatologic Emergencies** 16
3 **Endocrinologic Emergencies** 32
4 **Environmental Emergencies** 38
5 **Gastrointestinal Emergencies** 49
6 **Gynecologic Emergencies** 61
7 **Head and Neck Emergencies** 70
8 **Hematologic/Oncologic Emergencies** 85
9 **Infectious Disease Emergencies** 93
10 **Metabolic Emergencies** 127
11 **Neurologic Emergencies** 133
12 **Obstetric Emergencies** 148
13 **Orthopedic Emergencies** 157
14 **Pediatric Emergencies** 168
15 **Psychiatric Emergencies** 181
16 **Pulmonary Emergencies** 186
17 **Rheumatologic/Allergic Emergencies** 194
18 **Toxicologic Emergencies** 198
19 **Trauma** 218
20 **Urogenital Emergencies** 243
21 **Wounds** 251

Appendix A: Advanced Cardiac Life Support (ACLS) Algorithms **259**

Appendix B: Radiographic Evaluation of Common Interventions **270**

Appendix C: Goldberg Acid-Base Map **272**

Appendix D: Common Medications **275**

Appendix E: Dermatomes **276**

CONTRIBUTORS

Bikram S. Dhillon, M.D.
Assistant Clinical Professor of Medicine
University of Illinois School of Medicine
Department of Emergency Medicine
Illinois Masonic Medical Center
Chicago, Illinois

Lance Kreplic, M.D.
Assistant Professor of Internal Medicine
University of Illinois School of Medicine
Research Director
Department of Emergency Medicine
Christ Medical Center
Oak Lawn, Illinois

Matthew A. Kopp, M.D.
Chicago Medical School

Ned Magabgab, M.D.
Assistant Professor of Emergency Medicine
Chicago Medical School
Director of Occupational Medicine
Department of Emergency Medicine
Mount Sinai Medical Center
Chicago, Illinois

Jack Stump, M.D., FAAEM
Attending Physician
Rogue Valley Medical Center
Medford, Oregon

Joan Surdukowski, M.D.
Assistant Professor of Emergency Medicine
University of Connecticut
Associate Director of Emergency Medicine
Director of Emergency Medical Services
Midstate Medical Center
Meridien, Connecticut

Stephen H. Thomas, M.D.
Instructor of Internal Medicine
Harvard Medical School
Associate Director of Boston Medflight
Department of Emergency Medicine
Massachusetts General Hospital
Boston, Massachusetts

Thomas Widell, M.D., FACEP
Assistant Professor of Emergency Medicine
Chicago Medical School
Director of Emergency Medical Services
Department of Emergency Medicine
Mount Sinai Medical Center
Chicago, Illinois

Les S. Zun, M.D., MBA, FACEP, FAAEM
Associate Professor of Emergency Medicine
Chicago Medical School
Chairman, Department
of Emergency Medicine
Mount Sinai Medical Center
Chicago, Illinois

PREFACE

Derived from the popular National Medical Series (NMS), *NMS Emergency Medicine Clinical Manual* is the first in a series of books intended to present need-to-know information in an easily retrievable format, with an emphasis on diagnosis and treatment. Designed to serve as an aid for the immediate management of patients in the emergency department, *NMS Emergency Medicine Clinical Manual* employs alphabetical organization (of chapters as well as the disease entities within each chapter) to speed information retrieval. A template has been developed to convey the salient points about each disease entity consistently and quickly:

KY **Key information:** Crucial facts concerning the entity

HX **Patient history:** Major symptoms and patient complaints

PX **Physical examination:** Major findings on physical examination

DD **Differential diagnosis:** Major differential diagnoses to consider

LB **Laboratory studies:** Studies to consider ordering and likely findings

IM **Imaging studies:** Studies to consider ordering and likely findings

TX **Therapy:** Appropriate options for management of the patient

DI **Disposition:** Appropriate follow-through for the patient

In addition, the book features several pragmatic figures for quick reference, including five advanced cardiac life support (ACLS) algorithms and an acetaminophen poisoning nomogram.

The highly condensed format of this book renders it impossible to thoroughly discuss all of the potential therapeutic strategies and diagnostic procedures, or the risks associated with each; however, an attempt has been made to avoid ambiguity. Readers working in an emergency department should have access to additional resources, including Emergency Physicians with extensive training in the discipline. The authors welcome comments and suggestions for future editions.

ACKNOWLEDGMENTS

The editors would like to thank the contributing authors and the staff at Lippincott Williams & Wilkins. Special thanks to Melanie Cann, Senior Development Editor at LWW, for her patience and professionalism.

CHAPTER 1

Cardiovascular Emergencies

ABDOMINAL AORTIC ANEURYSM (AAA)

HX Typically, the patient is an elderly man with severe, constant, lower abdominal and/or back pain that is not relieved by position; pain may be present in the lower back, scrotum, or perineum

PX Findings may include:

- Hypotension (suggestive of a severe leak or impending rupture)
- Unequal extremity pulses, abdominal tenderness in the suprapubic region with radiation to the lumbar area, and a pulsatile abdominal mass

DD • **If signs of shock:** hemorrhagic pancreatitis, perforated viscus, mesenteric infarction
- **If no signs of shock:** renal colic, diverticulitis, lumbar disk disease or compression fracture, small bowel obstruction, appendicitis, peritonitis

LB CBC, SMA-7, PT, PTT, T&C (10 U)

IM EKG, lateral abdominal radiograph (demonstrates a bulging calcified aorta), ED US (can diagnose an aneurysm but cannot determine if it is leaking), CT (diagnostic but can only be used in the stable patient)

TX • ABCs, supplemental O_2, monitoring
- Place two or more large-bore IV lines; maintain SBP at 90–100 mm Hg with IV fluids or blood transfusion; consider using MAST

DI • **Unstable patients:** OR for immediate surgery
- **"Stable" patients:** Surgical evaluation in the ED; consider ICU admission with evaluation for surgery

ACUTE AORTIC DISSECTION

HX Typically, the patient is an elderly man with a history of hypertension who experiences the sudden onset of severe chest pain with a "tearing" quality that radiates to the back

PX Rales, diastolic murmur of aortic insufficiency, differences in left and right or upper and lower extremity BPs and pulses, abdominal tenderness and/or pulsatile mass, neurologic deficits caused by compromised arterial supply, signs of CVA (if carotid arteries are involved) or myocardial ischemia (if coronary arteries are involved), and signs of pericardial tamponade

1

DD New-onset angina, stable or unstable angina, variant (Prinzmetal's) angina, MI, pericarditis, pericardial effusion or tamponade, pneumonia, pulmonary embolus, pneumothorax, chest wall pain, biliary disorders, GI disorders (e.g., gastritis, dyspepsia, peptic ulcer, esophagitis, esophageal spasm)

LB CBC, SMA-7, PT, PTT, T&C (6–8 U)

IM EKG, CXR (may show mediastinal widening, prominent ascending aorta, enlargement of the aortic knob, and/or pleural effusion), CT or aortography (if the patient is stable), transesophageal echocardiography (if available in the ED), bedside US (to check for pericardial effusion)

TX • **Supportive care:**
    ABCs, IV fluids, supplemental O$_2$, monitoring, ß Blocker (to lessen the force of contraction): esmolol (500 µg/kg IV over 1 minute, followed by infusion at a rate of 50 µg/kg/min) or propranolol (1 mg/min, to total of 10 mg)
    Nitroprusside (to lower SBP to 100–120 mm Hg): begin at 0.5 µg/kg/min IV; observe for organ perfusion and neurologic status; do not overshoot
• **Definitive therapy:**
    Daly (Stanford) type A (DeBakey I & II) requires immediate surgery
    Daly (Stanford) type B (DeBakey III) can be treated medically or surgically

DI ICU or OR

ACUTE MYOCARDIAL INFARCTION (AMI)

HX • Chest pain may be substernal, severe, steady, "squeezing," "heavy," "tight," or "pressure-like," often radiates to the left side of the jaw or shoulder, and is unrelieved by nitrates
• Associated symptoms include nausea, vomiting, dyspnea, diaphoresis, palpitations, weakness, and sense of impending doom

PX • **General:** Anxious, pale, or diaphoretic patient; precordial bulge, gallop, S$_3$, S$_4$, murmur, and JVD (suggestive of right-sided failure); rales (suggestive of left-sided failure)
• **Anterior MI:** Hypertension, tachycardia, bradycardia (if 2° AV block or complete heart block develops)
• **Inferior MI:** bradycardia (if the inferior wall is involved)

DD New-onset angina, stable or unstable angina, variant (Prinzmetal's) angina, aortic dissection, pericarditis, pneumonia, pulmonary embolus, pneumothorax, chest wall pain, biliary disorders, GI disorders (e.g., gastritis, dyspepsia, peptic ulcer, esophagitis, esophageal spasm)

Table 1.1 Location of Cardiac Ischemia or Infarction as Suggested by Findings in Various EKG Leads

Location of Ischemia or Infarct	Leads in Which Abnormalities Are Seen
Inferior wall	II, III, aVF
Lateral wall	I, aVL, V_5, V_6
Anterolateral region	V_1 to V_6, I, aVL
Anterior wall	V_1, V_2
Anteroseptal region	V_1 to V_4
Right ventricle	V_3R to V_6R
Posterior wall	V_1, V_2, V_7 to V_9

Reprinted with permission from Plantz SH, Adler JN: *NMS Emergency Medicine.* Baltimore, Williams & Wilkins, 1998, p 45.

LB
- Cardiac enzymes (CK-MB fraction elevates in 4 hours, peaks in 24 hours), troponin
- Pulse oximetry or ABG, CBC, SMA-7, LFTs prn

IM • **CXR**

ST segment elevations in leads II, III, and aVF (inferior wall); V_1–V_3 (anteroseptal); I, aVL, and V_4–V_6 (lateral); or V_1–V_6 (anterolateral)

ST segment depression in leads V_1–V_3 (posterior)

Nonspecific ST and T wave abnormalities in subendocardial MI

TX • **ABCs, IV fluids, supplemental O_2, monitoring, aspirin:** 160 mg PO (swallowed or chewed)
- **Thrombolytic therapy** should be provided within 30 minutes of ED presentation to all patients with AMI who do not have contraindications to such therapy (Table 1.2), and who present within 6 hours of the onset of symptoms and have ST segment elevation on EKG. Thrombolysis is a dangerous treatment and should only be initiated under the supervision of the ED attending physician. The choice of agent and dosing regimen for thrombolysis depends on local practice and current research; suggested guidelines are given in Table 1.3. Physicians should be prepared for hypotension and reperfusion arrhythmias following the administration of thrombolytic therapy.
- **Emergent angioplasty** may be considered (if readily available)
- **Adjunctive therapies** include:

  β **Blockers,** especially for tachycardia [e.g., metoprolol (5 mg IV q5min × 3)]

Table 1.2   Contraindications to Thrombolytic Therapy

Absolute	Relative
Suspected aortic dissection or pericarditis	CVA
CVA	Conditions placing the patient at high risk of intracardiac thrombus (e.g., atrial fibrillation, mitral valve stenosis)
Cerebrovascular surgery within the previous 2 months	
Cerebrovascular neoplasm or aneurysm	Major surgery within the previous 2 months
Active bleeding in the GI tract or other noncompressible site; hemorrhagic diathesis	Puncture of, or recent injury to, a noncompressible vessel within the previous 2 weeks
Major surgery within the previous 2 weeks	Uncontrolled hypertension
	Prolonged CPR
Pregnancy or 2 weeks postpartum status	Metastatic cancer
	History of GI bleeding
Allergy to thrombolytic agent	Hemorrhagic retinopathy
Unstable angina	

Reprinted with permission from Plantz SH, Adler JN: *NMS Emergency Medicine.* Baltimore, Williams & Wilkins, 1998, p. 48.

> **NTG:** SL or spray × 3 q5min while starting IVs; add NTG paste or initiate IV drip at a rate of 10–50 µg/min and titrate to pain and SBP
>
> **Magnesium sulfate** (consider if ventricular arrhythmia develops): 1–2 g IV
>
> **Anxiolytic** [e.g., alprazolam (0.25 mg PO)]
>
> **Heparin:** thrombolytic therapy protocol may dictate timing of heparin; common dosing is 5000 U IV load or 100 U/kg load and a 1000–1200 U/hr drip
>
> **Rescue angioplasty or CABG:** consult with a cardiologist

DI CCU

ARRHYTHMIAS

Asystole

KY Asystole is normally caused by profound myocardial injury that results in cardiac arrest. The outcome is usually fatal. Causes include MI, hypoxia, hyperkalemia, hypokalemia, acidosis, drug overdose, hypothermia, and trauma.

PX No heartbeat or pulse

DD Fine VF

Table 1.3   Suggested Regimens for Thrombolytic Therapy

Front-loaded tPA

1. Gently reconstitute two 50-mg vials with 50 ml diluent. Add both (100 mg, 100 ml) to 100 ml D_5W (0.5 mg/ml).
2. Start a dedicated IV line and use an infusion pump. Withdraw a 15-mg bolus (30 ml) from the bag and inject. (The initial bolus is often administered by the physician.)
3. Administer ASA (160 mg PO and start the infusion at a rate of 50 mg (100 ml) over 30 minutes, followed by 35 mg (70 ml) over the next 60 minutes. Dosing for patients < 65 kg is 1.25 mg/kg tPA given over 90 minutes (15% IV bolus administered by physician, 50% over 30 minutes, and 35% over the next 60 minutes).
4. Inject 20 ml NS into an empty IV bag at the end of the dose and infuse to ensure that all tPA is delivered.
5. Heparin may be administered during tPA infusion (100 U/kg as an IV bolus, followed by infusion at a rate of 1000–1200 U/hour).

Streptokinase

1. Withdraw 10 ml NS from a 250-ml NS bag, and reconstitute two 750,000-IU vials with 5 ml NS each. Add both reconstituted vials (1.5 MU) to the 250-ml bag (6000 IU/ml).
2. Start a dedicated IV line with an infusion pump.
3. Administer ASA (160 mg PO, swallowed or chewed) and infuse the streptokinase over 60 minutes.
4. Inject 20 ml NS into the empty IV bag at the end of the dose and infuse to ensure that all streptokinase is delivered.
5. Heparin is no longer clearly indicated after streptokinase infusion, but a dose of 12,500 U SQ q12hr may be considered.

Anistreplase

1. Reconstitute in 5 ml sterile water.
2. Infuse 30 U IV over 5 minutes.
3. Heparin is not indicated.

LB Chem-7 (if quickly available), ABG

IM No cardiac activity on EKG; must be confirmed in two leads

TX • ABCs, IV fluids, supplemental O_2, monitoring
- Consider immediate transcutaneous pacing
- Epinephrine: 1 mg IV push, repeat q3–5min (peds 0.01 mg/kg)
- Atropine: 1 mg IV, repeat q3–5min (peds 0.02 mg/kg) to a total of 0.04 mg/kg
- Consider transvenous pacing — *passes*

DI ICU

ATRIAL FIBRILLATION (AF)

KY AF, the most common arrhythmia, is frequently seen in elderly patients. In AF, multiple ectopic foci stimulate irregular ventricular responses. The engorged and poorly contracting left atrium predisposes to thrombus formation, emboli, and stroke. Causes include CAD, MI, CHF, cardiomyopathy, thyrotoxicosis, rheumatic heart disease, hypertension, alcohol ingestion, and pulmonary embolism.

HX • Long-standing arteriosclerotic heart disease (possibly asymptomatic)
  • Palpitations and skipped beats possibly accompanied by weakness and a feeling of faintness (in paroxysmal AF)

PX • Rhythm is irregularly regular, with a rate of 80–180 bpm (80–120 bpm in chronic AF)
  • Pulse deficit (i.e., some beats may not be transmitted to peripheral circulation)

DD Multifocal atrial tachycardia, supraventricular tachycardia, sinus tachycardia

LB Digitalis level, SMA-7, CBC

IM EKG shows small irregular baseline undulations accompanied by irregular QRS complexes and no clear P waves

TX Immediate therapy is not usually required if the heart rate is < 120 bpm. Therapeutic interventions may include:

  • **Anticoagulation therapy** should be considered for AF > 48–72 hours' duration prior to pharmacologic therapy or cardioversion
  • **ABCs, IV fluids, supplemental O₂, monitoring**
  • **β Blockers** (e.g., esmolol, metoprolol, propranolol) or **calcium channel blockers** (e.g., diltiazem, verapamil) for rate control; these two classes of drugs may cause hypotension
  • **Digoxin** (modify dose for patients already taking digoxin)
  • **Immediate cardioversion** after sedation for unstable patients (i.e., those with chest pain, dyspnea, hypotension, CHF, mental status changes, or cardiac ischemia): 100 J, increased to 200 J, 300 J, and 360 J as needed

DI Telemetry or CCU

Atrial flutter

KY Atrial flutter occurs when there is an ectopic focus originating from a small area in the atrium.

HX Heart palpitations, with or without other symptoms

PX Cardiac rate is usually about 150 bpm (2:1 block) or 75 bpm (4:1 block) and is usually regular; rate and rhythm may be irregular, alternating between 2:1 and 4:1 block

DD AF, heart block

LB Chem-7

IM • EKG shows characteristic "sawtooth" flutter waves with an atrial rate of 250–350/min
 • AV block is usually present (commonly 2:1, but 4:1 and alternating blocks are not uncommon)

TX • **ABCs, IV fluids, supplemental O$_2$, monitoring**
 • **β Blockers** or **calcium channel blockers** to control the rate (see Arrhythmias, Atrial Fibrillation)
 • **Cardioversion:** unstable patients can usually be converted with 50 J of synchronized energy, increased as needed

DI Telemetry or CCU

Bradyarrhythmias [sinus bradycardia, sinus arrest, 2° AV blocks (types I and II), 3° AV block]

HX Chest pain, shortness of breath, AMS; athlete

PX Heart rate < 60 bpm; may be regular or irregular; some patients (e.g., athletes) may have normal resting heart rates of < 60 bpm (treat the patient, not the monitor)

DD Normal resting heart rate, MI, drug toxicity, electrolyte abnormality

LB SMA-7, consider drug levels (e.g., digitalis)

IM EKG

TX Bradycardia algorithm (see Appendix A)

Paroxysmal supraventricular tachycardia (PSVT)

KY PSVT is characterized by a sudden increase in heart rate (usually to 140–200 bpm) and is caused by the impulse reentering the AV node. PSVT is seen in patients with accessory tracts that bypass part of the normal conducting system (e.g., Wolff-Parkinson-White syndrome). Other causes include mitral valve prolapse, hyperthyroidism, and atherosclerotic heart disease.

HX • Heart palpitations, sometimes accompanied by weakness, dizziness, or feeling faint
 • Patient may have a history of hyperthyroidism or atherosclerotic heart disease

PX Heart rate is 120–280 bpm (usually 160–200 bpm) and regular

DD Digitalis toxicity (i.e., PSVT with a 2:1 block), VT

LB SMA-7, digitalis level

IM EKG shows narrow-complex QRS without P waves; wide complexes may be apparent with aberrant conduction or retrograde reentrant conduction

TX • ABCs, IV fluids, supplemental O_2, monitoring
  • Appropriate vagal maneuvers (e.g., carotid massage)
  • Tachycardia algorithm (see Appendix A)

DI Stable patients without a dangerous underlying cause for the PSVT who respond well to treatment can usually be discharged; others require admission, often to telemetry

Premature ventricular contractions (PVCs)

KY PVCs are caused by one or more ectopic foci in the ventricle. They are exacerbated by ischemia, electrolyte abnormalities, digoxin toxicity, and sympathomimetic drugs.

HX Chest pain, palpitations, sensation of irregular heart beat

PX Rhythm is irregularly irregular, or regularly irregular if in bigeminy or trigeminy

DD PACs

LB SMA-7

IM EKG shows a wide QRS complex with no P wave and a deflection opposite the normal QRS

TX No treatment is usually necessary unless PVCs are frequent (> 6/min), multifocal, or occurring in runs. In the setting of myocardial ischemia or MI with these criteria, administer lidocaine (1 mg/kg as an IV bolus and 2–3 mg/min as an IV drip). Consider magnesium sulfate in the setting of MI.

DI Telemetry or ICU

Pulseless electrical activity (PEA)

KY PEA is a common arrest rhythm. The electrical activity of the heart is insufficient to cause muscle contraction. Outcome is poor unless a reversible cause can be identified and treated. Reversible causes include hypovolemia from hemorrhage, hypoxia, cardiac tamponade, tension pneumothorax, hypothermia, massive pulmonary embolism, drug overdose, hyperkalemia, and acidosis.

PX • No pulse is present, but an impulse is seen on the cardiac monitor
   • Signs of reversible causes

LB SMA-7, CBC, ABG

IM Cardiac rhythm is present on the monitor

TX PEA algorithm (see Appendix A)

DI ICU

Ventricular fibrillation (VF)

KY VF is the most common cause of cardiac arrest. Electrical activity of the heart is chaotic, and no heart beat is present. Causes include severe ischemia, heart disease, and AMI.

HX Ischemic heart disease or MI

PX No pulse

DD Asystole

LB Consider SMA-7, ABG, drug screen

IM EKG shows irregular waves in more than one lead

TX VF/VT algorithm (see Appendix A)

DI ICU

Ventricular tachycardia (VT)

KY VT is defined as three or more consecutive PVCs from an ectopic focus in the ventricle, at a rate > 100 bpm. There are two types of VT— "stable," in which the patient has a pulse, and "unstable" or "pulseless." VT causing symptomatic cardiac ischemia or pulmonary edema is considered unstable. Causes include MI, hypertrophic cardiomyopathy, drug toxicity, hypoxia, alkalosis, and electrolyte abnormalities.

HX VT usually occurs in the setting of severe ischemic heart disease or MI

PX Rhythm is regular; rate is 150–200 bpm

LB Consider SMA-7, ABG, drug screen

IM • **Typical VT:** EKG shows wide QRS complexes in a sustained manner or in short bursts, a heart rate > 100 bpm, a regular rhythm, and a (usually constant) QRS axis

- **Atypical VT (torsade de pointes):** EKG shows gradual alteration in amplitude and direction of electrical activity

TX • VF/VT algorithm (see Appendix A)
- Atypical VT: magnesium sulfate (2 g IV over 2 minutes, followed by 1 g/hr IV), followed by transcutaneous "overdrive" pacing or isoproterenol

DI CCU

CHEST PAIN

HX • **Elicit description of pain:** character, location, radiation, duration, onset (sudden or gradual), precipitating events, associated symptoms, aggravating and alleviating factors, timing of previous episodes
- **Obtain PMH:** previous CAD or MI, significant medications, diabetes, smoking, elevated cholesterol, alcohol or drug abuse (including cocaine), or a significant family history

PX See differential diagnosis for specific findings

DD Table 1.4 gives the typical clinical picture for the major causes of chest pain; other causes include valvular disease, pleurisy, esophagitis, hiatal hernia, peptic ulcer, costochondritis, and radiculitis.

LB CBC, SMA-7, cardiac enzymes, pulse oximetry or ABG

IM EKG, CXR (Table 1.5)

TX • ABCs, IV fluids, supplemental O_2, monitoring
- Treat underlying cause

DI • Patients with minor causes of chest pain (e.g., costochondritis, uncomplicated pneumonia in an otherwise healthy person): discharge
- All other patients: admission to ICU/CCU, telemetry, or surgery

CONGESTIVE HEART FAILURE (CHF)

HX Dyspnea, PND, orthopnea, nocturia, edema, chest pain, previous cardiac disease

PX Respiratory distress, tachycardia, tachypnea, hypotension, JVD, hepatojugular reflux, rales, murmurs, pulsatile liver, cyanosis

DD • Constrictive pericarditis, cardiac tamponade, MI, pulmonary embolism, COPD
- Acute left ventricular dysfunction (caused by tachyarrhythmia, bradyarrhythmia, or AMI)

Table 1.4   Clinical Features of the Common Causes of Chest Pain

Cause	History	Physical Examination
Pulmonary embolism	Sudden pleuritic pain accompanied by dyspnea, with a history of risk factors (e.g., immobilization, leg pain and swelling)	Tachypnea, tachycardia, and edema in the thigh or calf
MI	Sudden substernal or precordial, dull, tight, or pressure-like pain that radiates to the neck, jaw, or arms, is unrelieved by NTG, lasts more than 30 minutes, and is accompanied by nausea, vomiting, and diaphoresis	Signs of shock, arrhythmias, paradoxical splitting of S_2, gallops, and murmurs
Unstable angina	Chest pain that increases in severity or frequency, or that is precipitated by minimal exertion, or a first episode of squeezing pain occurring at rest, lasting less than 30 minutes and unrelieved by NTG	Anxious appearance, diaphoresis
Acute aortic dissection	Sudden, excruciating retrosternal pain that radiates to the back, accompanied by a history of hypertension	Differences in pulses in arms and legs, hemiparesis, pulsatile mass
Pneumonia	Gradual pleuritic pain with productive cough accompanied by fever	Rales and consolidation on physical examination
Pneumothorax	Sudden onset of sharp pleuritic pain in young, slender patients or patients with COPD	Decreased breath sounds on one side
Acute pericarditis	Gradual pleuritic retrosternal pain that is relieved by leaning forward and is accompanied by fever	Distant heart sounds and friction rub

- Chronic left ventricular dysfunction (caused by chronic fluid overload as seen in valvular heart disease)

LB Pulse oximetry, ABG, CBC, SMA-7, CPK with isoenzymes, sputum for Gram stain and C&S

Table 1.5   Radiographic Findings in Patients with Chest Pain

Cause of Chest Pain	Findings on CXR
Pneumothorax	Air in pleural space
Pneumonia	Lung infiltrates
MI	Pulmonary congestion or edema (if accompanied by heart failure)
Dissecting aneurysm	Widened mediastinum; occasionally globular heart from pericardial effusion and pleural effusion
Pulmonary embolism	Elevated hemidiaphragm; rarely Hampton's hump or Westermark's sign

IM CXR, EKG

TX • **ABCs, IV fluids, supplemental O$_2$, monitoring**
  • **Mechanical ventilation:** CPAP may help avoid intubation; PEEP if patient requires intubation
  • **Keep patient upright** if possible
  • **Place Foley catheter** for monitoring I/Os; IV to keep open
  • **Anticipate BP drop** as patient's failure improves
  • **Medications**
      Furosemide: 10–80 mg IV over 1–2 minutes q30min, may repeat several times, double dose each time if there is no response
      NTG: spray or SL × 3, while monitoring BP; then NTG paste or IV titrated to effect and BP
      Morphine sulfate: 1–4 mg IV, repeat q5–10min for effect
      Digoxin (if AF): loading dose 0.25–0.5 mg IV, followed by 0.25 mg IV q6hr to a total dose of 1.0 mg (8–12 µg/kg lean body weight; 6–10 µg/kg in patients with renal failure)
      Dobutamine (2.5–10 µg/kg/min) or **dopamine** (1–20 µg/kg/min): titrate for urine output and BP
      Bronchodilators: albuterol or metaproterenol, 2.5 mg in NaCl nebul q30–60min
      Nitroprusside: for hypertension, 0.1–10 µg/kg/min IV, increase by 5 µg/min to a maximum dose of 400 µg/min

DI • **Patients with new-onset CHF** or pulmonary edema: admission to the ICU (if the patient has evidence of pulmonary edema) or a medical floor (with appropriate monitors) if the patient is improved and stable after ED management
  • **Patients with chronic CHF** and a mild worsening of symptoms who respond to IV diuretics: discharge following adjustments in the chronic drug regimen, consultation with the patient's physician, and assurance of follow-up within 24–48 hours

HYPERTENSIVE EMERGENCIES

HX Headache, nausea, vomiting, visual disturbances, chest pain, shortness of breath, orthopnea, confusion, stupor, or abdominal pain

PX • Sustained elevated BP (SBP > 140 mm Hg or DBP > 90 mm Hg)
• Signs reflective of end-organ damage [e.g., neurologic deficits (e.g., seizure, coma), fundal abnormalities, acute renal failure]
• Rales, pulmonary edema, dyspnea
• Murmurs
• Signs of hemorrhage, thrombosis, or embolus

DD AMI, CHF, thoracic aortic dissection, coarctation of the aorta, renovascular disease, primary aldosteronism

LB CBC, SMA-7, UA

IM EKG, CXR, head CT

TX • **ABCs, IV fluids, supplemental O_2, monitoring**
• **Antihypertensives:** lower symptomatic BP or asymptomatic BP of 220/120 mm Hg with one of the following drugs (specific disease state recommendations are given in Table 1.6):
  Labetalol: 20–30 mg IV, double dose q30min until adequate response or 300 mg given (infuse at 0.5–2.0 mg/min)
  Nitroprusside: infuse 0.3–10 μg/kg/min (avoid in pregnancy)
  Hydralazine: 5–15 mg administered as an IV bolus
  NTG: infuse 5–100 μg/min
  Phentolamine: 5–10 mg as IV bolus q5–15min

DI • Uncomplicated hypertension: home (follow-up within 1 week)

Table 1.6 Therapeutic Recommendations for Specific Disease States in Hypertensive Emergency

Disease State	Recommended Agents
Hypertensive encephalopathy	Nitroprusside or labetalol
CNS events	Nitroprusside
Myocardial ischemia	NTG, labetalol, or nifedipine
CHF	Nitroprusside or NTG
Eclampsia/preeclampsia	Hydralazine or magnesium
Interaction between MAO inhibitor and food or another drug	Phentolamine or labetalol
Antihypertensive withdrawal	Labetalol or nitroprusside
Renal failure	Nitroprusside or labetalol
Cocaine	Benzodiazepine
AAA	Nitroprusside, ± labetalol

- Hypertensive urgency: home with oral medication if treated in ED (follow-up within 1 week)
- Hypertensive emergency (e.g., stroke, dissecting aortic aneurysm, acute pulmonary edema or CHF, hypertensive encephalopathy, acute myocardial ischemia, eclampsia): ICU

PULMONARY EMBOLISM

HX • Risk factors include prolonged bed rest or travel, elderly patient, CHF, carcinoma, CVA, pregnancy, oral contraceptive use, postoperative status, leg trauma, obesity
- Patients often present with anxiety, chest pain, dyspnea, agitation, hemoptysis, and syncope

PX Tachycardia, tachypnea, low-grade fever, hypotension, rales, rub, decreased breath sounds, and evidence of phlebitis or DVT

DD MI, angina, pneumonia, pleural effusion, pneumothorax, musculoskeletal chest pain, pleurisy, pericarditis

LB • **Baseline labs,** including PT and PTT; consider D-dimer
- **ABG:** hypoxia (90% of patients have $Po_2 < 80$ mm Hg), decreased Pco_2, alkalosis, A-a gradient may be normal in 5%–50% of patients

IM • **CXR:** usually abnormal; nonspecific abnormalities may include elevated hemidiaphragm, infiltrate, or small pleural effusion
- **EKG:** Normal (15%), tachycardia and nonspecific ST-T wave changes most common, $S_1Q_3T_3$ pattern (12%), incomplete right BBB
- **V̇/Q̇ scan:** multiple segmental or lobar perfusion defects with normal ventilation; a normal scan excludes pulmonary embolism; patients with low and intermediate probability scans often require pulmonary arteriography to confirm the diagnosis
- **Doppler studies:** if diagnosis is suspected but not confirmed by V̇/Q̇ scan, Doppler studies of the lower extremities may be indicated
- **Pulmonary angiography:** intraluminal filling defects and/or arterial cutoffs suggest pulmonary embolism

TX • **Manage airway** and maintain adequate oxygenation with supplemental O_2
- **Manage pain** as needed
- **Heparin:** 5000- to 10,000-U bolus followed by continuous IV infusion at a rate of 1000 U/hr; patients with a high probability V̇/Q̇ scan require immediate anticoagulation
- **Stat thoracic surgery consult** for consideration of embolectomy; thrombolysis or embolectomy is necessary if hypotension is present

(requiring vasopressors) in a patient with angiographically documented pulmonary embolism
- **Thrombolytic therapy** with tPA (100 mg over 2 hours), streptokinase (250,000 IU load over 30 minutes followed by 100,000 U/hr × 24 hours), or urokinase (4400 IU/kg load over 10 minutes, followed by 4400 IU/kg/hr × 12–24 hours)

DI ICU or CCU for patients with suspected or documented pulmonary embolism, if necessary

SYNCOPE

HX Ask about events immediately preceding the episode:
- Associated symptoms (e.g., chest pain, palpitations, prodrome, dyspnea, headache, incontinence)
- History of cardiac, pulmonary, or endocrine disease, or a prior history of syncope or seizure disorder

PX
- **Evaluate vital signs** and check for orthostatic hypotension
- **Perform a cardiovascular examination** (carotid bruits suggest cerebral ischemia)
- **Evaluate neurologic status,** including mental status, sensory and motor function, reflexes, and cerebellar signs (pinpoint or dilated pupils may suggest a "toxidrome")
- **Heme check stools**

DD
- Common causes of syncope include vasovagal syncope (a diagnosis of exclusion), hypoglycemia, arrhythmia, and drugs; less common causes include oxygen deficit (as a result of COPD, anemia, pulmonary embolism, or CO poisoning), cardiac disease (valvular disease or ischemia), CVA or TIA (mostly vertebrobasilar), CNS infection or sepsis, hyperventilation syndrome, and GI hemorrhage

LB Finger-stick glucose, CBC, SMA-7, T&C, drug screen, pulse oximetry; consider ABG

IM EKG and CXR; CT if neurologic cause is suspected

TX As indicated by findings and/or test results

DI
- Patients with syncope as a result of seizure, vasovagal episode, corrected hypovolemia, or hypoglycemia who improve in the ED and have no complications can usually be safely discharged
- Patients, especially elderly patients, with syncope caused by arrhythmia, valvular disease, CVA, SAH, pulmonary embolism, aortic dissection, MI, or in whom the cause is unclear should be admitted to a monitored bed

CHAPTER 2

Dermatologic Emergencies

BACTERIAL SKIN INFECTIONS

Cutaneous abscess

KY Localized induration and fluctuance occurs as a result of inflammation of the soft tissue and accumulation of pus.

HX Swelling, redness, tenderness, throbbing pain, and fever

PX
- **Folliculitis:** infected hair follicles
- **Furuncle:** infection of dermal gland with erythema, induration, and tenderness
- **Carbuncle:** large abscess in neck, back, or thigh with pain and fever
- **Anorectal abscess:** localized induration, fluctuance, and inflammation near the rectum or anus
- **Cellulitis:** warm, tender, erythematous skin, usually with smooth border

DD Carcinoma, tumors, syphilis, tuberculous ulceration

TX
- **Folliculitis:** topical antibiotics and cleansing
- **Furuncle, carbuncle, anorectal abscess:** local heat and I&D
- **Cellulitis:** consider antibiotics in special circumstances (e.g., diabetes, immunocompromise)

DI
- Usually home, except perhaps operative admission for patients with anorectal abscess with fistula
- Admission if signs of sepsis are present or if patients have diabetes or are immunocompromised

Impetigo

KY This infection by *Staphylococcus aureus* or GABHS is common in children, usually in the summer. *S. aureus* causes the bullous form. Complications include glomerulonephritis ($\leq 1\%$) but not rheumatic fever.

HX Fever (rarely)

PX Painful lesions on face, buttocks, and extremities, which begin as papules and vesicles that develop into honey-colored crusts. Flaccid bullae define the bullous form.

DD Herpes, tinea, scabies, contact dermatitis

LB Consider CBC and blood culture

TX Antibiotics (do not prevent glomerulonephritis); appropriate regimens include:

- Cloxacillin: 50–100 mg/kg/day qid × 10 days or
- Erythromycin: 40 mg/kg/day qid × 10 days or
- Cefaclor: 20 mg/kg/day tid × 10 days

DI Home

Meningococcemia

KY Without prompt diagnosis and treatment, meningococcemia may lead to shock and death in hours. This disease usually occurs in late winter and early spring. Meningitis develops in 50% of cases.

HX Fever, headache, malaise, myalgias, arthralgias, rash, and AMS

PX Maculopapular tender lesions; ecchymosis and purpura, which indicate DIC and shock (mucous membranes involved); AMS; focal neurologic signs; tachycardia; tachypnea; hypotension; cyanosis; petechiae; and arthritis

DD Sepsis, Rocky Mountain spotted fever, Henoch-Schöenlein purpura, gonococcemia, endocarditis, HUS, influenza

LB CBC, PT, PTT, fibrin split products, fibrinogen, SMA-7, ABG, cultures, LP; expect thrombocytopenia, lactic acidosis, prolonged PT and PTT, low fibrinogen, elevated FDPs

IM CXR; consider brain CT and LP

TX
- **Penicillin G:** 24 MU/day IV q2–4hr (peds: penicillin G 250,000 U/kg/day IV q2–4hr up to 20 MU or ampicillin 200–400 mg/kg/day IV qid)
- **Penicillin-allergic patients:** chloramphenicol; cefuroxime; or cefamandole, cefotaxime, ceftizoxime, or ceftriaxone
- **Inotropic support and IV fluids:** steroids and heparin are controversial
- **Prophylaxis:** rifampin for household, nursery, and day care contacts or for individuals in contact with oral secretions: 600 mg q9–12hr × 8 (peds 10 mg/kg q9–12hr × 8)

DI ICU

Rocky Mountain spotted fever

KY This condition is caused by *Rickettsia rickettsii*, which is transmitted by female ticks [*Dermacentor variabilis* (dog tick) in the southeastern

United States; *D. andersoni* (wood tick) in the western United States]. The overall mortality (including with treatment) is ≤ 5%.

HX Abrupt high fever, headache, nausea, myalgias, and rash on second through fourth digits

PX • Red macules that blanch on wrists and ankles, which spread to trunk and face and become petechial lesions on palms and soles
 • Splenomegaly

DD Drug eruptions, infectious mononucleosis, rubeola, *Mycoplasma,* roseola, enteroviruses, erythema infectiosum, erythema multiforme, anaphylactoid purpura, meningococcemia, gonococcemia

LB Weil-Felix test, CBC, SMA-7, blood culture

IM Consider CXR

TX • Tetracycline for adults and children > 9 years of age × 4 days (until afebrile)
 • If patient appears seriously ill, use chloramphenicol: 100 g/kg/day q6hr up to 3 g/day

DI Usually home

Scarlet fever

KY Scarlet fever, a disease of children, leads to a sore throat and rash. The etiologic agent is GABHS. Complications include glomerulonephritis, rheumatic fever, pneumonia, otitis, and lymph node infection.

HX Fever, sore throat, and malaise followed in 12–24 hours by rash

PX • Papular, paper-like eruptions in hyperemic base on chest; pinhead-sized lesions
 • Injected pharynx, petechiae on palate (red "strawberry tongue"), desquamation
 • Circumoral pallor
 • Pastia's lines in antecubital area

DD Rubeola, rubella, infectious mononucleosis, roseola, syphilis, TSS, SSSS, Kawasaki syndrome, drug hypersensitivity

LB Throat culture

LB Consider CXR

TX • Penicillin VK: 250 mg PO qid × 10 days (peds 25–50 mg/kg/day PO qid × 10 days) or
 • Erythromycin: 250 mg PO qid × 10 days (peds 40 g/kg/day PO qid × 10 days) or
 • Penicillin G: 1.2 MU IM (peds 600,000 U IM)

DI Home

DERMATITIDES

Contact dermatitis

KY This cutaneous reaction to an external surface may be immediate or delayed.

HX Exposure to soaps, perfume, plants, nickel, chemicals, and detergents

PX Erythema, papules, vesicles, pruritus, and eyelid and genital swelling

TX • Topical corticosteroids and oral antihistamines
  • Severe cases: prednisone (40–60 mg PO qid × 7 days)

DI Home

Rhus (Toxicodendron) dermatitis

KY Etiologic agents are plants of the genus *Rhus*. Poison sumac has 7–13 leaflets per leaf, and poison ivy and poison oak have U- or V-shaped leaves with three leaflets. The rash is spread by clothes, animals, and fingernails; the blister fluid does *not* contain allergens.

HX Exposure to *Rhus;* the rash occurs 1–10 days postexposure

PX Erythema, pruritus, papulovesicles in a linear pattern, vesicles, and bullae

DD Herpes simplex, bullous pemphigoid, seborrheic dermatitis, atopic dermatitis, nummular eczema, lichen simplex chronicus, xerosis, stasis dermatitis

TX • **Mild cases:** calamine or steroid creams, oral antihistamines for pruritus
  • **Severe cases, with larger surface area involvement:** Domeboro compresses tid, potassium permanganate baths, and oral antihistamines. Consider oral prednisone (usually given for long course): 40–60 mg per day tapered over 2–3 weeks

DI Home

Seborrheic dermatitis

KY This chronic, superficial, inflammatory condition, which is most common in men and adolescents, affects the hairy regions of the body, usually the eyebrows, face, and scalp. The disorder occurs as a result of sebaceous gland dysfunction.

HX Minimal pruritus, waxing and waning symptoms, bilateral and symmetrical

PX Erythema, greasy yellow scales on the scalp, face, axilla, groin, buttocks, and body folds; possible excoriation

DD Tinea, dandruff, atopic dermatitis, eczema, rosacea, lupus, psoriasis

TX Shampoo with coal tar, sulfur, or salicylic acid; face may be treated with hydrocortisone 1% cream bid

DI Home

ERYTHEMA NODOSUM

KY The multiple, bilateral, cutaneous lesions initially begin as erythematous nodules and become bruise-like areas. Inflammatory eruptions are nonulcerating and nonscarring. Etiologic factors include oral contraceptives, collagen vascular disease, and infections.

HX The typical patient is a woman 20–40 years of age who complains of fever, malaise, chills, and arthralgias

PX Raised, warm, tender, brightly erythematous nodules located on anterior shins and extensor surfaces of the thighs and forearms; hilar adenopathy; episcleral lesions (diameter: 1–15 cm)

DD Superficial thrombophlebitis, cellulitis, septic emboli, erythema induratum, nodular vasculitis, cutaneous polyarteritis nodosa, lymphoma, sarcoidosis granulomata

LB ESR (elevated), CBC, throat culture, stool culture, skin test for mycobacteria (if indicated)

TX
- Bed rest, leg elevation, elastic stockings, and aspirin (600 mg PO q4hr) or indomethacin (75–150 mg/day tid)
- Resolution in 3–8 weeks
- If pain is severe, potassium iodide: 400–900 mg qd bid–tid × 3–4 weeks
- Corticosteroids are necessary for severe, refractory cases

DI Outpatient management

FUNGAL INFECTIONS

Candidiasis

KY *Candida albicans* causes a variety of infections. Cutaneous manifestations include folliculitis, blastomycetica, erosio interdigitalis, balanitis, intertrigo, paronychia, onychomycosis, diaper rash, perianal candidiasis, esophagitis, vaginitis, oral thrush, and hematogenously disseminated candidiasis. Candidiasis is most commonly seen in patients who are pregnant, taking antibiotics, diabetic, or immunocompromised.

HX Most patients present with a rash that itches and burns. Patients with severe cases may complain of fever and malaise.

PX • **General findings:** maculopapular or nodular skin rash
    Oral: white, raised, painless patches
    Vulvovaginal: whitish, "cottage cheese"–like discharge; erythematous patches in the vagina and on the labia, vulva, and perineum
    Esophagitis: dysphagia, odynophagia, retrosternal pain
    GI: ulcerations, pain
    Ungual: nails elevated on a base of crusty material
• **Severe cases:** tachycardia, hypotension, AMS, hepatosplenomegaly

DD Bacterial infections, viral and fungal rashes

LB KOH prep to check for pseudohyphae and yeast forms

IM A contrast esophagram may show ulcerations

TX • **Oral:** nystatin (2-ml suspension): 100,000 U/ml qid × 5–7 days after lesions disappear
• **Ungual:** nystatin, clotrimazole, or miconazole topical cream; keep area dry
• **Vulvovaginal:**
    Miconazole: 2% cream or 100-mg suppository vag qhs × 7 days
    or
    Clotrimazole: one 100-mg suppository vag qhs × 7 days or
    Ketoconazole: one 200- to 400-mg tab qd x 14 days or
    Fluconazole: one 200-mg tab qd PO × 14 days
• **Severe infections:** amphotericin B

DI Usually home; admission to medical floor for systemic infections or immunocompromise

Tinea

KY A superficial fungal infection of the skin that may occur on virtually all areas of the body but is most common on the scalp, groin, and feet. It develops as a result of excessive heat and moisture.

HX Pruritus, burning, scaling, maceration, vesicles, and bullae

PX Keratin accumulation between the toes and in the axilla, groin, and body folds

• **Tinea capitis:** occurs on the scalp; can cause hair loss
• **Tinea corporis:** occurs on the trunk and extremities; lesions have a sharp, raised margin with central clearing
• **Tinea cruris:** involves the perineum, thighs, and buttocks, but spares the scrotum
• **Tinea pedis ("athletes foot"):** occurs in the interdigital spaces
• **Tinea unguium:** thick, crackled, opaque, and crumbled nails

- **Tinea versicolor:** brown, yellow macules that coalesce to form patches anywhere on the body

DD Psoriasis, intertrigo, hyperkeratosis, contact dermatitis, eczema, dyshidrosis, seborrheic dermatitis, candidiasis, pityriasis rosea, lupus, erythema annulare, syphilis

LB Wood's light (fluorescent lesions), KOH smear to check for branching hyphae and spores

TX
- **Tinea capitis:** griseofulvin (10 mg/kg/day PO × 4–8 weeks) with close monitoring of LFTs; selenium sulfide 2.5% shampoo
- **Tinea corporis, tinea cruris, tinea pedis, tinea versicolor:** topical miconazole or clotrimazole (bid–tid × 1–2 weeks); for palms and soles, also give ASA
- **Tinea unguium:** griseofulvin (1 g PO qd × 6–12 months) with close monitoring of LFTs

DI Outpatient therapy

LIFE-THREATENING DERMATOSES

Erythema multiforme/Stevens-Johnson syndrome

KY Erythema multiforme is an acute, self-limited hypersensitivity reaction involving the skin and mucous membranes. Stevens-Johnson syndrome is similar, but bullous lesions are present with systemic and mucous membrane involvement. Mortality is 50%.

HX Exposure to drugs, herpes, hepatitis, influenza, fungal infections, collagen vascular disease, and flu-like prodrome

PX
- **Erythema multiforme:** target lesions are papules or vesicles surrounded by normal skin and then a halo of erythema; macules and bullae on the soles, palms, and extensors of extremities, and on the back of the hands and feet
- **Stevens-Johnson syndrome (potentially fatal):** mucous membrane and multisystem involvement, with headache, tachycardia, tachypnea, hematuria, diarrhea, bronchitis, and pneumonia

DD TEN, urticaria, necrotizing vasculitis, drug reaction, contact dermatitis, viral exanthems, Rocky Mountain spotted fever, meningococcemia, syphilis

LB CBC, cultures, SMA-7, LFTs, Ca

IM CXR as needed

TX
- **Discontinue offending agent**
- **Mild forms:** resolution in 2–3 weeks

- **Severe cases:** prednisone (80–120 mg IV qd), wet compresses of potassium permanganate solution or silver nitrate 0.05%
- Ophthalmology consult for corneal lesions

DI Admission for severe cases, usually to the ICU

Staphylococcal scalded skin syndrome (SSSS)

KY Children, primarily 6 months to 6 years of age, are affected. The exotoxin is produced by *S. aureus*.

HX Prodrome of fever, malaise, and skin tenderness

PX • Mucous membranes not involved
  - Painful erythema and blistering of skin, positive Nikolsky's sign, bullae and vesicles that begin around mouth

DD TEN, drug reactions, Kawasaki syndrome, meningococcal or possibly Gram-negative sepsis, Rocky Mountain spotted fever, streptococcal scarlet fever, erythema multiforme

LB Biopsy blister, *S. aureus* culture from nose or oropharynx

IM CXR as needed

TX • Nafcillin (50–100 mg/kg/day IV) or dicloxacillin (50 mg/kg/day PO)
  - Management of fluids and electrolytes

DI Admission

Toxic epidermal necrolysis (TEN)

KY In this disease, which primarily affects adults, the skin sloughs off in large sheets. TEN is thought to represent a severe form of erythema multiforme, and mortality exceeds 50%.

HX Flu-like prodrome, precipitated by drugs or blood products. The skin is painful, hot, and red. Blisters develop, and sloughing of skin occurs.

PX Mucous membrane involvement, entire thickness of epidermis desquamates from dermis; positive Nikolsky's sign

DD SSSS, drug reactions, Kawasaki syndrome, meningococcal or Gram-negative sepsis, Rocky Mountain spotted fever, streptococcal scarlet fever, erythema multiforme

IM CXR as needed

TX • **Removal of precipitating agent**
  - Management of fluid and electrolytes similar to burns

- Dermatology and ophthalmology consult for eye involvement
- Corticosteroids (controversial)

DI ICU

Toxic shock syndrome (TSS)

KY This acute multisystem illness is associated with *S. aureus* infection; an exotoxin produced by *S. aureus* is the presumed cause. Complications include coagulopathy as well as respiratory and myocardial depression.

HX
- Fever, rash, headache, arthralgia, vomiting, diarrhea, and involvement of any three organ systems
- Associated with tampons and nasal packing

PX
- Diffuse, blanching, macular erythroderma; hypotension (SBP < 90 mm Hg); pharyngitis; conjunctivitis; vaginitis; renal, hepatic, or hematologic dysfunction; mucous membrane inflammation; and CNS or musculoskeletal hyperemia
- Full-thickness desquamation of hands and feet in 1–2 weeks; hair and nail loss 1–2 months later

DD Kawasaki syndrome, Rocky Mountain spotted fever, scarlet fever, TEN, drug reactions, SSSS, meningococcal sepsis

LB CBC, cultures, SMA-7, LFTs, Ca

TX
- IV nafcillin, vancomycin, or clindamycin
- Drainage of staphylococcal infection
- Early corticosteroids

DI All symptomatic patients: admission

PAPULOSQUAMOUS ERUPTIONS

Pityriasis rosea

KY This idiopathic skin eruption, which is believed to be caused by a virus, is characterized by widespread papulosquamous lesions. A self-limited condition (usual duration: 4–7 weeks), it most commonly occurs in individuals who are 10–35 years old.

HX Fever, pruritus, lymphadenopathy, and malaise

PX Oval, salmon-colored, scaling patches on trunk and neck that follow cleavage lines; "Christmas tree" pattern on back. A "herald patch," 2–6 cm in diameter, occurs before the rash appears.

DD Tinea corporis, psoriasis, drug reaction, 2° syphilis, viral exanthems, eczema, lichen planus

TX • Symptomatic treatment involves antihistamines, lukewarm oatmeal baths, and topical steroids
 • UV light has been used, but its efficacy has not been proven

DI Home

Psoriasis

KY This chronic, genetically determined, epidermal proliferative disease is most common in Caucasians.

HX Usually occurs in individuals who are 11–29 years old

PX • Papules with white scales on extensor surface, scalp, palms, or soles; nails pitted and discolored
 • Pustular psoriasis, which can be fatal, is manifested by fever, malaise, or leukocytosis

DD Tinea, candidiasis, pityriasis rosea, 2° syphilis, seborrhea

TX • Sunlight or UV radiation; oatmeal bath for itching; tar shampoos; wet dressings (may relieve pruritus)
 • Severe cases: methotrexate and PUVA
 • Pustular form: penicillin (500 mg PO qid x 10 days) plus topical antibiotic ointment; referral to a specialist

DI Home

Urticaria

KY This condition, which may be recurrent, is characterized by an itchy rash and single or multiple superficial raised pale macules with red halo. Acute urticaria lasts for ≤ 6 weeks, and chronic urticaria for > 6 weeks.

HX Allergic reaction to food, drugs, contrast dye or stimuli (e.g., sunlight, exercise, temperature extremes)

PX • Pruritus, erythematous, edematous raised wheals, raised papules that move from one area to another and blanch
 • Signs of possible anaphylaxis include wheezing, rhinorrhea, hypotension, and laryngeal edema

TX • **If anaphylaxis:** epinephrine 1:1000 (0.2–0.5 ml SQ or IM q15min × 3) or 1:10,000 (1–2 ml IV)
 • **Other measures:**
   Antihistamines: diphenhydramine (25–50 mg IV, with 25–50 mg PO for home) or hydroxyzine (10–25 mg PO)
   Cool showers, colloidal oatmeal baths, and antipruritic lotion
 • **Severe cases:** cimetidine (300 mg IV) and prednisone (40–60 mg IV) or methylprednisolone (125 mg IV)

DI Severe cases require admission and observation; otherwise, outpatient management is sufficient

PURPURIC LESIONS

Henoch-Schönlein purpura

KY This disorder, which is most common in children 4–11 years of age, generally occurs in the spring. Henoch-Schönlein purpura is a vasculitis of the small vessels characterized by palpable purpura, arthritis, abdominal pain, and nephritis.

HX The disease often occurs after an infection. Onset is abrupt to gradual. Low-grade fever, malaise, and colicky abdominal pain may be present.

PX **Palpable purpura** on extremities, face, and ears; possible diffuse abdominal pain, arthritis, and edema on the face and ears

TX • Anti-inflammatory agents for fever and arthritis
  • Corticosteroids for angioedema and severe GI symptoms (prednisone: 1–2 mg/kg/day)
  • Resolution in 1–4 months

DI Discharge, unless complications occur

Idiopathic thrombocytopenic purpura (ITP)

KY ITP, which is caused by IgG antiplatelet antibody, is characterized by a decrease in the circulating number of platelets in the absence of disease or toxic exposure associated with low platelet counts. The acute form occurs in children 2–6 years of age, whereas the chronic form affects adults.

HX • Tendency for bruising, gingival bleeding, menometrorrhagia, menorrhagia, recurrent epistaxis, and neurologic symptoms secondary to intracerebral bleeding
  • A viral prodrome usually occurs in children, but there is no prodrome in adults

PX • Petechiae and purpura
  • Nonpalpable spleen (absence of an enlarged spleen is an essential diagnostic criteria)
  • Neurologic deficits secondary to intracerebral bleeding
  • Heme-positive stools

DD Lupus, urticaria, lymphoma, telangiectasis

LB PT, PTT, CBC, platelet count, fecal occult blood

TX • **Acute ITP:** prednisone (1–2 mg/kg/day × 4 weeks, then taper); IV gamma globulin (1–2 g/kg single dose); splenectomy may be considered

- **Chronic ITP:** prednisone (60 mg/day × 4–6 weeks, then taper); high-dose IV gamma globulin may sometimes be used for emergencies
- **Other therapies:** vincristine, vinblastine, danazol, plasmapheresis, azathioprine, cyclophosphamide, and interferon
- Aspirin is contraindicated; avoid gamma globulin if the patient has IgA deficiency
- Hematology consult

DI • Outpatient management, unless the patient is at risk for bleeding (platelet count < 20,000/mm³)
- Admission for active bleeding

Thrombotic thrombocytopenic purpura

KY This disorder, which is most common in individuals 10–40 years of age, is characterized by fever, change in mental status, renal insufficiency, and microangiopathic hemolytic anemia. Mortality is 80%.

HX Familial bleeding disorder, infection (including hemorrhagic *Escherichia coli*), drug history, easy bruising, epistaxis, menorrhagia, or prolonged postsurgical bleeding

PX • Flat, nonpalpable purpura in areas of pressure, petechiae < 3 mm, and ecchymosis > 3 mm; purpura may involve the mucous membranes and optic fundi
- Fluctuating neurologic symptoms, including stroke, seizures, and AMS
- Possible hematuria, proteinuria, jaundice, or pallor

LB CBC, PT, PTT, platelet count, T&C, SMA-7, UA; inpatient bone marrow biopsy

TX • Corticosteroids, aspirin, dipyridamole, anticoagulation; inpatient splenectomy and plasmapheresis
- Platelet count should be maintained at > 20,000/mm³ (1 U of platelets increases count by 5000–10,000/mm³)
- Hematology consult

DI ICU for septic shock and intracranial hemorrhage

VESICULAR LESIONS (HERPETIC)

Herpes simplex

KY Patients have multiple clusters of painful ulcers or vesicles on the skin or mucous membranes. Other manifestations include pneumonia, encephalitis, or disseminated infection.

HX Prodrome of flu-like symptoms and paresthesia

PX • Painful vesicles on the cornea, lips, penis, vulva, and buttocks
  • Lymphadenopathy

DD Chancroid, impetigo, aphthous stomatitis, herpes zoster, syphilitic chancre, trauma, Stevens-Johnson syndrome, Behçet's syndrome

LB • **All lesions:** Tzanck smear (multinucleated giant cells); viral culture of unroofed vesicles (only 50% will be positive in 2 days; remainder may take ≥ 6 days), which is not considered a reasonable method for following activity of recurrent disease near delivery
  • **Periorbital lesions or those involving the nose tip:** fluorescein staining (to check for herpetic keratitis), ophthalmology consult

TX • **Primary HSV:** acyclovir [400 mg PO tid or 200 mg PO q4hr (total of five times/day) × 7–10 days or until lesions form crust]; primary HSV proctitis: acyclovir (800 mg PO tid or 400 mg PO five times/day × 7–10 days)
  • **Recurrent genital herpes:** acyclovir (400 mg PO bid for up to 12 months)
  • Application of viscous lidocaine for pain
  • Good genital hygiene, sitz baths, and loose undergarments
  • If delivery is imminent, it must be by C-section

DI Usually home. Patients with periorbital or nasal lesions or keratitis require admission.

Herpes zoster (shingles)

KY Herpes zoster occurs as a result of reactivation of dormant VZV in the dorsal root ganglia.

HX History of varicella; prodrome of painful hyperesthesia, with tingling, itching, boring, knife-like pain; fatigue; headache; fever; and weakness

PX Unilateral painful dermatomal eruption, with multiple painful vesicles grouped on one or two dermatomes (commonly thoracic and trigeminal). Vesicles become pustular and/or hemorrhagic in 3–4 days, and crusts eventually form in 14–21 days.

DD Herpes simplex, Coxsackievirus, contact dermatitis, pyoderma

LB **Periorbital lesions or those involving the nose tip:** fluorescein staining (to check for herpetic keratitis)

IM CXR as needed

TX • Acyclovir: 800 mg PO five times/day × 10 days; 5–10 mg/kg IV q8hr for urinary retention, severe cases, or immunosuppression
  • Analgesics for pain; Burrow's solution compresses tid

- Steroid use (controversial)
- Ophthalmology consult prn

DI Home except in severe cases

Varicella (chickenpox)

KY Varicella, a common, highly contagious childhood exanthem, is characterized by crops of vesicles on the skin and mucous membranes. The disease is caused by VZV. Transmission is by respiratory droplet or direct contact, and incubation is typically 14–16 days. Until the lesions are crusted over, patients remain contagious.

HX Exposure to VZV, prodrome of flu-like symptoms (e.g., fever, malaise, anorexia, headache)

PX Lesions progress from macules to papules to vesicles on trunk, face, scalp, and extremities, and crusting eventually develops. The hallmark of the disease is lesions of various stages on one part of the body with pruritus.

DD Herpes simplex, herpes zoster, Coxsackievirus, contact dermatitis, pyoderma, scabies, drug rash, impetigo, papular urticaria

TX
- Oral analgesia, oral antihistamines, tepid compresses
- Acyclovir (5–10 mg/kg IV q8hr or 20 mg/kg PO five times/day) for urinary retention, severe cases, or immunosuppression
- Treatment of complications (e.g., pneumonia, encephalitis, cellulitis)

DI Home except in severe cases

VIRAL EXANTHEMS

Roseola

KY Roseola, a disease of infants and young children (6 months–3 years of age), usually causes a high fever followed by a rash. The incubation period is 5–15 days. Patients with roseola are at risk for febrile seizures.

HX Fever for 3–4 days followed by rash, anorexia, irritability, and listlessness

PX
- Pink macules or papules, which blanch and are slightly elevated; the rash begins on the trunk and spreads to the neck and extremities, with no desquamation
- Lymphadenopathy in cervical and posterior auricular regions
- Spleen may be enlarged

DD Sepsis, UTI, rubeola, otitis media, enterovirus infection, meningitis, drug eruption, bacterial pneumonia

LB CBC, UA

TX Supportive

DI Home (usually)

Rubella (German measles)

KY This illness, which affects both children and adults, is sometimes associated with fetal anomalies when pregnant women are infected in the first trimester. Congenital defects occur in 24% of exposed pregnant patients. Other complications include thrombocytopenia, encephalitis, and arthritis.

HX
- **Children:** rash heralds onset
- **Adults:** flu-like prodrome, symptoms resolve 24 hours after rash, fever; incubation period of 14–21 days,

PX
- Red maculopapules on face, neck, trunk, and extremities for 1–5 days
- Lymphadenopathy (suboccipital, postauricular, and posterior cervical) 1 week before the rash

DD Drug eruptions, infectious mononucleosis, rubeola, *Mycoplasma,* roseola, enteroviruses, erythema infectiosum, Rocky Mountain spotted fever, anaphylactoid purpura

LB Immediate antibody titer for pregnant women who are exposed

TX Supportive

DI Home

Rubeola (measles)

KY Rubeola, an acute viral exanthem, classically manifests as a confluent erythematous maculopapular rash that begins on the head and spreads to the trunk and extremities. This very contagious reportable disease has an incubation period of 10–14 days. Complications include otitis, encephalitis (15% mortality), and pneumonitis (pneumonia may be fatal).

HX Malaise, photophobia, sore throat, nausea, vomiting, and diarrhea

PX
- **Day 1:** cough, conjunctivitis, coryza, and fever
- **Day 2:** Koplik spots (red spots with blue-white centers on buccal mucosa)
- **Days 3 to 5:** maculopapular red lesions on forehead, neck, face, trunk, and extremities

DD Drug eruptions, infectious mononucleosis, *Mycoplasma pneumoniae,* rubella, erythema infectiosum, roseola, enteroviruses, Rocky Mountain spotted fever

TX • Supportive
  • Immunization (children < 1 year and immunocompromised children exposed to rubeola within 6 days): ISG (0.25 L/kg IM)

DI Home; patients are not contagious on the fifth day following the rash (children: no school for 4 days)

CHAPTER 3

Endocrinologic Emergencies

ADRENAL CRISIS

KY Acute adrenal insufficiency (adrenal crisis) occurs in patients with or without chronic adrenal insufficiency precipitated by acute infection, sepsis, adrenal hemorrhage, acute stress or illness (e.g., trauma, MI, hypothermia, surgery, burns) or abrupt withdrawal of chronically used steroids.

HX Weakness and confusion with appropriate PMH; prominent GI symptoms (e.g., anorexia, nausea, vomiting, abdominal pain)

PX • Acute illness with hypotension and circulatory collapse; temperature elevation
 • Hyperpigmentation, disorientation, confusion, or unconsciousness

DD MI, heart failure, hypovolemia, sepsis, pulmonary embolism, shock, CVA, ischemic bowel, bowel obstruction

LB SMA-7, CBC, plasma cortisol and ACTH levels (before and after dexamethasone-containing infusion) [laboratory evaluation simultaneous with treatment; see treatment]

IM EKG, CXR, CT prn

TX • If adrenal crisis is suspected, treatment should be initiated without waiting for confirmation
 • Airway, IV fluids, Foley catheter, supplemental O_2, monitoring
 • Cosyntropin (synthetic ACTH): 0.25 mg IV or hydrocortisone 100–300 mg IV
 • D_5NS (containing dexamethasone 4 mg): 1 L IV infused over 1 hour; needs to be repeated q6–8hr
 • Continue D_5NS IV 2–3 L over next 8 hours to restore BP
 • Avoid treatment of hyperkalemia with insulin and calcium—total body stores are usually low, and hyperkalemia will resolve with IV fluids and glucocorticoid replacement

DI ICU

ALCOHOLIC KETOACIDOSIS

HX After recent drinking binges and decreased food intake, chronic alcoholics complain of abdominal distress accompanied by nausea and vomiting that leads to decreased alcohol consumption. Patients often present 1–2 days after last alcohol use.

PX Tachycardia, ketotic breath, dehydration, Kussmaul's respirations, tachypnea, and abdominal findings are variable; neurologic states range from normal to lethargy or stupor

DD Pancreatitis, PUD, gastritis, hypoglycemia, other causes of anion gap metabolic acidosis

LB CBC, SMA-7, phosphate and lactate levels, serum ketones, ABG, possibly LFTs

IM CXR or abdominal films if clinically indicated

TX
- Thiamine: 100 mg IV (before glucose administration)
- D_5NS or NS to replace fluid losses; specific electrolytes prn
- Insulin not needed
- $NaHCO_3$ if blood pH < 7.10

DI Admission to floor or ICU depending on stability

DIABETIC KETOACIDOSIS (DKA)

KY DKA results from a relative deficiency of insulin with concurrent excess of stress hormones.

HX Omission of daily insulin and/or presence of stress (e.g., infection, CVA, MI, trauma, pregnancy, hyperthyroidism, nausea, vomiting, abdominal pain, pancreatitis, emotional upset)

PX
- Dehydration, hypotension, and tachycardia
- Gastric dilation, paralytic ileus, and abdominal tenderness
- Neurologic manifestations ranging from normal orientation to coma

DD Hypoglycemic coma, nonketotic hyperosmolar coma, alcoholic ketoacidosis, lactic acidosis

LB
- CBC, SMA-7 (recheck q2–4hr, more frequently prn), ABG, phosphate level, serum ketones, UA, culture as appropriate; glucose and serum ketones are usually elevated, potassium levels that are slightly elevated will drop with treatment, and anion gap acidosis will improve with therapy

IM EKG, CXR

TX
- Airway, IV fluids, supplemental O_2, monitoring
- NS: 1 L/hr IV × 2–3 hours; initial bolus prn
- Insulin: run 50 ml through tubing to saturate binding sites before administering; then begin 10 U/hr IV (peds 0.1 U/kg/hr); when glucose

≤ 250 mg/dl, slow infusion to 2–4 U/hr and change IV fluids to D₅1/2NS

- NaHCO₃ if pH < 7.0
- Consider potassium and phosphate replacement

DI ICU

HYPOGLYCEMIA

KY Hypoglycemia is generally accepted as serum glucose levels of less than 35–55 mg/dl. This condition may be caused by postprandial or reflex endogenous insulin release, fasting, hepatic disease, drugs (e.g., propranolol, salicylates, insulin, sulfonylureas), and alcohol.

HX Most commonly, hypoglycemia occurs in patients with diabetes who use insulin and fail to eat after an insulin dose. Patient complaints include fatigue, anxiety, hunger, confusion, combativeness, and headache.

PX Diaphoresis, pallor, tremulousness, tachycardia, and palpitations; perhaps moderate hypothermia; neurologic manifestations ranging from mental confusion to coma

DD Ketoacidosis, drug interaction, islet cell tumor, hormonal deficiency states, all potential causes of AMS

LB Dexi stick, SMA-7

TX
- Dextrose 50% solution: 50 ml IV; consider continuous 5%, 10%, or 20% glucose infusion
- Glucagon: 2 mg IM, if IV unavailable; provide complex carbohydrates

DI Home, unless prolonged hypoglycemia or sulfonylurea ingestion; otherwise, admission

NONKETOTIC HYPEROSMOLAR COMA

KY This syndrome of profound dehydration results from osmotic diuresis. Fluid deficits are high (9–12 L). The condition can occur in young adults or elderly patients, two-thirds of whom have no diabetic history but a diabetogenic stressor (e.g., drugs, infection, surgery, MI). Mortality approaches 50%.

HX Antecedent polyuria and polydipsia; history of AMS (lethargy to coma), with progression of symptoms over hours to days

PX
- Dehydration, postural hypotension, reflex tachycardia due to cardiovascular collapse
- Neurologic findings include seizures, AMS, focal deficits, aphasia, nystagmus, tremors, and hyperreflexia

DD DKA and other causes of AMS (e.g., hepatic failure, sepsis, drug ingestion, dehydration, uremia, CVA)

LB
- SMA-7 (glucose average values ~ 1000 mg/dl), CBC, UA, ABG, blood and urine culture, amylase, LFTs, coagulation studies
- Serum osmolarity = 2[Na] + glucose/18 + BUN/2.8

IM CXR, EKG

TX
- ABCs, IV fluids, supplemental O_2, monitoring
- Immediate fluid resuscitation with 1–2 L NS over first hour, then 1 L/hr for first few hours
- Potassium replacement if no hyperkalemia or renal failure
- Hyperglycemia will decrease with fluid resuscitation. However, consider low-dose insulin for patients who are hyperkalemic, acidotic, or in renal failure. Regular insulin: 0.15 U/kg bolus then 0.1/kg/hr until glucose falls to 250 mg/dl

DI ICU

THYROID DISORDERS

Hypothyroidism and myxedema coma

KY Hypothyroidism is a clinical condition resulting from decreased circulating levels of free thyroid hormone. Severe hypothyroidism, or myxedema coma, commonly occurs in elderly females, with hypothyroidism plus a precipitating event (e.g., hypothermia, shock from any cause, hypoglycemia, sepsis). Mortality approaches 50%, even with treatment.

HX
- History of hypothyroidism, treated Graves' disease, and cessation of thyroid replacement therapy
- Patients may complain of weakness, cold intolerance, constipation, muscle cramps, arthralgias, paresthesias, weight gain, menorrhagia, depression, and hoarseness

PX Dry skin, dull facial expressions, husky voice, bradycardia, hypothermia, decreased BP, increased DBP, periorbital puffiness, swelling of the hands and feet, reduced body and scalp hair, delayed relaxation of DTRs, macroglossia, anemia, hyponatremia, enlarged heart, AMS

DD Nephrotic syndrome, chronic nephritis, depression, neurasthenia, CHF, amyloidosis, dementia, nephritis, sepsis, CVA

LB CBC, SMA-7, ABG (to look for hypercarbia in particular)

IM EKG (may show low voltage)

TX
- Airway, IV fluids and glucose, supplemental O_2, monitoring
- Passive rewarming for hypothermia

- Hormone therapy: thyroid replacement (T_4: 300–500 mg slow IV); consider hydrocortisone [300 mg (adrenal insufficiency is often a concomitant finding)]
- Treatment of precipitating causes

DI ICU

Thyroid storm

KY This condition occurs in individuals with undiagnosed or undetected thyrotoxic Graves' disease or toxic multinodular goiter. Its abrupt onset is usually precipitated by infection, trauma, vascular accident, or diabetic complications.

HX
- Severe weakness preceding weight loss a few weeks prior to presentation; heat intolerance and eye complaints from bulbar palsy
- History of thyroid disease
- Nervousness, increased sweating, palpitations, dyspnea, increased appetite, tremor, and emotional lability

PX
- Fever; wide pulse pressure; neurologic manifestations ranging from restlessness to coma and increased DTRs; and cardiovascular effects, including AF and CHF
- Possible occurrence of ophthalmopathy; goiter; warm, moist skin; and weight loss

DD Heat stroke; drug toxicity, including NMS and withdrawal syndrome; psychosis; pheochromocytoma; CHF

LB CBC, SMA-7, LFTs, Ca level (often elevated), TFTs (T_4 RIA, free T_4 index)

IM Consider CXR

TX
- Airway, IV fluids, supplemental O_2, monitoring
- Propranolol to block hormone action: 1–2 mg IV q15min prn to 10 mg total dose
- SSKI to prevent hormone release: 3–5 gtt PO/NG tube q8hr
- PTU to inhibit hormone synthesis: 900–1200 mg PO/NG tube (loading dose)
- Acetaminophen and cooling blanket for hyperthermia
- Treat CHF (see Chapter 1, Cardiovascular Emergencies, Congestive Heart Failure)

DI ICU

WERNICKE-KORSAKOFF SYNDROME

KY This potentially fatal disorder, which is caused by thiamine deficiency, carries a mortality range of 15% to 20%. Wernicke's encephalopathy is associated with one or more findings of the triad of global confusion, ataxia, and ophthalmoplegia. Korsakoff's psychosis consists of irreversible memory deficit marked by amnestic apathy and confabulation.

HX Most commonly, patients are chronic alcoholics and those with a history of genetic defects in transketolase. The administration of glucose to thiamine-deficient individuals can theoretically precipitate symptoms.

PX Nystagmus and ophthalmoplegia, followed by disorientation and ataxia; abnormal mental status, including progression to coma, hypotension, hypothermia, and circulatory collapse

DD Alcohol intoxication or withdrawal, acute or chronic subdural hematoma, intracranial trauma, metabolic or drug-induced encephalopathies, CNS infection, vascular accident, tumor, demyelinating disease, hypothermia

LB The diagnosis is clinical. Concomitant Mg deficiency is common. Labs (e.g., CBC, chemistry) are used to rule out other pathologic etiologies.

IM Consider CXR

TX • Monitoring, serial neurologic examinations
• Thiamine: 100 mg IV
• Alcohol abstinence and adequate diet

DI Admission to acute care service

CHAPTER 4

Environmental Emergencies

COLD-RELATED CONDITIONS

Cold-induced tissue injuries

KY Frostbite is the destruction of tissue as the result of freezing. Immersion foot is tissue injury at temperatures of 0°C to 10°C with prolonged exposure to a wet environment.

HX Frozen part is cold and lacks sensation. Patients with immersion foot complain of numbness, pain, and paresthesias.

PX • Initially the skin is pale, waxy white, or mottled blue, and may range from rock-solid to firm on palpation
  • Early findings include coolness, pallor, sensitivity, and edema; later, cyanosis, mottling, or erythema may develop
  • Vesicles or bullae with clear to bloody fluid may be present, and maceration with secondary bacterial or fungal infection may occur
  • A superimposed burn injury may be present due to rewarming

DD Devascularizing injury, envenomation, thermal or chemical burn

IM Consider CXR

TX • **Frostbite:**
      No rubbing, warming, or manipulation of frozen parts should occur on transport to ED
      Removal of all wet, nonadherent apparel; placement under a warm blanket
      Rapid thawing of frostbitten part in 40°C water bath
      Tetanus prophylaxis
      Analgesia for pain control: ibuprofen (400 mg PO bid)
      Ascorbic acid: 1 g PO bid
      Removal of clear blisters (hemorrhagic blisters should be left intact); aloe vera q6hr
      Smoking cessation
  • **Immersion foot:**
      Rewarming, elevation, avoidance of manipulation and pressure
      Local skin care: cleansing, topical antibiotics (Neosporin and silver sulfadiazine cream), and dressing of denuded areas

DI All but the most superficially injured frostbite patients should be admitted, and surgical consultation should be obtained. Patients who are discharged should be reexamined within 24 hours.

Hypothermia

Hypothermia is a decline in core body temperature to $\leq 35°C$. Several mechanisms may contribute to heat loss: conduction (loss by direct contact), convection (body-to-air loss), radiation (loss to air), and evaporation (sweating).

PX
- **Mild hypothermia:** apathy, confusion, lethargy, fatigue, incoordination, shivering, slurred speech, tachycardia, and tachypnea
- **Moderate hypothermia:** cessation of shivering ($< 32°C$); decreased pulse rate, BP, and respiratory rate; disorientation, stupor, inappropriate behavior, polyuria, rhonchi, and wheezing may occur. AF, PAT, T-wave changes, PVCs, or Osborne waves
- **Severe hypothermia ($< 28°C$):** coma, dilated unreactive pupils, absent or weak pulses, barely detectable respirations, absent reflexes, muscle rigidity, hypotension; bradycardia, asystole, or VF; flat EEG

DD Endocrine, metabolic, toxic, traumatic, or vascular conditions that cause CNS depression

LB CBC, SMA-7, ABG, amylase, coagulation studies, UA, serum Ca, Mg, phosphate, lactate, cardiac enzyme levels, LFTs, toxicology screening, pulse oximetry

IM EKG, CXR

TX
- Airway, IV fluids, supplemental O_2, monitoring (continuous temperature monitoring with a rectal probe)
- Removal of wet, nonadherent clothing and placement under warm blankets
- Active rewarming for neonates and adults with moderate and severe hypothermia: warm IV fluids ($45°C$); humidified O_2 ($42°C$–$45°C$)
- Active core rewarming for severe hypothermia with peritoneal lavage fluid ($45°C$), blood warming by hemodialysis or femorofemoral cardiopulmonary bypass pump, and pleuromediastinal lavage via thoracostomy or thoracotomy
- Correction of underlying metabolic derangements; consider stress-dose steroid or thyroid hormone if the patient is unresponsive to aggressive warming or underlying endocrinopathy exists

DI
- **Mild hypothermia:** observation until the patient is asymptomatic and normothermic
- **Very young and very old patients or those with underlying pathology:** admission
- **Moderate-to-severe hypothermia:** ICU

ELECTRICAL INJURIES

HX Nausea, vomiting, paresthesias, AMS, and pain

PX • Pallor, ileus, burned and necrotic tissue, skeletal fractures, joint dislocations (especially posterior shoulder), and spinal compression fractures may be present
- CNS manifestations include amnesia, AMS, irritability, depression, emotional lability, motor deficits, seizures, and coma
- Arrhythmias and respiratory depression may occur
- Small entrance wounds commonly found on the hands and upper extremities may demonstrate charring, depression, edema, and inflammatory changes
- Large exit wounds may be multiple and have an explosive appearance

LB • Standard trauma evaluation as appropriate
- CBC; SMA-7; CPK, including isoenzymes to evaluate for cardiac injury and rhabdomyolysis
- Urine dip to check for rhabdomyolysis (positive for RBC in presence of myoglobin); if positive, order UA that includes urine myoglobin
- Coagulation studies, LFTs, amylase, lipase, and Ca should be considered

IM EKG (continuous monitoring)

TX • ABCs, with stabilization of the cervical spine; standard ACLS and ATLS protocols as indicated (see Appendix A); IV fluids, supplemental O_2, monitoring
- Indwelling urinary catheter
- NG suctioning, tetanus prophylaxis, and possible antibiotic (e.g., cefazolin)
- Treatment of rhabdomyolysis: aggressive fluid resuscitation, mannitol, and diuretics to enhance urinary output. The addition of $NaHCO_3$ (usually 3 amp in 1 L D_5W) to the IV line alkalinizes the urine and prevents myoglobin precipitation in the renal tubules.

DI • **Exposure to > 600 V:** probable admission to a monitored bed or ICU
- **Low-voltage, nonsystemic injuries:** discharge after evaluation, observation, and management in the ED
- **All serious injuries:** consultation and/or transfer to a burn center (essential)

HEAT-RELATED CONDITIONS

KY An inability of the body's normal regulatory mechanism to cope with heat stress leads to a spectrum of conditions, including cramps due to sweat-induced hyponatremia without volume depletion; heat exhaustion with volume depletion; and heat stroke involving CNS temperature elevation with CNS findings.

HX **Heat exhaustion:** weakness, dizziness, anxiety, lack of muscle coordination, palpitations, headache, vomiting, muscle cramps, and diarrhea

Heat stroke: malaise or flu-like prodrome; changes in CNS function

PX • **Heat exhaustion:** agitation; confusion; oliguria; elevated temperature; cool, clammy skin; tachycardia, and hypotension
• **Heat stroke:** AMS, confusion, coma, ataxia, focal neurologic signs, seizures, tachypnea, tachycardia, and high core temperature (> 40°C)

DD Meningitis, thyroid disease, drug intoxication, NMS

LB Orthostatic BP, rectal temperature, CBC, ABG, SMA-7, CPK, UA, LFTs, coagulation studies, Ca, Mg, P, uric acid, urine myoglobin

IM EKG, CXR

TX • Airway, IV fluids, supplemental O$_2$, monitoring
• Rapid cooling (cooling is necessary until temperature drops to 38.5°C–39°C): spritz the patient with lukewarm water and use a fan
• Foley catheter
• Correction of acid–base, electrolyte, and coagulation abnormalities
• Rhabdomyolysis: alkaline diuresis [NaHCO$_3$ (3 amp in 1 L D$_5$W)]
• Midazolam (2.5–10.0 mg IV) for shivering
• Diazepam or phenobarbital for seizures (phenytoin is ineffective)

DI • **Heat exhaustion:** admission to floor
• **Heat stroke:** ICU

HIGH-PRESSURE INJECTION INJURIES

KY Although high-pressure injection injuries may appear innocuous, they may have devastating consequences if treatment is delayed or inadequate. A detailed peripheral neurologic/motor/sensory examination of the affected part should be performed. The index finger is the most commonly injured extremity. Consultation with a hand or plastic surgeon is always warranted.

HX Penetration of skin through high-pressure exposure

PX • The extremity or body part is initially pain-free, followed by an acute inflammatory process that causes swelling and intense pain
• Usually a small pinhole entrance wound with an expressible drop of injectate is present
• Pallor, pulselessness, and paresthesia may occur

DD Envenomation by reptiles, insects, and arachnids; tenosynovitis, presence of foreign body

LB Allen test, preoperative labs (e.g., CBC, chemistry, PT, PTT, UA)

IM Radiograph to rule out the presence of a foreign body and gas; Doppler evaluation of peripheral pulses and palmar arches

TX • Soft, bulky dressing without undue compression, splinting of extremity in neutral position, and elevation on pillows (no IV or BP measurements in affected arm)
  • Broad-spectrum antibiotics; tetanus prophylaxis
  • Consult with plastic surgeon

DI Admission for possible surgical exploration

INSECT AND SPIDER BITES AND STINGS

Bee, wasp, and ant stings

KY The order Hymenoptera includes bees, wasps, hornets, yellow jackets, and ants. Their stings may result in local inflammatory reactions, immediate and delayed (10–14 days after sting) hypersensitivity reactions, atypical reactions, and direct systemic toxicity. Anaphylactic reactions may be fatal.

HX Pruritus, pain, and slight erythema and edema at sting site

PX • **Local reaction:** redness, edema at sting site, and possible presence of stinger or venom sac
  • **Toxic reaction:** ≥ 10 or more stings: vomiting, diarrhea, light-headedness, syncope, headache, fever, muscle spasms, and edema
  • **Anaphylactic reaction:** generalized urticaria; facial flushing; itching eyes; dry cough; chest or throat constriction; wheezing; dyspnea; cyanosis; abdominal cramps; diarrhea; nausea and vomiting; vertigo; fever; chills; pharyngeal stridor; shock; LOC; involuntary bowel and bladder action; and bloody, frothy sputum or pulmonary edema

TX • **Airway, IV fluids, supplemental O$_2$, monitoring**
  • **Local reaction:**
      If a stinger is present, it should be scraped out (not squeezed), and the wound washed with soap and water to minimize infection
      Analgesics may be indicated
      Ice pack applied to site and elevation of affected limb to delay absorption and limit edema
      Prednisone (to reduce swelling): 20–40 g PO qd × 3 days
      Medications for pruritus: diphenhydramine (25–50 mg PO q6–8hr)

- **Systemic reaction:**

  Epinephrine HCl (1:1000): 0.3–0.5 ml SQ (peds 0.01 ml/kg SQ, no more than 0.3 ml); in more severe reactions, a second injection should be given in 10–15 minutes along with diphenhydramine: 25–50 mg IM/IV

  O₂ via mask or ET tube should be administered as indicated; if bronchospasm develops, give albuterol: 2.5 mg in 3 ml nebul and repeat

  Crystalloid infusions for hypotension; persistent hypotension requires dopamine: 200 mg in 250 ml NS at 5 µg/kg/min (titrated to effect)

  Methylprednisolone: 80–120 mg IV (or prednisone: 40–60 mg IV) initially, then prednisone (to limit urticaria and edema): 10–40 mg PO qd × 5–7 days

- **Delayed reaction:**

  Oral steroids

  Brompheniramine maleate [2–4 mg qid (peds 1–2 g qid)] or diphenhydramine if needed

  Antibiotics may be necessary in secondary infection

DI • **If epinephrine is required:** monitoring in ED for several hours to ensure that symptoms do not intensify

- **If reaction is severe:** admission with cardiac monitoring for 24–48 hours

Black widow spider bites

KY Female black widow spiders (*Latrodectus mactans*), which have a globular abdomen and a leg span of 2.5 cm, are poisonous to humans. These spiders are shiny black with a red "hourglass" design on the ventral surface of the abdomen.

HX • The bite produces a brief, sharp pain. Deep, burning, aching, or numbing pain near the bite location such as an arm or leg may begin over 30 minutes; the pain may be located in the back, neck, chest, abdomen, or flanks.

- Vomiting, headache, chest tightness, hypertension, salivation, and lacrimation may occur.

PX • Two minor puncture wounds, with no necrosis or significant swelling

- Possible halo lesion consisting of a circular area of pallor surrounded by a ring of erythema
- Rigid and tender abdominal muscles, diaphoresis, hypertension, and periorbital ecchymosis

DD Almost any illness that causes pain must be considered; MI and acute abdomen must be ruled out

LB CBC, SMA-7, UA, CPK

IM EKG, CXR

TX • Airway, IV fluids, supplemental O_2, monitoring
• Tetanus prophylaxis, pain relief
• Antivenin use:
  For severe pain or dangerous hypertension
  Contraindicated in patients allergic to horse serum and ill-advised in patients taking β-blocking agents
  Skin test before administration of antivenin
• Nitroprusside, nifedipine, and/or hydralazine for control of hypertension
• Calcium and methocarbamol are of questionable value

DI • Patients with mild-to-moderate symptoms who are controlled by oral analgesics: discharge
• Patients who received antivenin without complications: discharge after 8–10 hours of asymptomatic observation
• Patients < 14 and > 65 years of age, those with history of hypertension, those requiring parenteral narcotics, and those who are pregnant: admission

Brown recluse spider bites

KY The brown recluse spider (*Loxosceles reclusa*), which measures 1.5 cm leg-to-leg, is fawn to dark brown. It has a violin-shaped, dark brown-to-yellow marking on its cephalothorax, with the larger end toward the head.

HX The bite feels like a pinprick; the area itches, tingles, and swells, becomes red, tender, and blanches within a few hours after the bite
  Weakness, nausea, arthralgias, and myalgias may occur
  Systemic loxoscelism manifests as severe illness, high fever, rash, and hemolytic anemia with hemoglobinuria

PX Fever, chills, malaise, rash, and blebs or purpura; necrosis with induration and eschar within hours

DD Other bites and stings, erythema multiforme, diabetic ulcer, herpes simplex, poison oak and ivy (*Rhus* dermatitis)

LB CBC, UA, coagulation studies, LFTs, serum amylase, SMA-7

IM Consider CXR

TX • Standard initial wound care plus ice compresses
• Best treatment unknown; primary treatment is "benign neglect;" antipruritic or antianxiety drugs are comforting; give analgesics for pain; NSAIDs are contraindicated
• Dapsone (leukocyte inhibitor): 100 mg PO bid; erythromycin: 250 mg PO qid
• Platelet or RBC administration for systemic arachnidism
• Methylprednisolone (of questionable benefit): 1–2 mg/kg IV qid
• Plastic surgery referral; corrective surgery is delayed 6–8 weeks until necrosis is clearly demarcated
• Consult regional poison control center or toxicologist

DI Admission for significant systemic symptoms; after discharge, daily evaluation for 3–5 days

Mosquito and fly bites

HX History of exposure; pruritus, erythema, and wheal

PX • Wheal, itching, erythema, edema, or pain
• Hypersensitivity reactions may produce nausea, vomiting, fever, malaise, generalized edema, and necrosis with resulting scarring

TX • Primarily symptomatic
• Oral antihistamines may relieve pruritus; topical antihistamines may cause contact dermatitis
• Trimeprazine tartrate is useful in mosquito bites
• Cold compress may decrease local edema
• Severe local reactions: topical steroids are helpful. In severe cases, oral or parenteral steroids can be given.
• Severe systemic reactions require treatment for anaphylaxis as for Hymenoptera stings (see Insect and Spider Bites and Stings; Bee, Wasp, and Ant Stings)

DI Home

SMOKE INHALATION

KY Smoke inhalation–related injuries are a common cause of morbidity and mortality in patients exposed to fires. Treated textiles can create cyanide when burned, and combustion produces CO.

HX Hoarseness, dysphagia, dyspnea, neck pain, dizziness, seizures, and chest pain

PX Cough, conjunctivitis, tearing, singed nasal hairs, rhinitis, pharyngitis, tachycardia, tachypnea or bradypnea, hypotension, arrhythmias, drooling, hoarseness and stridor (laryngospasm), laryngeal edema, wheezing (bronchospasm), rhonchi, rales, cyanosis, respiratory arrest, confusion, ataxia, or coma

DD Arson, attempted murder, or attempted suicide

LB ABG, CoHb levels, pulse oximetry, toxicology screen, whole blood cyanide level, ethanol level; bedside spirometry, laryngoscopy prn

IM EKG, CXR, other radiographs appropriate for trauma, head CT prn

TX
- ABCs with ACLS and ATLS protocols as indicated (see Appendix A)
- Consider early ET intubation; humidified O_2 with racemic epinephrine for relief of upper airway symptoms
- Removal of clothing and irrigation of eyes and skin prn
- Treatment of CO poisoning (see Chapter 18, Toxicologic Emergencies, Carbon Monoxide Poisoning)
- Treatment of cyanide toxicity

DI
- Patients with CO poisoning: possible transfer for HBO
- Patients with significant surface burns or physical injuries: possible transfer to a burn or trauma center
- Other patients: ICU, telemetry, or floor bed admission may be appropriate, depending on the severity of clinical findings and the coexistence of surface burns or traumatic injuries

SNAKEBITE

KY Treatment is often determined by the type of snake encountered. When this is not known, the patient's symptoms may suggest the identity of the snake and permit assessment of the severity of the bite. Reference information regarding snakes indigenous to the area may be helpful.

HX Encounter with a venomous snake; alcohol is usually involved

PX
- **Fang marks** (one or two) may be present at the site, with pain, edema, and erythema
- **Systemic effects** include increased or decreased temperature, nausea, vomiting, diarrhea, pain, restlessness, and increased or decreased heart rate
- **Neurotoxic symptoms** include dysphagia, convulsions, psychosis, muscle weakness, paresthesia, fasciculation, and in extreme cases, paralysis
- **Hemopathic manifestations** such as local bleeding, ecchymosis, bleeding from kidneys, peritoneum, rectum, or vagina are seen with pit viper bites

LB CBC, T&C, PT, PTT, SMA-7, UA, wound culture

TX • ABCs, IV fluids, supplemental O_2, monitoring; treatment of arrhythmias per ACLS protocols (see Appendix A)
   • Placement in supine position to rest and decrease metabolism, with placement of injured body part in dependent position
   • Tetanus booster
   • Transfusions prn if bleeding is severe
   • Antihistamines for itching or urticaria
   • Antivenin (type determined by type of snake encountered): generally given within 4 hours of the bite; after 12 hours, the value is uncertain; check for hypersensitivity
   • Copperhead bites, which are self-limited, do not require antivenin unless the snake is unusually large, multiple bites are present, or the victim is small or debilitated
   • Compartment syndrome may develop in the injured extremity; fasciotomy should be performed with pressure ≥ 30 mm Hg

DI • Asymptomatic patients: discharge after 8–12 hours of observation (generally)
   • Patients with mild-to-moderate envenomation: admission to a floor bed
   • Patients with a severe bite who are receiving antivenin: ICU

SUBMERSION INJURIES

KY Drowning is death from suffocation due to submersion in a fluid. Near-drowning implies survival (at least temporarily) after such suffocation. Prompt resuscitation is the most important factor affecting morbidity and mortality. Prognosis is very difficult to predict based on initial presentation, so all patients should receive aggressive resuscitation.

HX Coughing, choking, or vomiting after submersion; respiratory distress or arrest

PX • **Signs and symptoms:** increased pulse, BP, and respiratory rate; hypothermia, with cool, clammy, pale, or cyanotic skin; vomitus, water, or foreign material in the mouth; rhonchi, rales, or wheezing; gastric distention (common)
   • **Severe hypoxia:** presence of decorticate or decerebrate posturing or flaccid paralysis, unreactive pupils, and other cranial nerve findings, as well as decreased or absent vital signs; brain stem reflexes and DTRs may be apparent

DD Head and/or spinal trauma, drug or chemical intoxication, cardiac arrest, stroke, cerebral air embolus, attempted suicide or murder, hypothermia

LB CBC, ABG, Chem-7, UA, platelet count, LFTs, coagulation studies, cardiac enzymes; consider toxicology screen

IM EKG; consider CXR, cervical spine radiograph, and head CT

TX • **Life support:**

ABCs, ACLS and ATLS protocols (see Appendix A); treatment of change in mental status (see Chapter 11, Neurologic Emergencies)

Intubation if Po_2 < 50 mm Hg or Pco_2 > 50 mm Hg on 100% O_2 by mask or if the patient is in respiratory arrest

PEEP; if the patient is unresponsive to 100% O_2 and PEEP, consider extracorporeal membrane oxygenation

• **Other measures:**

Bronchodilators prn (albuterol 2.5 mg nebul)

Isotonic crystalloid solution IV for hypotension

Foley catheter, CVP, and NG tube

Pharmacologic treatment of agitation and seizures; hyperventilation, elevation of head by 30°, osmotic diuretics, barbiturates, and steroids for increasing ICP

DI • **Asymptomatic patients,** or those who become so after 4–6 hours of observation with a normal physical examination, room air ABG analysis, and CXR: home with a responsible relative or friend

• **All other patients:** admission. The level of care (floor versus ICU) depends on severity and progression of clinical and laboratory findings. Indications for transfer include lack of ICU facilities and lack of a pulmonary specialist capable of performing bronchoscopy.

CHAPTER 5

Gastrointestinal Emergencies

ACUTE ABDOMINAL PAIN

KY Abdominal pain is associated with several common diagnoses (listed in descending order of frequency): etiology unknown (42%), gastroenteritis (31%) [presence of vomiting (gastritis) and diarrhea (enteritis)], gastritis, PUD, gallbladder disease, diarrhea, and pancreatitis. Other causes of abdominal pain are UTI, diverticulitis, PID, appendicitis, ectopic pregnancy, ovarian cyst and torsion, bowel obstruction, renal colic, AAA, and DKA.

- **Visceral abdominal pain** (autonomic fibers) is crampy, intermittent, and colicky; common causes are early appendicitis, bowel obstruction, and renal colic.
- **Somatic abdominal pain** (pain fibers in parietal peritoneum) is constant, sharper, and more localized and often results from late appendicitis, liver disease, and peritonitis from any cause.

HX
- **Characteristics of pain:** location, onset, duration, quality, severity, radiation
- **Associated symptoms:** nausea, vomiting, diarrhea, urinary difficulties, and vaginal discharge or bleeding
- **Important factors in PMH:** previous episodes, use of drugs and alcohol, and menstrual history

PX
- **General:** Abnormal vital signs and temperature; possible pallor, shock, rales, diminished breath sounds
- **Abdomen:** splinting, guarding, and pulsatile masses; auscultation for bowel sounds; percussion for peritoneal irritation; palpation of all four quadrants, initially away from most tender region, for masses, rebound, point tenderness, Murphy's sign, iliopsoas sign, obturator sign, hernia
- **Back:** possible CVA tenderness
- **Rectum:** possible masses, tenderness, blood
- **Genital:** males: scrotal masses and tenderness; females: vaginal discharge, bleeding, cervical motion tenderness, adnexal fullness, and focal tenderness

DD
- **Lower lobe pneumonia** may mimic abdominal pain
- **Common etiologies for tenderness** (according to abdominal region):
  RUQ: hepatitis, cholecystitis, cholangitis

LUQ: gastritis, PUD
Epigastric: PUD, pancreatitis
RLQ: appendicitis, PID, ectopic pregnancy
LLQ: diverticulitis, PID, ectopic pregnancy
Suprapubic: cystitis, hernia, torsion
Diffuse or any quadrant: aneurysm, pancreatitis (mostly peri-umbilical), bowel obstruction, ureteral calculus, perforation/peritonitis, irritable bowel syndrome, gastroenteritis, inflammatory bowel disease, mesenteric ischemia
CVA/flank: ureteral calculus, pyelonephritis

LB CBC, SMA-7, UA, cardiac enzymes

IM EKG, chest and abdominal radiographs; CT of abdomen prn

TX • Airway, IV fluids, supplemental O_2, monitoring prn
• Treatment for specific condition
• NG tube for obstruction or bleeding
• NPO
• Analgesia as indicated
• Appropriate consult (e.g., surgery, OB-GYN); immediate surgical intervention for major emergencies, including perforated viscus, abdominal aortic aneurysm, appendicitis, and strangulated hernia; generally, abdominal pain lasting > 6 hours or occurring in the elderly requires a surgical consult

DI Admission for all but mildest cases to floor, ICU, or OR

APPENDICITIS

KY This disorder usually results from hyperplasia of lymphatic tissue or fecaliths, leading to luminal obstruction. Mucus accumulates, intraluminal pressure increases, and obstruction of lymphatic drainage occurs, causing pain. Incidence peaks in the second and third decades.

HX The typical case involves diffuse abdominal pain that lasts several hours and low-grade fever, followed by pain localizing to the RLQ. The pain is accompanied by anorexia, nausea, and occasional vomiting.

PX • Temperature rarely > 37.8°C without perforation
• Abdomen: guarding, maximum tenderness at McBurney's point, sometimes hyperesthesia, percussion, rebound, psoas sign, obturator sign
• Rectum: tenderness in RLQ

DD • **Most common misdiagnoses (in descending order of frequency):** mesenteric lymphadenitis, PID, twisted ovarian cyst, mittelschmerz, gastroenteritis

- **Less common erroneous causes:** diverticulitis, perforated ulcer, cholecystitis, ectopic pregnancy, kidney stone, bowel obstruction, pyelonephritis, endometriosis, mesenteric infarction

LB CBC (WBC shows slight elevation with left shift), UA, β-hCG, SMA-7 (if nausea and vomiting are present); LFTs, amylase, lipase

IM Plain film of abdomen may show appendicolith; perhaps abdominal CT for appendicitis

TX
- Airway, IV fluids, supplemental O_2, monitoring prn; NPO
- If diagnosis is unequivocal: surgical consult

DI OR. If diagnosis is unclear, admission for observation or discharge with clear instructions for return for reexamination either in 8 hours or if pain increases

CHOLECYSTITIS

KY Most cases (95%) are caused by gallstones (cholelithiasis) passing through the cystic duct. Biliary colic involves pain lasting < 6 hours, and cholecystitis is pain of longer duration, indicating obstruction with secondary infection and fever. The condition is common in women who are > 40 years of age, obese, or multiparous.

HX Commonly, a sudden onset of RUQ pain after a fatty meal. Initially colicky pain, which is then constant and radiating to the back and/or the right scapular region; it is accompanied by nausea and vomiting

PX
- Slight fever; decreased bowel sounds, RUQ tenderness often with guarding and rebound, occasionally palpable gallbladder, Murphy's sign
- Restlessness with biliary colic; avoidance of motion in cholecystitis

DD Appendicitis, perforated ulcer, acute pancreatitis, hepatitis, RLL pneumonia, PUD

LB CBC (WBC, 10,000–15,000/mm³), SMA-7 with LFTs (increased bilirubin, mild elevation of ALT, AST, alkaline phosphatase), amylase (amylase elevation suggests pancreatitis secondary to biliary tract disease), UA

IM US, radionuclide (HIDA) scan if high suspicion and US normal

TX
- Airway, IV fluids, supplemental O_2, monitoring prn
- NG tube decompression
- Acute cholecystitis: surgical consult

DI
- **Resolved uncomplicated biliary colic:** discharge
- **Acute cholecystitis:** surgical admission for possible immediate surgery

CIRRHOSIS

KY Alcoholic destruction of liver is the most common cause of cirrhosis. Hepatic metabolism is altered, coagulopathy occurs, and the detoxifying ability of the liver is lost. Because of fibrosis, blood is shunted from hepatic artery to portal vein, resulting in portal hypertension and varices. Complications include bleeding esophageal varices, hepatic encephalopathy, hepatorenal syndrome, and spontaneous bacterial peritonitis.

HX • Malaise, lethargy, weight loss, fluid retention, pruritus, weakness, muscle wasting, anorexia, nausea, vomiting, diarrhea, and fever
• Chronic alcohol consumption
• Viral, gallbladder, or inflammatory bowel disease
• Other chronic or childhood diseases
• Coagulopathy
• Exposure to hepatotoxic agents (e.g., carbon tetrachloride) or drugs (e.g., acetaminophen, allopurinol, phenytoin)

PX Evaluate vital signs
• Skin: spider angioma, palmar erythema, hyperpigmentation, and jaundice
• Chest: gynecomastia
• Abdomen: ascites and hepatosplenomegaly
• Rectum: bleeding
• Extremities: asterixis ("liver flap"), pedal edema, and polyneuropathy
• Neurologic signs: cerebellar dysfunction, tremors, and AMS

DD • **Jaundice:** hemolysis, obstructive jaundice, viral hepatitis, hepatotoxic ingestions, septicemia
• **AMS:** hepatic encephalopathy, viral hepatitis, Reye's syndrome, hepatotoxic or other drug ingestions, intracranial bleeding

LB CBC (anemia and thrombocytopenia), chemistries (elevated bilirubin, alkaline phosphatase, hyponatremia, hypokalemia, decreased albumin), coagulation studies (elevated PT), serum ammonia; toxicology screen prn

IM CXR, EKG; brain CT prn

TX • **General measures:** ABCs; IV fluids, O_2, protein restriction, cautious use of potassium-sparing diuretics, and correction of fluid and electrolyte abnormalities
• **Decreased mental status:** thiamine (100 mg IV), 50% dextrose (1 amp)
• **Bleeding esophageal varices:** two large-bore IV lines, volume replacement with NS and packed cells, NG suction, IV vasopressin drip (20 U in 200 ml NS) at 0.5 U/min, and tamponade with Sengstaken-Blakemore tube or emergency portal decompression prn

- **Hepatic encephalopathy:**
    Neomycin (to suppress bacteria responsible for ammonia production): 1 g PO or by NG q6hr
    Lactulose (to prevent ammonia diffusing from bowel): 30 ml PO/PR tid. (Lactulose in contact with colonic bacteria creates low pH, which traps ammonia in colon as nondiffusible ammonium ions.)
- **Spontaneous bacterial peritonitis:** cefotaxime (2 g IV q6hr)

DI All but mildest cases: admission; for complications/surgical consultation for bleeding varices: ICU

DIARRHEA

KY Diarrhea is an increase in stool liquidity, frequency, and urgency. Most acute cases result from viral diseases or food poisoning from *Staphylococcus* or *Clostridium* toxins.

HX Similar symptoms in family members or friends; intake of unusual foods, drugs (particularly antibiotics), or alcohol; history of previous episodes, surgery, systemic illnesses, and recent travel; and weight loss

PX
- Vital signs: evaluate and check for orthostatic BP
- Dehydration or cachexia
- Abdomen: bowel sounds increased except in surgical abdomen; tenderness localized or diffuse, masses
- Rectum: tenderness and blood

DD Viral or bacterial infection (commonly *Shigella, Salmonella,* or *Campylobacter*), parasitic infection (amebiasis, giardiasis), inflammatory bowel disease (Crohn's disease or ulcerative colitis), food poisoning, acute surgical abdomen (e.g., small bowel obstruction, perforated appendicitis, ulcer, diverticulitis, mesenteric infarction), drugs

LB CBC, chemistries, UA, stool specimen for wet mount, Gram/Wright stain for WBCs (suggests bacterial etiology), O&P, culture prn

IM KUB

TX
- IV fluids and electrolytes for dehydration
- Clear liquids for 48 hours, then expand the diet as tolerated
- Antibiotics are generally not indicated for acute diarrhea; if a bacterial cause is suspected, give empiric therapy with TMP-SMX (one DS tab bid) or ciprofloxacin (500 mg PO bid × 7 days)

DI
- Discharge
- Admission for severe dehydration or surgical abdomen (see Acute Abdominal Pain)

DIVERTICULAR DISEASE

KY Diverticula are herniations of the mucosa or submucosa through the muscular layer of the colon (usually the sigmoid colon), near vasculature. Diverticula are prevalent in elderly individuals. Diverticulosis refers to the presence of diverticula with or without symptoms, and diverticulitis is inflammation of diverticula, with significant signs and symptoms. Complications include perforation, bleeding, obstruction, and abscess and fistula formation.

HX • **General:** previous attacks, bloody bowel movements, and dark-colored stools
  • **Diverticulosis:** intermittent, crampy LLQ pain, which is worse after eating and relieved by bowel movement or flatus, and may be accompanied by either constipation or diarrhea
  • **Diverticulitis:** constant, severe, usually LLQ pain, accompanied by altered bowel habits; anorexia; nausea and vomiting; and fever

PX • Vital signs: fever and tachycardia indicate infection; hypotension indicates sepsis or perforation
  • Abdomen: LLQ tenderness, mass, signs of peritonitis (e.g., rebound, guarding)
  • Rectum: blood, mass
  • Pelvic area: mass

DD Irritable bowel syndrome, inflammatory bowel disease, colorectal cancer, appendicitis (rare), sigmoid volvulus, TOA, ischemic colitis, angiodysplasia (bleeding)

LB CBC, chemistries, blood and urine cultures, PT, T&C prn

IM CXR to check for free air under the diaphragm, indicating perforation; abdominal radiographs (flat and upright)

TX • **Diverticulosis:** high-fiber diet and anticholinergic agent [e.g., dicyclomine (20 mg PO qid)]
  • **Mild diverticulitis:** same treatment as for diverticulosis, plus clear liquid diet and aerobe/anaerobe coverage with amoxicillin or cephalexin plus metronidazole (500 mg PO qid) or ciprofloxacin (500 mg PO bid × 7 days)
  • **Severe diverticulitis:** IV with LR, NG suction, and cefoxitin 1 g IVPB q6hr

DI • **Diverticulosis** and **mild diverticulitis:** outpatient surgical follow-up
  • **Diverticulitis:** admission and surgical consult

GASTROINTESTINAL BLEEDING

KY GI bleeding, which may be occult, overt, or massive, is referred to as upper or lower, depending on whether it is proximal or distal to the suspensory ligament of Treitz. The most common cause of upper GI bleeding is PUD, and the most common cause of lower GI bleeding is diverticulosis.

HX
- Vomiting blood (hematemesis) with or without abdominal pain; black tarry stools (melena) suggest upper GI bleeding; bright red bloody stools (hematochezia) indicate lower GI bleeding
- Previous episodes or a history of ulcers, alcohol abuse, liver disease, bleeding problems, or the use of aspirin or other anti-inflammatory agents and anticoagulants may be noted
- Severe bleeding may manifest as weakness, pallor, syncope, or if the patient is in shock, as hypotension, tachycardia, and diaphoresis

PX
- Vital signs: hypotension, tachycardia, and orthostatic changes
- HEENT: epistaxis, bleeding, palpebral pallor consistent with anemia
- Skin: stigmata of alcoholism and pallor
- Abdomen: distention, bowel sounds, masses, tenderness, and rebound
- Rectum: frank bleeding or occult blood

DD
- **Upper GI bleeding:** PUD, erosive gastritis, erosive esophagitis, esophageal varices, Mallory-Weiss tear, neoplasm, hemoptysis, pharyngeal bleeding, epistaxis
- **Lower GI bleeding:** diverticulosis, neoplasm, polyps, infection, vascular malformation, hemorrhoids, trauma

LB CBC, PT, PTT, T&C (4–6 U) prn, chemistries; NG tube (bright red blood or coffee-ground material)

TX
- **Airway, IV fluids, supplemental O$_2$, monitoring prn**
- **Upper GI bleeding:**
  - NG tube and saline lavage
  - Sengstaken-Blakemore tube
  - Pharmacologic intervention with vasopressin or octreotide
  - Consider emergent EGD for unstable patients
  - Suspected perforation: antibiotics (e.g., cefoxitin); surgical consult regarding EGD
- **Hemodynamic instability (upper or lower GI bleeding):**
  - O$_2$, cardiac monitoring, two large-bore IV lines, NS or LR wide open, and Foley catheter for I/O measurement

Table 5.1 Characteristics of Inflammatory Bowel Disease

	Crohn's Disease*	Ulcerative Colitis
Area of colon affected	"Stem-to-stern" (mouth to anus) Segmental (skip areas) Ileum (most common)	Contiguous (no skip areas) Rectosigmoid colon (95% of cases)
Epidemiology (peak incidence)	(15–22 yr; 55–60 yr) Common in Europeans, Jews; more frequent in Caucasians than African Americans Family history in 10%–15% of patients	(10–20 yr; 20–30 yr) Family history: 1°-relative with disease: 15× greater risk
Bowel involvement	All layers Thick bowel wall; narrow lumen Creeping fat: mesenteric fat over bowel wall "Cobblestone" mucosal appearance Fissures; fistulas; abscesses	Mucosa and submucosa Mucosal ulceration Epithelial necrosis Mild: fine, granular, friable mucosa Severe: spongy, red, oozing ulcerations Cryptococcal abscesses Toxic megacolon
Clinical features	Fever, chronic diarrhea without gross blood, RLQ pain	Bloody diarrhea, abdominal pain, ± vomiting, fever If toxic megacolon: toxic appearance ± mass
Treatment	Antidiarrheal medications	*No* antidiarrheal medications

*Crohn's disease is also known as regional enteritis, terminal ileitis, and granulomatous ileocolitis.

> If class III hemorrhage (30%–40% blood loss indicated by decreased capillary refill and decreased SBP), then transfusion with packed cells (O-negative if hypotensive after 2 L NS and type-specific blood is not available)

DI Unstable cases: admission, usually to ICU; persistent bleeding or unstable vital signs: ICU and immediate surgical/GI consult

INFLAMMATORY BOWEL DISEASE

KY This disorder encompasses two conditions, Crohn's disease (regional enteritis) and ulcerative colitis. Inflammatory bowel disease accounts for the most ED visits for complications of a previously diagnosed GI disease, including hemorrhage, intestinal obstruction, bowel perforation, and toxic megacolon (Table 5.1).

HX
- **Crohn's disease:** chronic diarrhea, anorexia
- **Ulcerative colitis:** occasional constipation, rectal bleeding, bloody diarrhea, and tachycardia. Frequency of bowel movements, severity of abdominal pain, rectal bleeding, past history of hospitalizations, and family history of similar disease should be considered.
- **Both conditions:** abdominal pain, fever, and weight loss

PX
- Fever, tachycardia, and decreased BP; dehydration
- Abdomen: distended, tender, tympanitic, rigid, possible rebound, and presence of mass (toxic megacolon)
- Rectum: blood

DD
- **Bleeding:** bacterial diarrhea (e.g., *Shigella, Campylobacter*), amebiasis, gay bowel syndrome, HIV infection, ischemic colitis
- **Abdominal pain:** gastroenteritis, appendicitis, cholecystitis, intestinal obstruction, aneurysm, mesenteric occlusive disease, diverticulitis

LB CBC, chemistries

IM Abdominal series

TX
- **General management:** airway, IV fluids, supplemental O_2, monitoring prn, correction of volume and electrolytes; consult with primary care physician concerning the patient's condition and need for admission in cases of known disease
- **Ulcerative colitis:** for toxic megacolon: aggressive fluid management, NG tube to decompress stomach, and surgical consult; if the patient's condition is not fulminant, prednisone (30 mg PO bid) should be considered
- **Crohn's disease (regional enteritis)**
  Fulminating symptoms without previous steroid use: ACTH (120 U/day continuous IV)
  Fulminating symptoms with no previous steroid use; hydrocortisone (100 mg IV q6–8hr) or methylprednisolone (20 mg IV q6–8hr)
  Sulfasalazine: 5 g/day; diphenoxylate: 5 mg PO qid
  Metronidazole (10–20 mg/kg/d) should be considered

DI Admit for pain control; for patients with toxic megacolon, hemorrhage, obstruction, or perforation: ICU and surgical consult

INTESTINAL OBSTRUCTION

KY The most common causes of mechanical obstruction of the small bowel (listed in order of descending frequency) are adhesions from previous surgery, hernia, and carcinoma. Obstruction of the large bowel usually results from fecal impaction or carcinoma. Paralytic ileus, or decreased motility of intestine, is due to dysfunction of structures touching the bowel (e.g., ureteral distention, retroperitoneal hemorrhage).

HX The most frequent symptom is crampy abdominal pain, with spasms lasting several minutes. Vomiting and abdominal distention are common. Previous surgery and abdominal infection such as PID should be considered.

PX • Abdomen: scars and hernias; bowel sounds are decreased, come in rushes, and are frequently high-pitched or tinkling; distention and tympany may be present; palpation reveals diffuse tenderness
  • Rectum: possible impacted feces or tumor, occult blood
DD • Perforated ulcer, pancreatitis, appendicitis with peritonitis, cholecystitis, renal and biliary colic
  • With distention: uremia, mesenteric thrombosis, peritonitis
  • Large bowel obstruction: peritonitis, colitis with distention, ileus (i.e., postoperative), uremia

LB CBC, SMA-7

IM Upright CXR, flat and upright abdominal films (small bowel obstruction: "stepladder" appearance of bowel gas, with AFLs; large bowel obstruction: gas round or square in shape, with haustra markings)

TX Airway, IV fluids, supplemental O_2, monitoring prn; NG tube to decompress stomach if the patient is vomiting; surgical consult

DI Admission

PANCREATITIS

KY This disease involves the aberrant activation of enzymes in pancreatic ducts resulting in autodigestion of portions of the gland. Alcoholism is the most common cause, and cholelithiasis is the second most common etiologic factor. The Ranson criteria for predicting severity on admission are: age > 55 years, WBC > 16,000/mm^3, glucose > 200 mg/dl, LDH > 350 IU/L, AST > 250 U/L. Within 48 hours, the criteria are: BUN is > 5 mg/dl, PaO_2 < 60 mm Hg, Ca < 8 mg/dl, Hct falls > 10%, base deficit > 4 mEq, fluid sequestration > 6 L. Mortality with three or more positive findings (Ranson criteria) is 95%.

HX • Constant severe abdominal pain, often radiating to the back because of retroperitoneal irritation; bending over gives relief because it moves peritoneal organs away from the retroperitoneum; nausea and vomiting are common
  • The patient may have a history of alcohol or drug use, gallbladder disease, endocrine disorders, and previous attacks

PX Fever and tachycardia in severe cases. Observe for sequelae of alcoholism. Abdomen: guarding, decreased bowel sounds, diffuse tenderness, and often with signs of peritoneal irritation; periumbilical ecchymosis (Cullen's sign) and/or flank ecchymosis (Grey Turner's sign) in hemorrhagic pancreatitis

DD Acute cholecystitis, PUD, alcoholic gastritis, alcoholic ketoacidosis, perforated viscus, bowel infarction; serum amylase elevation occurs in cholecystitis, bowel obstruction, perforated peptic ulcer, mesenteric thrombosis, ruptured aortic aneurysm, ruptured tubal pregnancy, and advanced renal insufficiency

LB CBC (low Hgb and Hct may suggest hemorrhagic pancreatitis), SMA-7, Ca (glucose elevation, Ca decrease secondary to precipitation of Ca soaps), serum amylase and lipase (usually elevated; lipase more sensitive)

IM CXR (effusion and/or free air), KUB (gallstones; calcifications in chronic pancreatitis; localized ileus, with "sentinel loop")

TX
- Airway, IV fluids, supplemental O_2, monitoring prn; NPO
- Analgesia with meperidine (50–100 mg IM q4–6hr prn) because less spasm of ampulla of Vater than morphine
- Antiemetic with prochlorperazine [10 mg IM (5–10 mg IV) q3hr prn] or hydroxyzine (50 mg IM q2–3hr prn)
- NG suction if ileus present

DI Admission to general floor; with hemorrhagic or other complications, ICU with surgical consult

PEPTIC ULCER DISEASE (PUD)

KY Disruption of balance between acid–pepsin and mucosal defense factors causes ulceration of gastroduodenal mucosa extending through the muscularis mucosa. Surgical complications are bleeding and perforation. *Helicobacter pylori* is involved in the etiology of PUD, and referral for further evaluation to a primary care physician is appropriate.

HX
- Exacerbations of abdominal pain after eating, when acid increases in response to food (gastric ulcer), or at night/early morning when food or antacids bring rapid relief and "pain later" (duodenal ulcer)
- Hematemesis and dark stools
- Perforation: sudden onset of severe constant abdominal pain radiating to back, chest, or shoulders
- Risk factors: positive family history, associated diseases, male gender, advanced age, smoking, and use of ASA or NSAIDs

- Few signs unless complications occur; bleeding or perforation may result in tachycardia and hypotension (check for orthostatic hypotension if bleeding is suspected); with perforation, shallow respirations and lying perfectly still
- Abdomen: bowel sounds with mild epigastric tenderness (mild case); guarding, rebound, and abdominal rigidity (perforation)
- Rectum: guaiac-positive stool or melena

DD Gastritis, gastroenteritis, biliary tract disease, esophagitis, pancreatitis, MI, angina, pneumonia

LB CBC, SMA-7. If bleeding or perforation is suspected, PT, PTT, T&C, cardiac monitor

IM EKG (if high-risk age group), upright CXR and/or flat and upright abdominal films (to detect free air)

TX • **IV fluids, supplemental O_2, monitoring prn**
- **Uncomplicated cases:** relief with antacids such as Maalox or Mylanta (30 ml PO) or combinations with viscous lidocaine (10 ml PO); sometimes cimetidine (300 mg bolus IVPB and 900 mg continuous infusion over 24 hours) or ranitidine (50 mg IV q6hr) prn
- **Bleeding:** O_2, IV of isotonic solution (LR or NS), NG tube, saline nasogastric lavage, blood products, mechanical or pharmacologic intervention, GI consult (see Gastrointestinal Bleeding)
- **Perforation:** O_2, NG tube, large-bore IV lines, Foley catheter, surgical consult

DI • Uncomplicated cases: home with H_2 receptor antagonist [e.g., cimetidine (800 mg qhs), ranitidine (300 mg qhs), famotidine (40 mg qhs)] prn, or a protein-pump inhibitor (omeprazole). May add OTC antacid such as Mylanta PO qid (primarily ac and qhs)
- Pain, bleeding, or comorbid disease, or PUD in elderly patients: admission to general floor
- Continued bleeding or perforation: immediate surgical or GI consult and preparation for OR or EGD

CHAPTER 6

Gynecologic Emergencies

DYSFUNCTIONAL UTERINE BLEEDING

KY Abnormal uterine bleeding, which is associated with anovulatory cycles, may occur in the absence of other detectable organic lesions. Metrorrhagia is heavy bleeding between periods, and menorrhagia is prolonged, increased menstrual bleeding. The bleeding is usually related to anovulation with estrogen overstimulation of endothelium unopposed by progesterone, with subsequent breakdown.

HX Patients are adolescent and perimenopausal women, with delayed menses, who complain of bleeding that soaks more than one tampon or pad an hour for several hours

PX Thorough pelvic examination, which includes visual inspection and bimanual examination, to look for evidence of injury; mass; foreign body, especially in prepubescent girls; or infectious process

DD Fibroids, endometriosis, polyps, foreign body, carcinoma, coagulopathy, threatened abortion, ectopic pregnancy

LB CBC, PT, PTT, pregnancy test

IM Consider transvaginal US for positive pregnancy test, adnexal tenderness, or palpable adnexal mass

TX
- **Bleeding lesions (cervical or vaginal):** silver nitrate sticks or suture with 0-0 chromic in figure-of-eight stitch
- **Brisk bleeding:** conjugated estrogen (25 mg IV q4hr × 4 doses)
- **Women < 35 years of age:** control with combination oral contraceptive
- **Postmenopausal women:** OB-GYN consult; endometrial biopsy is necessary to rule out endometrial hyperplasia, and D&C may be required to control bleeding

DI Admission for patients with severe anemia or those who are hemodynamically unstable; surgery may be necessary

DYSMENORRHEA

KY The incidence of dysmenorrhea, which affects 90% of women with a positive family history, peaks in the mid-20s. Primary dysmenorrhea, which is believed to be mediated by prostaglandins, has no organic pathology. Secondary dysmenorrhea, which occurs at menarche or after 30 years of age, has an organic cause. Common etiologic factors include endometriosis, fibroids, polyps, and uterine abnormalities.

HX Painful menstruation, with midline abdominal cramps that radiate to the back or thighs; diarrhea, headache, nausea, and vomiting

PX Pelvic examination to rule out organic causes, with visual inspection and bimanual examination, looking for vaginal or cervical discharge; evidence of trauma; mass; foreign body; or infectious process

DD Vaginal or cervical trauma, cervical or uterine mass, uterine fibroma, pelvic endometriosis

LB Hct, Hgb, pregnancy test

IM Consider pelvic US or CT

TX • Pain control: NSAIDs (ibuprofen, naproxen), with bed rest and moist heat
  • Consider OCPs

DI Most patients can be discharged home, with OB-GYN referral for close follow-up and possible workup, including direct laparoscopy

ENDOMETRIOSIS

KY Endometriosis, the abnormal implantation of endometrial tissue anywhere in the peritoneal cavity, is caused by retrograde tubal transmission of menstruation products.

HX Dyspareunia, dysmenorrhea, infertility, chronic pelvic pain, and abnormal vaginal bleeding

PX • Large cystic ovarian mass, immobile uterus, and tender nodules on uterosacral ligaments or in posterior cul-de-sac
  • Rupture of "chocolate cysts" or endometriomas on ovaries may present as an acute abdomen

LB Pregnancy test; CBC; T&C

IM Consider pelvic US or CT

TX OB-GYN referral for combination pill ("pseudopregnancy"), danazol ("pseudomenopause"), or progesterone therapy

DI Outpatient workup, unless laparoscopy is necessary or the patient is acutely ill, in which case admission is necessary

MITTELSCHMERZ

KY Mittelschmerz, or midcycle pain, results from ovulation.

HX Adnexal pain at the time of ovulation; unilateral pain from leakage of blood from the graafian follicle

PX Sharp, localized, pain; peritoneal irritation

DD Acute appendicitis, ovarian torsion, hemorrhagic ovarian cyst, acute salpingitis, acute nephrolithiasis, pyelonephritis, diverticulitis, inflammatory bowel disease

LB Pregnancy test; also consider CBC with differential, UA, cervical Gram stain

IM Consider pelvic US or CT

TX NSAIDs; condition usually resolves in 24–48 hours

DI Home

OVARIAN CYST

KY Ovarian cysts often cause pressure with pelvic or abdominal discomfort. Rupture causes acute, often unilateral pain after exercise or intercourse.

HX Patients are usually asymptomatic unless rupture, hemorrhage, infection, or torsion occurs.

PX • Normally, ovaries of premenarchal and postmenopausal women are not palpable; if they are, malignancy must be ruled out.
   • Irritation of peritoneum can be absent, well localized, or diffuse.
   • Sudden enlargement of adnexal mass signifies intra-ovarian hemorrhage that requires surgery.

DD Dermoid cyst, serous cyst, corpus luteal cyst, endometrioma, malignancy, torsion, appendicitis, UTI, pyelonephritis, salpingitis, TOA, ectopic pregnancy

LB Pregnancy test, CBC with differential, UA; possibly culdocentesis

IM Pelvic US

TX • **Rupture of serous cyst:** spontaneous resolution
   • **Rupture of endometrioma and corpus luteum cyst:** laparotomy

DI Admission to gynecology floor for severe pain, evidence of severe infection, or severe anemia; outpatient management in all other cases

OVARIAN TORSION

KY This condition involves twisting of the ovary, resulting in severe pain. Complications include infertility, increased risk of ectopic pregnancy from a scarred fallopian tube, and infection and necrosis leading to peritonitis and shock.

HX
- Sudden onset; sharp, intermittent, unilateral pain; nausea, vomiting; low-grade fever; and dysuria
- Previous episodes of a similar nature, which probably represent spontaneous detorsion

PX Hypogastric tenderness without rebound, adnexal tenderness, and possibly a palpable mass

DD Ectopic pregnancy, appendicitis, salpingitis, ovarian cyst, nephrolithiasis, pyelonephritis

LB Pregnancy test, CBC, culdocentesis

IM Pelvic US (more common) or CT

TX Laparotomy

DI OR

PELVIC INFLAMMATORY DISEASE (PID)

KY The CDC has established *specific,* standardized criteria for the diagnosis of this genital tract infection. PID should be diagnosed only when these criteria have been satisfied. Complications of PID include infertility, abscess, dyspareunia, chronic pelvic pain, and increased risk of ectopic pregnancy.

HX
- Symptoms include pelvic pain, fever, dysuria, nausea, vomiting, and abnormal postmenstrual vaginal bleeding. Risk factors include IUD use, recent pelvic instrumentation, and a history of STD or previous episode of PID.

PX
- **Necessary physical findings for diagnosis** (per the CDC; *all three must be present*): abdominal tenderness, cervical motion tenderness, and adnexal tenderness
- **Additional requirements for diagnosis** (*one of these conditions must also be present*):
   Temperature > 38.2°C
   WBC > 10,000/mm^3
   Inflammatory mass by examination or US
   WBCs or bacteria on culdocentesis

Gram stain or antibody test (C-reactive protein) positive for *Neisseria gonorrhoeae* and culture positive for *Chlamydia trachomatis*
- **Other signs:** friable cervix, purulent discharge, Fitz-Hugh—Curtis syndrome (perihepatitis, inflammation around the liver from pus leaking from right fallopian tube)

DD Acute salpingitis, cervicitis, TOA, ectopic pregnancy, appendicitis, ovarian cyst, vaginitis, cystitis, pyelonephritis

LB CBC, UA, pregnancy test, antibody test, Gram stain, cervical cultures for *N. gonorrhoeae* and *C. trachomatis*

IM Consider pelvic US or CT for severe tenderness or lack of response to antibiotics in 48–72 hours

TX • **Outpatient antibiotics (one regimen):**
   Ceftriaxone (250 mg IM once) or cefoxitin (2 g IM once) plus probenecid (1 g PO once) or
   Spectinomycin (2 g IM once) and doxycycline (100 mg PO bid × 10–14 days) or
   Ofloxacin (400 mg PO bid × 14 days) plus either clindamycin (450 mg PO qid) or metronidazole (500 mg PO bid × 14 days)
- **Inpatient antibiotics (one regimen):**
   Cefoxitin (2 g IV q6hr) or cefotetan (2 g IV q12hr) in addition to doxycycline (100 mg PO/IV q12hr) or
   Clindamycin (900 mg IV q8hr) and gentamicin (2 mg/kg IV loading dose, then 1.5 mg/kg IV q8hr)

DI • **Admission for IV antibiotics** for most patients (those with TOA or pyosalpinx; temperature > 38°C; pregnancy; inability to tolerate anything by mouth; IUD; peritonitis; uncertain diagnosis; failure with outpatient antibiotics for 48 hours; and nulligravida), except in the mildest cases
- **After hospital discharge, continue doxycycline:** 100 mg PO bid for a total of 14 days

SEXUAL ASSAULT

KY Rape is nonconsensual sexual assault that may range from fondling of genitals to oral, anal, or vaginal penetration with various objects or any part of the body of the assailant. Child molestation is an illegal act performed on or with the body of a child with lewd intent. In 50% of cases of sexual assault, and in many cases of child molestation, the victim knows the assailant.

HX
- Victims of rape are usually threatened and in fear of bodily harm, and only one rape in four is reported. Children are often < 11 years of age.
- Pertinent details concerning the event should be obtained:
    Time, date, and place
    Identity of the assailant
    Site of penetration
    Occurrence of ejaculation
    Threats made and weapons used
    Use of alcohol and drugs
- Other important information should be obtained:
    Occurrence of bathing, douching, urination, defecation, teeth brushing, or changing of clothes since the assault
    Date of the last consensual sexual intercourse
    Date of the LMP
    Method of birth control
    PMH, including allergies

PX All evidence of trauma (e.g., lacerations, bruising, bite marks, scratches) should be carefully documented. Facial and extremity trauma are more common than genital trauma. Special attention should be paid to the neck, mouth, breasts, wrists, and thighs. The vagina and anus should be carefully inspected. Male victims of sodomy may have abrasions on the thorax or abdomen.

LB
- Cervical cultures for *Chlamydia* and *N. gonorrhoeae,* pregnancy test, RPR, hepatitis B, HIV serologies
- Wet mount to observe for sperm (sperm motility is lost in 12 hours; nonmotile sperm can be recovered within 72 hours); acid phosphatase decreases in 2–9 hours
- Evidence collection with appraisal kit, maintaining "chain of evidence," which usually includes the victim's underclothes along with pubic hair combings and fingernail scrapings as evidence
- Rectal or buccal smears if penetration is alleged to have occurred at that site

IM Radiographs for fractures; consider US or CT for intra-abdominal trauma and/or hemorrhage

TX
- **Rape counseling**
- **STD prophylaxis:** ceftriaxone (125 mg IM) and doxycycline (100 mg PO bid × 10 days)
- **Pregnancy prophylaxis:** norgestrel (two tab, plus two additional tab in 12 hours)
- **HIV prophylaxis:** per current CDC guidelines

- **Hepatitis prophylaxis:**
    Hepatitis B immune globulin: 0.06 ml/kg IM within 7 days of
        exposure; repeat in 1 month
    Hepatitis B vaccine: 1 ml IM; repeat in 1–6 months (adults)
    Tetanus prophylaxis if needed
    OB-GYN reevaluation for STD and pregnancy

DI Outpatient follow-up with primary care physician, referral to psychiatry to crisis intervention team

UTERINE LEIOMYOMA

KY These benign uterine fibroids are more prevalent in African Americans than Caucasians. High estrogen levels during pregnancy and postpartum stimulate leiomyoma formation.

HX Pelvic pressure and discomfort, urinary frequency, constipation, neuropathy, and secondary dysmenorrhea

PX Enlarged uterus

DD Pelvic malignancy, cervicitis, salpingitis, ectopic pregnancy, ovarian cyst

LB Pregnancy test; CBC; gynecologic consult to consider D&C to rule out carcinoma

IM Pelvic US

TX
- **Mild-to-moderate cases:** NSAIDs (e.g., ibuprofen, naproxen)
- **Severe cases:** admission for hysterectomy
- **Complications:**
    Degeneration of fibroids in pregnancy, which results in fever and
        ileus leukocytosis: IV fluids and analgesics
    Twisting of pedunculated fibroids, causing colicky pain: immediate surgery
    Infection and eventual abortion of fibroids, with severe pain, prolonged bleeding, cervical dilation, and mass in cervical canal:
        immediate myomectomy, hysterectomy, or D&C

DI • Admission to gynecology bed for severe pain or associated problems; outpatient workup in all other cases

VAGINAL INFECTIONS

Vaginitis (trichomoniasis)

KY Trichomoniasis ranges in severity, from asymptomatic conditions to association with PID. Coinfection with GC is present in 50% of patients with *Trichomonas vaginalis* infection.

HX Vaginal discharge with vulvovaginal discomfort or pruritus; patients may complain of dysuria or dyspareunia

PX Profuse foamy vaginal discharge, some vaginal inflammation; "strawberry cervix" is rare but suggestive

DD Vaginosis, vulvovaginal candidiasis, PID, UTI

LB Wet mount shows mobile trichomonads

TX • **Sexual partners should be treated**
  • **Pregnant patients:**
     First trimester: no metronidazole; clotrimazole (100-mg tab vag qhs × 2 weeks)
     Second and third trimesters: either clotrimazole or metronidazole; consider obstetrics consult
  • **Nonpregnant patients:** metronidazole (2 g PO single dose or 500 mg PO bid × 7 days)
  • **Treatment failures:** metronidazole (500 mg PO bid × 7 days)

DI Home

Vaginosis (bacterial)

KY The malodorous vaginal discharge that occurs with vaginosis may be polymicrobial, but it is usually associated with *Gardnerella vaginalis.*

HX Vaginal discharge, with fewer associated symptoms than with vaginitis

PX Malodorous white or gray vaginal discharge; little sign of vaginal inflammation

DD Vaginitis and vulvovaginal candidiasis

LB Discharge contains stippled epithelial cells coated with coccobacilli, clue cells

TX • **Pregnant patients:**

> First trimester: no metronidazole; consider no treatment if minimal symptoms; if symptomatic: amoxicillin (250 mg tid × 10 days)

> Second and third trimester: as with first trimester; possible use of metronidazole

• **Nonpregnant patients:** metronidazole (0.5 g PO bid × 7 days) or 0.75% vaginal gel (5 g vag bid × 5 days)

DI Outpatient management

Vulvovaginal candidiasis

KY This condition, which often occurs after antibiotic treatment, is more common in immunocompromised or debilitated patients. *Candida* may be part of the normal flora.

HX Vaginal pruritus and thick "cheesy" discharge, with occasional dysuria

PX Vulvar erythema and vaginal discharge, as in bacterial vaginosis

DD Vaginitis, vaginosis, UTI

LB KOH prep for hyphae

TX • Avoidance of intercourse for 3–4 days; antifungal vaginal tab or cream such as miconazole (200-mg suppositories vag qhs × 3 days) or clotrimazole (200 mg vag qhs × 3 days)

• Even shorter treatment also advocated: clotrimazole (500 mg vag once)

• Pregnancy: nystatin × 14 days

• Recurrent disease: treat for 7–14 days and consider diabetes, pregnancy, and HIV

DI Home

CHAPTER 7

Head and Neck Emergencies

DENTAL EMERGENCIES

KY Common dental problems include abscess, gingivitis, dry socket, postextraction bleeding, tooth fracture, and tooth avulsion. Dry socket is a painful open tooth socket that develops 2 to 3 days after extraction. ANUG, or "trenchmouth," (also known as Vincent's angina) is a result of neglect.

HX Dental surgery (e.g., extraction), poor dental hygiene, trauma

PX
- **General findings:** Possible parapharyngeal, sublingual, or buccal swelling and tooth pain; each tooth in area of pain should be percussed with a tongue blade and its gingival base inspected for possible abscess
- **ANUG:** extensive inflammation, swelling, necrotic areas, bleeding, pain, fetid breath, and lymphadenopathy
- **Tooth avulsion:** an avulsed tooth should be transported in the mouth, in contact with patient's saliva if possible, and handled as little as possible

TX
- **Abscess:** penicillin VK (250 mg qid × 5 days) or clindamycin (300 mg PO tid × 5 days) and analgesic (e.g., NSAIDs, codeine)
- **ANUG:** débridement and irrigation; antibiotic in refractory cases
- **Dry socket:** irrigation of debris and sedative dressing in socket
- **Postextraction bleeding:** gauze dressing on extraction site; one suture is sometimes necessary
- **Tooth fracture:**
  Ellis I (enamel fractured; no hot-cold sensitivity or pain): elective treatment
  Ellis II (enamel fractured with dentin exposed; hot/cold sensitivity): patients < 12 years of age: $CaOH_2$ paste and foil to fracture; patients > 12 years: elective dressing with follow-up in 24 hours
  Ellis III (enamel fractured with dentin and pulp exposed; bleeding and pain): moist cotton over pulp, emergent consultation
- **Tooth avulsion:** do not scrub the tooth, thus disrupting its periodontal ligament; reimplant it immediately. The probability of successful reimplantation of avulsed tooth decreases ~ 1%/min.

DI Dental consult and follow-up

EPISTAXIS

KY Epistaxis, or nosebleed, is hemorrhaging from the nostril, nasal cavity, or nasopharynx. Anterior epistaxis usually originates from Kiesselbach's plexus.

HX Determine the nature, onset, duration, and amount of bleeding; personal or family history of hypertension, epistaxis or bleeding disorders; medication history (especially warfarin); occurrence of illness (chronic or acute) or trauma; and possible foreign body insertion

PX Ecchymosis, purpura, spider angiomas, hemarthrosis, hepatomegaly, and hypertension. Examine nares to identify source.

LB Hgb, Hct, PT, PTT

IM Consider plain radiographs or CT of facial bones if trauma is suspected

TX
- **Severe episodes:** airway, IV fluids, supplemental O_2, monitoring
- **Protective wear:** gowns for both physician and patient; gloves and eye wear for physician
- **Direct external pressure** for 5 minutes to stop bleeding; then gentle nose blowing to clear out all clots. If bleeding is brisk, cocaine-soaked pledgets may be placed in the affected nostril for 10–15 minutes before attempting other therapy
- **Control of focal areas of anterior epistaxis:** application of silver nitrate or topical hemostatic agent
- **Persistent bleeding: use of an anterior nasal pack**

  An anterior pack consisting of petroleum jelly—impregnated gauze strip smeared with antibiotic ointment may be formed in a stair-step manner using a nasal speculum and bayonet forceps

  In the nose, the leading and terminal ends should protrude from the nasal orifice. Then a $2'' \times 2''$ piece of gauze should be taped over the involved nostril.

  A nasal tampon may also be used for anterior nasal packing. This pack should be left in place for a minimum of 24–48 hours, and the patient should be given penicillin or a first-generation cephalosporin.

- **Uncontrollable bleeding:** failure to control bleeding or inability to visualize an anterior source suggests a posterior hemorrhage, which mandates the application of a posterior pack or an epistaxis balloon. Analgesia is required for this procedure. Consider topical agents (e.g., cocaine or lidocaine/phenylephrine–soaked cotton swabs) or opiate analgesia (PO or IM).

DI • Admission for patients with posterior packing, bilateral nasal packing, a history of coagulopathy, and chronic, debilitating illness or recurrent epistaxis
  • Otolaryngologic consult for patients with epistaxis unresponsive to the described treatment measures and for those who are admitted
  • Patients who are discharged with anterior nasal packing should be placed on amoxicillin or penicillin and seen by an otolaryngologist in 1–2 days

FOREIGN BODIES

Object in external auditory canal

HX • Any knowledge of foreign body type and mechanism involved; any history suggestive of tympanic membrane perforation
  • Sometimes history of chronic otitis externa or pulling at the ears in children. Younger children frequently have no definite history of insertion of any object in the ears, but parents may be concerned because children complain of pain and there is drainage from the ear.

PX Visualization of the foreign body with a large ear speculum placed in the ear and canal under anesthesia or with adequate analgesia (a good light source should be used)

DD Chronic or acute otitis externa, cholesteatoma

TX • **Small foreign bodies:** gentle irrigation with a jet of lukewarm water directed behind the foreign body is often successful
  • **Vegetable material** (irritation may cause swelling of the foreign body with subsequent occlusion of the canal): removal with alligator forceps is usually effective
  • **Smooth objects** (e.g., beads): removal with a suction catheter with a soft funnel tip. Sometimes a right-angle hook can be passed behind the foreign body and then carefully withdrawn
  • **Insects:** kill with viscous lidocaine or mineral oil in canal; then remove with alligator forceps

DI • Consider an ENT consult to discuss examination and treatment by otolaryngologist in the OR for all young children with foreign bodies in the ear
  • Immediate referral to an otolaryngologist for removal of small alkaline batteries

Object in nasal passages

HX • History of chronic rhinorrhea may be present; parents or caregivers may have witnessed the insertion of a foreign body in the nose, or the patient may confess to such insertion
• Many cases involve no history of foreign body insertion, and patients present with unilateral or bilateral purulent, foul-smelling rhinorrhea, unilateral nasal obstruction, epistaxis, or complications (e.g., sinusitis, septal abscess, cellulitis, erosion of the soft palate, bronchial aspiration, or rarely cerebral tetanus)

PX Red, swollen nasal mucosa, possibly excoriated, perhaps with signs of infection; possible foul-smelling discharge; facial swelling and pain to palpation; sometimes fever

DD Unilateral or bilateral sinusitis, facial cellulitis, septal abscess

IM • Radiologic evaluation may be helpful in cases of radiopaque foreign bodies and for assessment of complications such as sinusitis
• CT scan may be necessary for foreign bodies that are not radiopaque or cannot be localized

TX • **Forced-air technique (attempt first):**
    Occlude the uninvolved nares, place one's mouth over the child's, and blow until resistance of the closed glottis is felt
    Exhale forcibly into the patient's mouth, thus expelling the foreign body from the nose
• **If forced-air technique is unsuccessful:**
    Use cocaine 4% for anesthesia and vasoconstriction
    Attempt to remove foreign body. Many smaller objects may be amenable to removal with either bayonet or alligator forceps; a phalange-tipped suction catheter is often best for removal of round, hard objects such as beads.
    Insert a #4 Fogarty catheter above and posterior to the foreign body, inflate the balloon with 1 ml of water, and apply traction to the catheter until the balloon is lodged against the foreign body. Care must be taken when inserting the catheter so as not to push the foreign body into the nasal pharynx.
• **Do not attempt to push the foreign body posteriorly into the nasal pharynx,** because aspiration may occur. Obtain an otolaryngologic consult if these techniques are unsuccessful (see treatment)

DI • Otolaryngologic consult for complications associated with the foreign body (e.g., cellulitis, sinusitis) or if removal attempts are not successful

Sinusitis: treatment with antibiotics and close outpatient follow-up

Facial cellulitis: admission to medical floor and treatment with parenteral antibiotics

- Urgent otolaryngology consult for small alkaline battery in the nares for > 1–2 hour

Object in upper airway

HX • **Adults:** history of swallowing a piece of chicken or fish with the sensation of having a bone caught in the throat
- **Young children:** cough, stridor, hoarseness, wheezing, choking, or respiratory distress may be present

PX • Audible stridor, wheezing on auscultation, and inability to speak
- Perform a complete oropharyngeal examination, looking for the presence of a foreign body. Consider nasopharyngoscopy.

DD Croup, epiglottitis, trachomatis, asthma, bronchitis, pneumonia

IM CXR, both inspiratory and expiratory; lateral neck radiograph. Consider fluoroscopy

TX • **First priority:** immediate cricopharyngeal airway management (the most common site of upper airway obstruction is at the level of the cricopharyngeal muscle)
- **Young children** with an established or suspected hypopharyngeal or subglottic foreign body: laryngoscopy or bronchoscopy with foreign body removal performed under general anesthesia in the OR
- **Adults:** direct laryngoscopy using a blade, curved clamp, or McGill forceps for removal of fish or chicken bones; if this technique is unsuccessful, removal using a flexible bronchoscope with a channel for biopsy forceps may be effective

DI • Otolaryngologic consult for children with subglottic foreign bodies and adults with hypopharyngeal foreign bodies that cannot be removed by means of direct laryngoscopy
- Home with follow-up as necessary for all other patients if they are in no acute distress after foreign body removal

INFECTION OF THE MOUTH AND SALIVARY GLANDS

KY Cellulitis of odontogenic origin usually involves the middle and lower half of the face and neck. Ludwig's angina, a serious infection with potential for airway obstruction, involves the submaxillary, sublingual, and submental space with elevation of the tongue.

HX Pain (increased on eating), gingival swelling, massive facial swelling, toxic appearance, and compromised airway

PX
- **Pain** (to percussion with a tongue blade) indicates involvement at the apex of the tooth
- **Tender swelling of the gingiva** adjacent to a tooth suggests either a periodontal abscess or an extension of a periapical abscess to the cortex of the bone into the subperiosteal space
- **Facial cellulitis with closure of the eye** indicates potential spread of infection to the periorbital spaces and increased potential for cavernous sinus thrombosis
- **Signs of Ludwig's angina** include board-like swelling of the jaw, brawny induration, difficulty swallowing, stiffness of tongue movements, and trismus; respiratory compromise may occur as the tongue is elevated, and the oropharynx may become occluded

DD Tumor, TB, cervical lymphadenitis, submaxillary and parotid gland disease, autoimmune disease

LB CBC, blood cultures, and electrolyte determination if significant dehydration is present

IM Lateral soft tissue radiograph of the neck; consider CT scan

TX Penicillin (15–20 MU qd) or clindamycin (600–900 mg IV tid) or cefazolin (1–2 g IV tid)

DI Admission to medical floor or ICU for patients with extensive trismus, facial cellulitis with closure of the eye, suspected extension of infection to the fascial planes of the head and neck, Ludwig's angina, or impending Ludwig's angina

NECK MASS

KY Neck masses may be congenital or acquired, infectious or neoplastic, or benign or malignant. In children, most neck masses are relatively common and minor, whereas the incidence of neoplastic lesions is high in adults.

HX
- Assessment for the presence of the seven cardinal symptoms of head and neck disease: dysphagia, odynophagia, referred pain with swelling, hoarseness, stridor, speech disorder, and globus phenomena
- Other important historical features: use of tobacco, alcohol, previous radiation exposure of the neck, current or recent illnesses, current or recent injuries, infections of the head and neck, and other associated local and systemic symptoms

PX
- Scalp, face, skin, nose, ears, oral cavity, dental structures, and pharynx: thorough evaluation
- Nasopharynx, base of the tongue, and larynx: examination by digital palpation and indirect mirror visualization or nasopharyngoscopy
- Neck mass: examination and palpation for location, size, shape, consistency, mobility, and tenderness

DD
- Extensive and age-dependent
- The "80% rule" may be helpful:
  - 80% of isolated neck masses in children are benign
  - 80% of nonthyroid neck masses in adults are neoplastic
  - 80% of neoplastic masses are malignant
  - 80% of these malignant masses are metastatic
  - 80% of the primary tumors are located above the clavicle

LB CBC, Monospot, thyroid studies; needle aspiration of a neck mass in the ED is *not* recommended

IM Radiographic studies: posteroanterior and lateral views of the chest, sinus series, and lateral view of the neck

TX
- Supportive measures: airway, IV fluids, supplemental O_2, monitoring prn
- Suspected tumor in adults > 40 years of age with a history of tobacco or heavy alcohol use: referral to otolaryngologic surgeon within a short time period
- Children: treatment according to the most likely cause of the mass, with referral to their primary MD within 2 weeks if the mass does not resolve or changes shape
- Signs or symptoms of airway compromise or suspected deep neck space infection: otolaryngology consult

DI
- Admission for patients with a compromised airway or a suspected deep neck space or mediastinal infection. Toxic-appearing children or adults who are unable to swallow or tolerate oral fluids adequately should be admitted for IV antibiotic therapy and hydration.
- Outpatient workup for most patients

PERITONSILLAR ABSCESS

HX Pain, dysphagia, muffled voice, progressive inability to swallow, drooling, earache, and respiratory difficulty

PX Dehydration, unilateral enlargement of a tonsil, and trismus; erythematous soft palate and uvula pushed toward the opposite side of the abscess

DD Squamous cell carcinoma, lymphoma, leukemia, vascular lesion

LB Monospot, CBC, serum electrolyte determination, throat culture

IM Consider a soft tissue radiograph of the neck

TX
- Penicillin (1–2 MU IV q4hr) or clindamycin (600 mg IV tid)
- IV rehydration prn
- I&D
- Otolaryngologic consult

DI
- Otolaryngologic follow-up within 24 hours for patients with early peritonsillar abscess
- Admission for all other patients

RED EYE

KY Common causes of red, painful eye include corneal abrasion, corneal laceration, corneal ulceration, foreign body, and conjunctivitis. Less common causes include uveitis and glaucoma.

- **Corneal abrasion** may result from foreign bodies under the eyelid, accidental trauma, and contact lens use.
- **Corneal laceration** may result from high-energy impact injuries (e.g., from foreign bodies that embed in or penetrate the globe).
- **Corneal ulceration** is local ulceration caused by bacterial, viral, or fungal infection of the cornea; foreign bodies; burns; or abrasions. One common cause is leaving a contact lens in place beyond the recommended time frame.
- **Foreign body.** An object lodged under the eyelid may scratch or lacerate the cornea with continued blinking; an object traveling at high velocity may embed in or penetrate the globe.
- **Conjunctivitis** may be **viral** (common agents include adenovirus, enterovirus, HSV, coxsackievirus), **bacterial** (common agents include *Staphylococcus aureus, Haemophilus influenzae, Streptococcus pneumoniae, Neisseria gonorrhoeae*), or **allergic (contact)** [common agents include chemicals and cosmetics].
- **Anterior uveitis** is inflammation of the vascular tunic of the eye involving the iris (iritis) or ciliary body (iridocyclitis). Fifty percent of cases result from systemic disease (e.g., sarcoidosis, Behçet's syndrome).
- **Glaucoma.** Angle closure of the anterior chamber resulting from movement of the iris toward the cornea prevents outflow of aqueous humor. If outflow is not restored, the increased pressure may lead to irreversible optic nerve damage and blindness.

HX
- **Corneal abrasion.** The onset of symptoms is acute. Symptoms may include sharp pain or a scratching sensation (i.e., a foreign body sensation that worsens with blinking).

- **Corneal laceration.** Symptoms are similar to those of corneal abrasion, but may also include scotoma (i.e., partial vision loss) from an intraocular foreign body.
- **Foreign body.** Symptoms may include a sharp, scratching pain (as with corneal abrasions) or a sense of an object under the lid. Embedded or intraocular objects usually produce a dull, diffuse monocular ache. Patients may note decreased vision depending on the location of the foreign object.
- **Conjunctivitis**
    Viral. Symptoms (often bilateral) include diffuse conjunctival erythema and scleral injection, profuse itching, and copious watery discharge. Symptoms of an upper respiratory tract infection may be present. Other family members or close contacts may be affected.
    Bacterial. Symptoms (usually unilateral, but may become bilateral) include diffuse conjunctival erythema and scleral injection, a scratchy foreign body sensation, and a mucopurulent discharge.
    Allergic (contact). Symptoms (usually unilateral, but may become bilateral) include progressive pruritus, erythema, and scleral injection of the affected eye.
- **Anterior uveitis.** Symptoms include the acute onset of deep, burning eye pain, photophobia, and poor visual acuity.
- **Glaucoma.** Symptoms may be chronic, subacute, or acute. Patients with acute angle closure describe severe monocular pain with blurred vision, photophobia, "halos" around lights, monocular headache, nausea, and vomiting.

PX The physical examination may include the following:

- **Visual acuity evaluation** using the Snellen eye chart
- **Tonometry** (IOP usually > 50 mm Hg in glaucoma)
- **Fluorescein staining** and **Wood's lamp evaluation** to evaluate for scleral or corneal abrasions and foreign bodies
- **Slit-lamp examination** of cornea and sclera (may reveal foreign body, dendritic pattern in HSV conjunctivitis, hazy anterior chamber in glaucoma, inflammatory cells and flaring in iritis)

DD Direct ocular trauma, corneal infection (keratitis), chronic eyelid inflammation (blepharitis), dry eye syndromes (e.g., Sjögren's syndrome), autoimmune disorders (e.g., ankylosing spondylitis, Reiter's syndrome, SLE), vascular conditions (e.g., temporal arteritis); see also Table 7.1

LB Tests as appropriate if systemic condition suggested; consider Gram stain of mucopurulent discharge

IM Consider orbital radiographs or CT to rule out intraocular foreign body

Table 7.1   Differentiation of Some Conditions Associated With Red Eye

	Condition		
Finding	**Conjunctivitis**	**Anterior Uveitis**	**Glaucoma**
Onset	Gradual	Gradual	Sudden
Pain	Mild	Moderate	Severe
Vision	Normal	Blurred	Blurred
Injection	Diffuse	Ciliary	Diffuse flush
Pupil	Normal	Small, occasionally irregular	Mid-dilated
Cornea	Clear	Clear	Hazy
Discharge	Watery or purulent	Minimal	Minimal
Pressure	Normal	Normal	Increased

TX
- **Corneal abrasion** is treated by **foreign body removal, cycloplegia** [i.e., cyclopentolate 1% or homatropine 5% (2 gtt q12hr)], **analgesia** (with NSAIDs; avoid outpatient anesthetic drops because repeated use increases the risk of corneal ulcer), and **antibiotics** (bacitracin ointment applied directly to the eye and covered with an eye patch)
- **Corneal laceration.** Avoid direct outer pressure; apply a rigid eye shield.
- **Corneal ulcer.** Avoid eye patches and topical steroids. Cycloplegia involves cyclopentolate 1% or homatropine 5% (2 gtt q12hr as needed). Antibiotic therapy depends on the cause:

  Gram-positive: erythromycin 0.5% ointment every 3–4 hours or polymyxin B and trimethoprim drops every 1–4 hours

  Gram-negative: gentamicin 0.3% or tobramycin 0.3% (ointment or solution) every 4 hours

  HSV: vidarabine 3% ointment (0.5-inch applied 5 times daily), trifluridine 1% (2 gtt q2hr while awake), or idoxuridine 0.5% ointment (applied every 4–6 hours)

  VZV: acyclovir (800 mg PO 5 times daily)

  Fungal infection: IV amphotericin
- **Foreign body.** Removal can be attempted if the foreign body is located on the eyelid or outer surface; in patients with suspected embedded or intraocular foreign bodies, protect the eye with a rigid eye shield and refer the patient to an ophthalmologist for surgical removal of the object.
- **Conjunctivitis**

  Viral. Avoid topical anesthetics. Apply warm compresses and consider topical neomycin, polymyxin, or gentamicin to

prevent secondary bacterial infections [e.g., gentamicin 0.3% solution (1–2 gtt q4hr)].

Bacterial. Bacitracin or gentamicin ointments or solutions every 4 hours; if *N. gonorrhoeae* is suspected, treat with systemic ceftriaxone and frequent eye irrigation.

- **Anterior uveitis.** Treat the underlying disease process. Symptomatic treatment is with cycloplegics [e.g., cyclopentolate 1% (2 gtt q12hr) or homatropine 2% (2 gtt q12hr)] and steroids, such as prednisolone acetate 1% [2 gtt qid (consider only if infection has been ruled out)].
- **Acute angle closure glaucoma** requires emergent reduction of IOP.

  Hyperosmotic agents include mannitol 20% (1–2 g/kg IV over 45 minutes), glycerin 50% (0.1–0.15 g/kg PO), and isosorbide (1.5–2 g/kg PO).

  Carbonic anhydrase inhibitors include acetazolamide (500 mg IV and 500 mg PO administered once concomitantly, followed by 250 mg PO q6hr).

  β **Blockers** include timolol 0.5% (1 gtt q12hr), levobunolol 0.5% (1 gtt q12hr), and betaxolol 0.5% (1 gtt q12hr).

  Miotics include pilocarpine 2%–4% solution (1 gtt once).

  Corticosteroids [e.g., prednisolone 1% (1 gtt q4–6hr)] when infection is ruled out

  Antiemetics are administered as needed for hyperemesis.

DI All patients require a prompt ophthalmologic consult and/or evaluation within 24 hours.

- Patients with large corneal lacerations or intraocular foreign bodies require immediate ophthalmologic admission for surgical repair.
- Patients with suspected *N. gonorrhoeae* conjunctivitis require admission for systemic antibiotics and frequent irrigation.
- Patients with significant anterior uveitis may require medical admission to treat the underlying disease process.
- Patients with acute angle closure glaucoma may require ophthalmologic admission for surgical correction after acute intervention.

TEMPOROMANDIBULAR JOINT (TMJ) PROBLEMS

KY Jaw dislocation usually results from a weak capsule, and TMJ dislocation occurs after opening the mouth widely, yawning, or laughing. TMJ syndrome, an anatomic/occlusal problem, is associated with dull jaw pain that is usually unilateral, is exacerbated by opening the mouth, and is generally accompanied by a clicking sound.

HX Jaw pain and headache or earache

PX
- Dislocation (unilateral or bilateral), open mouth in forward position. Tenderness over the TMJ and surrounding area, which is intensified with mouth open, indicates TMJ syndrome.
- Popping and clicking can be felt by inserting the finger in the patient's ear during jaw opening and closing.

DD Toothache, headache, earache, neck ache, shoulder pain

IM
- TMJ dislocation: radiographs (also to rule out fracture)
- TMJ syndrome: radiographs in open and closed positions; tomograms and MRI may also be useful

TX
- **TMJ dislocation:**
    Conscious sedation with midazolam (3–6 mg IV) or diazepam (5–10 mg IV) titrated to achieve relaxation of masseter, temporalis, and pterygoids
    Reduction: grasp mandible with thumbs wrapped with gauze and press down and back. Deeper sedation using etomidate (0.3 mg/kg IV) or methohexital (1–2 mg/kg IV) and even potential paralysis and reduction in the OR may be necessary.
    Muscle relaxant and soft diet for 1 week
- **TMJ syndrome:**
    Moist heat for 15 min qid and soft diet for 2 weeks
    Anti-inflammatory medication and/or muscle relaxant

DI Follow-up with oral/maxillofacial surgeon

TONSILLITIS

HX Sore throat, fever, headache, dehydration, dysphagia, and myalgias

PX Erythema of the soft palate and tonsils, possible exudates, ulcerative lesions, petechiae, swollen cervical lymph nodes, and palpable liver and spleen

LB Throat culture, rapid screen for GABHS; CBC, Monospot; electrolyte levels if dehydration is a clinical problem

IM Lateral neck films if suspected abscess

TX
- **Positive for GABHS:** penicillin V (250–500 mg PO qid × 10 days) or erythromycin (250–500 mg PO qid × 10 days) or benzathine penicillin (1.2 MU IM once)
- **Negative for GABHS:** may await throat culture results and treat symptomatically

DI • Outpatient follow-up with primary care physician for patients who are not toxic with no suspected suppurative complications
- Admission should be considered for patients with complications of tonsillitis (e.g., peritonsillar abscess, cellulitis); an ENT consult is required

VERTIGO

KY Vertigo is the subjective sensation of motion, either of oneself or the external environment. There are two types of vertigo: central and peripheral.

- **Central vertigo** has an insidious onset, with mild and continuous symptoms that may last days to years.
- **Peripheral vertigo** has a sudden onset, with intense and paroxysmal symptoms that lasts for minutes to hours, but fatigues quickly when one fixes on an object

HX Sensation of motion, faintness, near-syncope, and unsteady gait

- **Central vertigo:** symptoms such as headache, visual disturbances, facial numbness, dysarthria, dysphasia, focal extremity weakness, and unilateral ataxia (i.e., a sense of being pulled to one side) suggest a central cause
- **Peripheral vertigo:** the relationship between symptoms to factors such as head motion, recent URI, drug ingestion, medication use, alcohol, nicotine, caffeine, stress, dental work, and head or neck trauma is important. Tinnitus, hearing loss, ear pain or fullness, and discharge from the external auditory canal suggest a peripheral cause.

PX • **Ear:** perform a visual inspection of auricle and mastoid area, looking for discoloration, erythema, and disfigurement; palpate and pull the auricle, testing for pain; check the tympanic membrane for perforation; determine whether hearing loss, if any, is conductive or sensorineural
- **Fistula test** (place the head at 60° backwards and apply pneumatic otoscopy to the external canal): exert positive pressure, and observe the eyes for movement; production of vertigo or nystagmus is a positive result
- **Hall-Pike maneuver:** check for nystagmus and a sensation of vertigo
    Central vertigo: nystagmus has no latency period or fatigability, is not suppressible, and has no positional component
    Peripheral vertigo: nystagmus is not continuous, has a latency period of 2–25 seconds, demonstrates fatigability, is usually suppressed by fixation, and has a definite positional component

- **Neurologic examination:** look for focal deficits; cranial nerve abnormalities may suggest specific disease or area of involvement; assess cerebellar function

DD Extensive (Table 7.2)

LB CBC and SMA-7 for selective screening; other lab tests, including RPR and TFTs, may useful for evaluation outside of the ED

IM Perform appropriate radiographs where indicated (e.g., in cases of trauma); consider EKG and CT if a central cause for the vertigo is suspected

TX • **Pharmacologic therapy:**

Acute therapy may include diazepam (2.5–5 mg IV) followed by meclizine (25 mg PO qid) prn or dimenhydrinate (50 mg PO q4hr)

Parenteral antiemetics are helpful, especially with occurrence of persistent nausea and vomiting [e.g., promethazine (12.5–25 mg IV/PO q8hr) or prochlorperazine (25 mg IV/PO q8hr)]

Antibiotic treatment of infectious causes of vertigo should be started in the ED

- **Surgical referral** is required for a cholesteatoma, perilymphatic fistula, otosclerosis, acoustic neuroma, or other CNS mass
- **Physical therapy** has been shown to improve symptoms in benign positional vertigo by desensitization with repetitive head motion
- **Antiplatelet or anticoagulation therapy** may be necessary in vascular insufficiency syndromes and nonhemorrhagic CVAs

DI • Otolaryngologic consult for many patients with peripheral vertigo; an immediate otolaryngologic consult is necessary for

---

Table 7.2 **Differential Diagnosis of Peripheral versus Central Vertigo**

Peripheral Vertigo	Central Vertigo	Multisystemic Causes of Nonvertiginous Dizziness
Otis media	Acoustic neuroma	Diabetes mellitus
Acute labyrinthitis	Encephalitis	Thyroid disorder
Meniere's disease	Meningitis	Anemia
Trauma	Vertebral basilar	Polycythemia
Benign positional	insufficiency	Hypertension
vertigo	Multiple sclerosis	Psychogenic conditions
Medications	Trauma	Dehydration/hypovolemia
Motion sickness	Drugs	
	Tumor	
	Toxins	

patients with a positive fistula test, trauma, mastoiditis, and purulent labyrinthitis
- Admission is necessary for all patients with central vertigo

VISION LOSS (SUDDEN)

HX Pain, location, trauma, symptoms at onset, and previous episodes

PX • **Ophthalmologic findings:** optic tract radiation impairment (visual fields by confrontation technique, homonymous hemianopia in contralateral field); hyphema, accommodation, light, and consensual response of pupils; retinal artery occlusion (pale retina with "cherry red spot" at macula); retinal vein occlusion (multiple hemorrhages, "blood and thunder" macular venous engorgement); visual acuity (Snellen eye chart), IOP (tonometer), slit-lamp examination
- **Other finding:** temporal arteritis (tenderness over temporal artery)

DD Retinal artery occlusion, retinal vein occlusion, uveitis, retinal detachment ("shade being drawn," decrease in peripheral visual field); glaucoma (halos around lights); macular dysfunction (distortion, spot in center of field); TIA (transient visual loss); CVA (sudden, painless, unilateral loss of vision); neoplasm; temporal arteritis (headache and pain in temporal region); ischemic optic neuropathy
- **Other ophthalmologic causes:** iritis (photophobia, tender eye); vitreous hemorrhage ("cobwebs," "floaters," peripheral light flashes)
- **Nonophthalmologic causes:** hypertension; diabetes; leukemia and thrombocytopenia

LB CBC, chemistries, ESR

IM Head CT, consider MRI

TX • **Retinal artery occlusion:**
Gentle digital massage on closed eye to reduce IOP
Acetazolamide: 500 mg IV
Breathing into paper bag to increase CO_2 and dilate arterioles
- **Glaucoma:** (see Red Eye)
- **Temporal arteritis:** prednisone (40 mg bid)

DI Immediate ophthalmologic consult and probable admission

CHAPTER 8

Hematologic/Oncologic Emergencies

Administration of blood products is required in the ED for some patients with abnormal bleeding (Table 8.1).

ANEMIA

KY In general, anemia is described as a drop in Hgb or Hct. Anemia may be caused by a large variety of diseases, and symptoms vary depending on the cause.

HX • **Insufficient production of RBCs:** from abnormalities of Hgb, Fe, and globin or from decreased production within bone marrow
- **Excessive destruction of RBCs:** from intrinsic synthesis anomaly, extrinsic destruction, or sequestration
- **Hemorrhagic anemia:** risks for bleeding, including cirrhosis, PUD, variceal hemorrhage, malignancy, infection, bleeding diatheses, and medications
- **Chronic anemia:**
    Symptoms may result from blood loss or production abnormality; existing underlying disease (e.g., angina, claudication, GI symptoms, syncope/near-syncope, focal neuropathy 2° to ischemia)
    Patients commonly present with malaise of gradual onset, DOE, and fatigue
- **Acute hemorrhage:** seek prior history of hemorrhage or bleeding disorder; determine location and estimate amount of bleeding; obtain history of NSAID or ethanol use and smoking

PX Pallor, tachycardia, orthostasis, wide pulse pressure, hypotension, murmur, icterus, petechiae, ecchymosis, and hepatosplenomegaly

DD • **Blood production disorders** (insidious onset of symptoms, low reticulocyte count):
    Hypochromic/microcytic (low MCV): Fe-deficiency anemia, thalassemia, sideroblastic anemia (e.g., lead poisoning)
    Macrocytic (elevated MCV): vitamin B_{12}, folate deficiencies, cirrhosis, thyroid disorders
    Normocytic (normal MCV): production disorder in marrow, including fibrosis, leading to aplasia and metaplasia; possible contribution from endocrine disorders, uremia, cirrhosis, chronic inflammation

Table 8.1   Some Transfusion Products Commonly Used in Emergencies

Product	Purpose	Dose	Comments
Cryoprecipitate	To replace fibrinogen and factor VIII; each unit contains ~ 200 mg of fibrinogen and 100 units of factor VIII in a volume of 10–15 ml	Transfuse to achieve a fibrinogen level of 100 mg/dl (approximately 10 units)	Each unit should increase fibrinogen 5–10 mg/dl
FFP	To provide factors V and VIII as well as other clotting factors	Transfuse 2 units at a time; repeat if bleeding persists	Monitor response by following PT
Platelets	To correct prolonged bleeding time associated with factor V deficiency and thrombocyto-penia	Transfuse to platelet count ~ 50,000/mm^3	Platelets should be considered whenever bleeding time is prolonged (> 9 minutes). Each unit should increase platelet count 5000–10,000/mm^3

- **Blood destruction disorders** (high reticulocyte count, hemolysis):
  - Intrinsic: G6PD and pyruvate kinase deficiencies; membrane anomalies (e.g., spherocytosis, spur cells), hemoglo-binopathies (e.g., thalassemia, sickle cell anemia)
  - Extrinsic: antigen—antibody reactions, autoantibody immune hemolysis, mechanical cell shearing on valve, environmental sources (e.g., drugs, toxins, hyperthermia, drowning), sequestration
- **Hemorrhagic anemia** (acute or chronic): PMH of NSAID or warfarin use may be helpful
- **LB** • CBC with differential; reticulocyte count and peripheral smear if anemia is not secondary to known recent hemorrhage
- Additional diagnostic tests are usually not useful in the ED
- Further laboratory evaluation may include Fe, TIBC, ferritin if hypochromic/microcytic anemia or Coombs' tests, serum bilirubins

and urine for free hemoglobin if hemolysis is found on smear; bone marrow biopsy may be required if the cause remains unknown, and endoscopic evaluation should be considered

IM Consider CXR to check for air under diaphragm consistent with perforation and for signs of high output and CHF

TX
- ABCs, IV fluids, supplemental O_2, monitoring (volume resuscitation initially with crystalloid)
- ED transfusion of appropriate blood products may be necessary for ongoing GI hemorrhage or DIC (see Table 8.1)
- Obtain GI consult for consideration of urgent endoscopy for active upper GI bleeding
- Chronic anemia and anemia secondary to chronic disease or Fe deficiency are usually well tolerated

DI
- Medical floor or ICU for patients with active bleeding, severe anemia, hypovolemia or shock, hemodynamic instability, any dangerous $2°$ problems (e.g., ischemia, CHF, change in mental status), and those who require transfusion
- Outpatient management and follow-up for patients with subacute or mild chronic anemia

DEEP VENOUS THROMBOSIS (DVT)

KY DVT is the presence of one or more clots within the deep veins of the pelvis or extremities. The major concern is embolization, most commonly to the lung, which can result in life-threatening pulmonary embolism. Although the risk for embolization is low with isolated calf DVT, up to 20% of clots in the calf may propagate proximally.

HX Risk factors include stasis (travel, sedentary/debilitated condition), hypercoagulability (cancer, surgery, pregnancy, OCPs, tobacco), vessel pathology (vascular disease, surgery, trauma), and previous DVT

PX Edema is the most reliable sign; palpable cords, calf firmness, warmth, tenderness, and Homans' sign may suggest DVT but are less specific

DD Cellulitis, lymphangitis, ruptured Baker's cyst, muscle strain, edema CHF, pelvic tumor, and pregnancy)

LB
- Baseline PTT, PT, CBC (tests ordered based on suspected location)
- IPG (sensitivity and specificity ~ 95% above knee) (not good for detection of calf vein thrombi)

IM
- Contrast venography, the gold standard test, is the most specific and most sensitive test; however, there is some discomfort and risk for morbidity

- Doppler US (sensitivity and specificity ~ 85%) is good for detection of popliteal and femoral but not calf vein thrombi

TX Heparin: approximately 75–100 U/kg bolus, then 10–20 U/kg/h maintenance (maintain PTT 1.5–2.5 times normal)

DI Treatment and admission to medical bed for patients with proximal DVT

DISSEMINATED INTRAVASCULAR COAGULATION (DIC)

KY DIC, the generation of fibrin and consumption of procoagulants and platelets, is always associated with severe underlying disease or injury. No single parameter is diagnostic, and repeated measures of coagulopathy are often required. Thrombocytopenia results from consumption of platelets in microvascular clots and platelet activation by circulating thrombin. Mortality is as high as 70%.

HX Infection (30%), surgery or trauma (25%), cancer (20%), hepatic disease, pregnancy, and other conditions (MI, environmental injuries, snakebite, and pancreatitis)

PX
- Hemorrhage, sometimes with thrombotic manifestations; bleeding from IV sites, hematuria and blood in NG aspirate, bloody sputum, ecchymosis, and petechiae
- Thrombotic manifestations include renal failure, bowel infarction, pulmonary insufficiency, cyanosis, hypoxemia, and AMS

DD Massive hepatic necrosis, vitamin K deficiency, HUS, ITP, warfarin overdose

LB
- Platelet counts of 50,000–100,000/mm³ are consistent with DIC; if platelet counts are persistently normal, the diagnosis of DIC is nearly excluded
- PT, PTT, thrombin time (generally prolonged)
- FDPs, fibrin D-dimer [elevated (FDP > 10 mg/dl, fibrin D-dimer > 0.5 mg/dl)]
- Fibrinogen levels [depleted (< 150 mg/dl)]
- Peripheral smear (evidence of microangiopathic hemolysis with schistocytes)

IM Consider CXR

TX
- ABCs, IV fluids, supplemental O_2, monitoring
- Management of severe hemorrhage with crystalloid, blood products, and platelets (see Table 8.1)
- Treatment of underlying disorder; evacuation of uterus in septic abortion; treatment of hypovolemia, hypothermia, hyperthermia, sepsis, acidosis, and hypoxia

- For patients at high risk for bleeding or actively bleeding with bio-chemical evidence of DIC:

  Replacement of fibrinogen, platelets, and clotting factors with cryoprecipitate (fibrinogen and factor VIII), FFP (clotting factors), and platelets (maintain platelets > 50,000/mm³) as appropriate (see Table 8.1); use whole blood if necessary

  Consider aminocaproic acid for refractory DIC: 5–10 g slow IV push, then 2–4 g/hr × 24 hours or until bleeding stops; use concurrent heparin treatment

- Consider management of thrombotic complications with heparin *except* for common ED presentations of DIC after surgery or trauma, with abruption, or when other bleeding risk is present. Use low-dose heparin: 500 U/hr ± 500–1000 U bolus; after 2–3 hours of infusion, consider FFP (2–3 U) and platelets (6–8 U).

- Monitor fibrinogen; consider cryoprecipitate if fibrinogen < 100 mg/dl (see Table 8.1).

- Consider hematology consult

DI ICU

HEPARIN OVERDOSE

HX Development of hemorrhage or necessity for reversal of anticoagulation

PX Spontaneous gingival hemorrhage, petechial rash, hematemesis from GI bleeding, hemoptysis, CVA

LB CBC, including platelets, PT, and PTT

IM Consider CXR

TX
- Protamine sulfate: consider if heparin (bolus or infusion) was given within 4 hours of the onset of bleeding. Protamine forms a heparin–protamine complex and reverses the anticoagulant effect of heparin; it neutralizes heparin within 5 minutes. The plasma half-life of heparin is 1–2 hours, and protamine is unlikely to be beneficial > 4 hours after the last heparin dose. Doses should be infused slowly over 1–3 minutes, and they should not exceed 50 mg in any 10-minute period.

  Recent heparin bolus: 1 mg IV for each 100 units of heparin administered

  Continuous heparin infusion: 1 mg IV for each 100 units given over the preceding 4 hours

  Discontinuation of heparin for > 30 minutes: 50% dosage reduction

Adverse effects: mild hypotension; anaphylactic reaction (uncommon); risk for allergic reactions in diabetic patients exposed to protamine through some insulin preparations

DI Admission, usually to ICU

SICKLE CELL CRISIS

KY Carriers of the sickle cell trait have less than 60% of the normal Hgb A and approximately 40% of the damaged Hgb S. They may present with painless gross hematuria, priapism, anemia, and rarely sickle cell crisis. Individuals with SS disease have ≥ 85% Hgb S and 90% sickling of RBCs, with a higher risk for sickle crisis, resulting in bony or visceral infarcts, hemolytic/aplastic anemia, and infection.

HX • Patients may present with severe pain in the back, abdomen, chest, or extremities and sometimes with associated fever and jaundice
• Recent illness (e.g., URI, gastroenteritis) or air travel may precede symptoms; recurrent splenic infarction is associated with increased risk for underlying infection
• Sequestration crisis is seen in children < 8 years of age

PX Underlying infection, organomegaly, joint effusion, and cardiotho-racic or abdominal catastrophe, jaundice (hemolytic crisis), shock (sequestration, aplastic crises)

DD • Chest: MI, pulmonary embolism, pneumonia, bony infarct
• Abdomen: visceral infarct, obstruction, infection
• Head: infection, CVA, bony infarct
• Extremities: infection, trauma, bony infarct

LB CBC, including WBC with differential and reticulocyte count, T&C, C&S to exclude infection; UA and urine culture
Vaso-occlusive crisis: Hct and reticulocyte count
Hemolytic crisis: Hct (low)
Sequestration crisis: CBC (low Hgb and pancytopenia)
Aplastic crisis: CBC (low Hct and reticulocyte count; possible evidence of infection)

IM CXR, abdominal plain film, or CT prn

TX • **Vaso-occlusive crisis:** supplemental O_2, hydration with 0.9 NS IV fluid, analgesics (NSAIDs, narcotics), folic acid, and antibiotic prn
• **Hemolytic crisis:** as for vaso-occlusive crisis, with transfusion of PRBCs
• **Sequestration crisis:** as for vaso-occlusive crisis; consider surgery: possible splenectomy
• **Aplastic crisis:** as for vaso-occlusive crisis, with transfusion prn

DI • Admission for transfusion, antibiotics, hydration, and pain control
  • Vaso-occlusive crisis only: if the condition is resolved in the ED, consider discharge home (with analgesia)

TRANSFUSION REACTION

KY The two types of transfusion reactions are the acute hemolytic transfusion reaction and the febrile transfusion reaction.

  • The **acute hemolytic transfusion reaction** is an antigen–antibody reaction to donor cells, leading to bronchospasm, shock, rash, DIC, and renal failure from products of cell destruction and inflammatory response. The severity of the reaction is related to the volume of blood infused.
  • The **febrile transfusion reaction,** which has an incidence of 0.5%–3% (more common in multiply transfused patients), is usually mild and self-limited. This reaction involves extravascular hemolysis secondary to an immune reaction to transfused platelets, leukocytes, or various plasma proteins.

HX Current transfusion and perhaps previous transfusions

PX • **Early symptoms:** sudden onset of anxiety, flushing tachycardia, and hypotension; associated chest and back pain, fever and dyspnea (common)
  • **Later symptoms:** chills followed by fever, headache, and malaise, during or within hours or 1–3 weeks post-transfusion

DD Bacteremia/sepsis, DIC, autoimmune disease, hemoglobinopathies, RBC enzyme defects, hemolytic reaction, pyogenic reaction to donor blood contaminants (bacteria)

LB • Notify the blood bank immediately after discontinuing the transfusion, and send unused donor blood and a sample of the patient's venous blood to the blood bank for repeat T&C; the blood cells of the patient should be examined for antibody, complement, and blood group antibodies using such tests as the direct and indirect Coombs' tests. A positive direct antiglobulin test indicates an acute hemolytic reaction.
  • Test urine for free Hgb (dipstick-positive); examine the patient's centrifuged plasma for pink coloration, indicating free Hgb

TX • Discontinuation of transfusion; maintenance of adequate renal output with use of IV fluids; mannitol and/or furosemide may be used after adequate volume replacement
  • Management of hypotension: NS or plasma expanders; maintain SBP of > 100 mm Hg; central venous monitoring may be indicated

- Monitoring of PT/PTT, platelets, fibrinogen, and FDPs for evidence of DIC or coagulopathy; manage with FFP, platelets, and/or cryoprecipitate (see Table 8.1)
- Symptomatic and supportive care: acetaminophen and diphenhydramine; meperidine (50 mg IV) is useful for treatment of chills

DI • Admission to appropriate level of care
- Observation for signs and symptoms of continued reaction; monitoring of PT/PTT, platelets, fibrinogen, and FDPs; checking for early DIC; restriction of PRBCs until complete antigen–antibody screening is complete

WARFARIN OVERDOSE

HX Development of hemorrhage or necessity for reversal of anticoagulation. Warfarins are present in many rodenticides.

PX Spontaneous gingival hemorrhage, petechial rash, hematemesis from GI bleeding, hemoptysis, CVA

LB CBC, including platelets; PT, PTT

TX • **Elimination measures:** activated charcoal if recent oral ingestion
- **Reversal of warfarin anticoagulation:** correction of coagulopathy either rapidly or slowly, depending on the severity or risk for bleeding and the need for reinstitution of anticoagulation.
  Emergent reversal: FFP (replacement of vitamin K-dependent factors) [15–20 ml/kg followed by 5–7 ml/kg q8–12hr]; vitamin K [10–50 mg IV or IM (peds 0.2–0.6 mg/kg IV or IM)]; dilute if given IV in 50 ml NS and infuse no faster than 1 mg/min. (There is a risk for anaphylactoid reactions and shock, and slow infusion minimizes risk. Some physicians prefer using a test dose and the IM route to avoid anaphylaxis.)
  Reversal over 24–48 hours: vitamin K (10–50 mg IM) [peds 0.2–0.6 mg/kg IM]; full reversal of anticoagulation results in resistance to further warfarin therapy for several days
  Temporary correction: lower doses of vitamin K (0.5–1.0 mg) will lower PT without interfering with reinitiation of warfarin

DI Patients with hemorrhage: ICU

CHAPTER 9

Infectious Disease Emergencies

ACQUIRED IMMUNODEFICIENCY SYNDROME (AIDS)

KY AIDS is caused by HIV, a retrovirus that infects CD4 (helper T) cells. Infection causes cell death and a decline in immune function, thus increasing malignancies and opportunistic infections. Research has demonstrated that HIV is transmitted via blood and blood products, semen, vaginal secretions, and through the placenta.

HX Presenting symptoms include fever; chronic infection; persistent lymphadenopathy; opportunistic infections; weight loss; malignancies; and mental status changes, including encephalopathy.

PX Possible findings:

- Constitutional: fever, cachexia, malaise
- Pulmonary: diffuse dry crackles, wheezes with prolonged expiration, coarse rhonchi with significant tracheobroncheolar lobar consolidation
- GI: oropharyngeal lesions, hepatosplenomegaly and tenderness, upper and/or lower GI bleeding
- Ophthalmologic: decreased visual acuity, perivascular retinal lesions (cotton-wool spots)
- Cutaneous: hypokeratinized, scaling skin; follicular, vesicular, or bullous lesions; ulcerations and/or macerations, capital and/or intertriginous alopecia
- Neurologic: cephalgia, disorientation, confusion, delirium, dementia, focal or generalized seizures, cranial nerve palsies, focal somatic findings, gait disturbance, limb ataxia
- Psychiatric: subdued, depressed mood, which may lead to suicidal ideation; AIDS psychosis, which may manifest as bizarre behavioral changes, delusions, and hallucinations

LB Customize for symptoms. Consider:

- ABG, CBC, SMA-7, LFTs, blood C&S × 2
- Sputum: Gram stain, C&S, AFB
- LP: samples for C&S, India ink for cryptococci, cryptococcal antigen, Giemsa stain, immunofluorescence or silver stain for *Pneumocystis carinii*
- Fungal C&S
- Fecal cells, O&P, culture

- VDRL, serum cryptococcal antigen, sulfadiazine levels, UCG, UA
- Confirmation of HIV may include ELISA or Western blot assay

IM CT with and without contrast, consider CXR

TX • **Antiretroviral therapy:** Treatment for HIV infection and exposure is changing rapidly. Currently, multiple antiviral agents are used in conjunction with symptomatic treatment. Consult current guidelines or an ID specialist prior to initiating therapy.
- **Opportunistic infections:**
    GI candidiasis: clotrimazole (40 mg/day PO) or ketoconazole (300 mg/day)
    CNS toxoplasmosis: pyrimethamine (25–50 mg/kg/day PO) plus sulfadiazine (100 mg/kg/day PO)
    Cryptococcal meningitis: amphotericin B (0.5 mg/kg/day IV)
    HSV: acyclovir (5 mg/kg IV over 1 hour q8hr or 200 mg PO five times/day)
    Herpes zoster: acyclovir (10–12 mg/kg IV q8hr infused over 1 hour)
    TB: isolation; then give INH (5 mg/kg/day up to 300 mg/kg/day) plus rifampin (10 mg/kg/day PO up to 600 mg/day) plus pyrazinamide (25 mg/kg/day PO up to 2.0 g/day). Consult an ID specialist, because additional drugs may be required.
    CMV: ganciclovir (induction: 5 mg/kg IV q12–24hr × 14–21 days; maintenance: 6 mg/kg IV 5 days/week or 1000 mg PO tid)
- **PCP,** which affects > 80% of patients with AIDS
    TMP-SMX [15–20 mg/kg/day (based on TMP) IV in three to four divided doses × 21 days]
    Consider prednisone (if $Po_2 \leq 70$ mm Hg on room air or A-a gradient ≥ 35 mm Hg) or pentamidine (4 mg/kg IV qd × 21 days) and consider steroids
    Pentamidine (if inadequate response to TMP-SMX) or dapsone (100 mg PO qd × 21 days) and trimethoprim (5 mg/kg PO qid × 21 days) [avoid dapsone in G6PD deficiency]
    Prophylaxis (previous PCP, CD4 < 200 cells/mm^3): TMP-SMX DS (160/800 mg PO qd) or pentamidine (300 mg in 6 ml sterile water via nebulizer over 20–30 minutes q4weeks); may pretreat with albuterol (2.5 mg in 5 ml NS)
- **Postexposure prophylaxis:** Consult current CDC guidelines.

DI ICU for clinical signs of sepsis or respiratory distress; most HIV patients with infections require admission at least to a medical bed for IV therapy

ANTIBIOTIC-ASSOCIATED AND PSEUDOMEMBRANOUS COLITIS

KY Disruption of the normal colonic flora, with overgrowth by *Clostridium difficile,* which results from reduction of other strains by oral or parenteral antibiotics, leads to this form of colitis. The *C. difficile*—generated toxin produces fever, abdominal cramping, and watery diarrhea. Implicated antibacterial agents include: clindamycin, erythromycin, ampicillin, penicillin, cephalosporins, chloramphenicol, tetracycline, and sulfonamides.

HX Severe abdominal cramping, watery, occasionally bloody diarrhea, and fever, and a history of current or recent antibiotic use

PX Clinical evidence of volume depletion, fever, diffuse abdominal tenderness, watery diarrhea, and possibly guaiac-positive stool

DD Abdominal visceral catastrophe, partial obstruction, enteritis, hepatitis, pancreatitis, parasitic enteritis, bacterial and viral gastroenteritis

LB Stool for toxin, C&S for O&P, and enteric pathogens (stool culture is not diagnostic, because *C. difficile* is part of the normal flora); endoscopy may reveal pseudomembranous plaques

IM Consider abdominal series (KUB and upright) if signs or symptoms of obstruction or perforation are present

TX • Hydrate (IV/PO); discontinue antibiotics; avoid antidiarrheals, because slow peristalsis allows organism multiplication and exacerbates symptoms
  • Consider metronidazole: 500 mg PO tid × 10 days
  • For severe symptoms, consider vancomycin (instead of metronidazole): 125 mg PO qid × 7–10 days

DI Admission for patients with severe symptoms to medical or surgical services

CHRONIC AMBULATORY PERITONEAL DIALYSIS (CAPD)–ASSOCIATED PERITONITIS

KY CAPD-associated peritonitis is a common problem. An eosinophilic peritonitis, this disorder may be evident in patients who have recently begun CAPD. Most likely it is an allergic reaction and requires no antibiotic treatment.

HX Patient notes cloudy or milky dialysate return followed by abdominal pain and fever

PX Tender abdomen and possibly peritoneal signs; fever and occasional dehydration if complicated by nausea and vomiting

LB CBC, SMA-7; Gram stain of peritoneal effluent, which usually shows organisms (most often Gram-positive), with WBC > 100/mm^3

TX Cefazolin (1 g IV/IM) plus cefazolin (250 mg) in each bag of dialysate × 10 days

DI Admission for toxic-appearing, dehydrated, or debilitated patients, or those unable to continue CAPD at home; other patients may be discharged home with appropriate resources

CYSTITIS AND PYELONEPHRITIS

KY *Escherichia coli* accounts for ≥ 80% of cases of uncomplicated UTI in women. *Staphylococcus saprophyticus* causes ≅ 10% of these infections. In complicated UTIs [abnormality of urinary tract (e.g., obstruction, reflux) or infection with antibiotic-resistant bacteria], *E. coli* accounts for ≅ 35% of cases, *Enterococcus faecalis* for ≅ 16%, *Proteus mirabilis* and *Staphylococcus epidermidis* for ≅ 13% each, and *Klebsiella* and *Pseudomonas* for ≅ 5% each. Uropathogenic *E. coli* causes uncomplicated pyelonephritis ≅ 80% of the time.

HX • **Cystitis:** fever, dysuria, frequency, urgency, retention, and hematuria
  • **Pyelonephritis:** high fever, nausea, vomiting, and back pain (suggestive)
  • Check for recent or ongoing catheterization

PX Fever, tachycardia, dehydration, and CVA tenderness, with possible debilitation and mental status changes, particularly in elderly patients with urosepsis

DD Cystitis versus pyelonephritis; PID, vaginosis, urethritis, renal calculus, renal infarction, renal thrombosis, GN, pancreatitis, cholecystitis, splenic infarct, appendicitis and other causes of abdominal pain; always rule out AAA for pyelonephritis

LB • Cystitis without complicating factors: urine dip or microscopic analysis of sediment (positive findings include elevated WBCs, nitrites, or bacteria)
  • Symptoms of > 1 week's duration; recurrent UTIs, pyelonephritis, or diabetes; and patients who are pregnant or elderly: urine culture
  • Toxic-appearing patients (if examination suggests pyelonephritis): CBC, SMA-7

IM Consider spinal CT or renal US for concomitant symptoms suggestive of nephrolithiasis and possible hydronephrosis

TX • **Symptomatic treatment:** phenazopyridine (100–200 mg PO tid) for relief of burning

- **Uncomplicated cystitis** (current recommendation): TMP-SMX DS (160/800 mg bid) or quinolone (bid × 3–5 days) [recommended for recurrent infections and current treatment failures]
- **Uncomplicated cystitis in pregnancy:** nitrofurantoin (second or third trimester only) [100 mg qid × 3–7 days] or amoxicillin (250 mg tid × 7–10 days)
- **Complicated cystitis:** quinolone (ofloxacin or ciprofloxacin) for 10–14 days
- **Candida cystitis:** amphotericin B; continuous bladder irrigation (50 mg/L sterile water via three-way Foley catheter at 1 L/day × 5 days) or fluconazole (100 mg PO or IV × 1 dose, then 50 mg PO or IV qd × 5 days)
- **Uncomplicated pyelonephritis** (patients who are able to tolerate oral medications; those who are not debilitated, indigent, immuno-suppressed, septic, or dehydrated from nausea and vomiting): TMP-SMX DS bid or quinolone × 14 days
- **Pyelonephritis or UTI requiring admission:** many IV regimens, including ampicillin (1 g q6hr) plus gentamicin (1 mg/kg q8hr) or quinolones (ofloxacin or ciprofloxacin) [200–400 mg q12hr] or cef-triaxone (1–2 g qd)

DI
- Admission for patients with complicated pyelonephritis
- Consider admission for patients with complicated UTI and for those who are debilitated, dehydrated, unable to tolerate oral med-ications, or toxic appearing

ENCEPHALITIS

KY Encephalitis, an infection that results in brain inflammation, may be viral or bacterial. Approximately 2000 cases occur each year in the United States. Many infectious causes are treatable, and early ID consul-tation is recommended.

HX
- Possible antecedent viral syndrome, vaccination, or travel to area with high incidence of encephalitis
- Presentation usually involves headache, fever, and progressive changes in mental status; seizures and focal neurologic deficits may be observed with progressive obtundation
- Immunocompromise is a predisposing factor, particularly with encephalitis due to mycobacteria, *Cryptococcus, Listeria,* and her-pes virus

PX
- Assess mental status carefully, documenting level and deficits
- Seek focal neurologic findings, papilledema

- Check for meningitic involvement (photophobia, neck stiffness, Kernig's signs, Brudzinski's signs)

DD Differential diagnosis for change in mental status (see Chapter 11, Neurologic Emergencies), particularly DKA, hyperosmolar hyperglycemic nonketotic coma, hypoglycemia, drug intoxication or a toxic syndrome, metabolic encephalopathy, Reye's syndrome, addisonian crisis, brain abscess, CVA

LB CBC, SMA-7; consider Ca, Mg, phosphate, osmolality, ammonia level, LFTs, ABG; C&S of urine, blood, sputum, and CSF; toxicology screen, LP [CSF may show pleocytosis, elevated protein, low glucose in cases of bacterial and tubercular infections (otherwise usually normal)]

> Most commonly, lymphocytes are increased, suggesting a viral etiology
>
> Increased neutrophils suggest bacterial or nonviral etiology
>
> Increased monocytes suggest infection with bacteria and mycobacteria

IM CXR; consider CT prior to LP

TX
- **Supportive measures:** airway, IV fluids, supplemental O_2, monitoring
- **ICP management:** hyperventilation, steroids, and mannitol prn
- **Antibiotic treatment:** do not delay antibiotic until after LP in most cases; consult the treatment recommendations for meningitis and Lyme disease in this chapter, as well as those for Rocky Mountain spotted fever (see Chapter 2, Dermatologic Emergencies, Bacterial Skin Infections). Treatment suggestions for toxoplasmosis and TB may also be applicable.
- **Arthropod-borne viruses:** see Lyme disease and Rocky Mountain spotted fever (Chapter 2, Dermatologic Emergencies, Bacterial Skin Infections)
- **HSV:** acyclovir (10 mg/kg IV q8hr × 10–21 days)
- **VZV-associated:** acyclovir (10 mg/kg IV q8hr × 10–21 days) [same as for HSV encephalitis]

DI Usually ICU

ENDOCARDITIS (INFECTIOUS)

KY Infectious endocarditis is an infection of the endocardial lining of the heart and valves. Individuals at high risk for disease include abusers of IV drugs, particularly cocaine; persons with prosthetic heart valves; and those with preexisting rheumatic valvular disease and mitral valve prolapse who undergo dental and surgical procedures. In individuals with a damaged heart, the mitral valve is commonly affected, and in drug abusers, the tricuspid valve is usually affected. Infective organisms include *Streptococcus* spp. (46% of cases) and *Staphylococcus aureus* (20%; highest in IV drug abusers); *Pseudomonas, Serratia marcescens,* and *Candida albicans* are increasing in incidence.

HX Low-grade fever for weeks to months; nonspecific complaints, including malaise, night sweats, unexplained rigors or weight loss, cough, and dyspnea; myalgias and arthralgias, including pain in chest, back, abdomen, and joints; IV drug abuse; recent GI, GU, or dental procedures; and heart disease

PX Chronic illness, with:

- **Cutaneous signs:** skin track marks, Osler's nodes (painful red nodules on fingers), Janeway lesions (nontender plaques on the palms and soles), subungual splinter hemorrhages
- **Ophthalmologic signs:** cotton-wool exudates, retinal hemorrhages, Roth's spots (retinal white spots surrounded by hemorrhage)
- **Lungs:** rales, other signs of CHF
- **Heart:** murmurs
- **Abdomen:** tenderness, splenomegaly
- **Neurologic signs:** AMS, meningismus

DD Septicemia, rheumatic fever, pericarditis, pneumonia, TB, meningitis, intra-abdominal infection, GN, CVA, SLE, cancer, CHF, pulmonary emboli, DIC

LB CBC, SMA-7, PT, PTT, blood culture × 3; UA; possible oximetry or ABG

IM EKG, CXR

TX **Supportive treatment:** ABCs, IV fluids, supplemental O_2, monitoring
- **Valvular disease and IV drug abuse:** nafcillin (2 g IV q4hr) plus gentamicin (1.5 mg/kg IV, then 1 mg/kg q8hr)
- **Prosthetic valve:** vancomycin (1 g IV q12hr) plus gentamicin (1.5 mg/kg IV, then 1 mg/kg q8hr) plus rifampin (300 mg PO q12hr)

DI Admission, usually to ICU

EPIGLOTTITIS

KY Epiglottitis is acute inflammation of the supraglottic, epiglottic, vallecula, aryepiglottic folds, and arytenoids. In children, *Haemophilus influenzae* type b is the usual cause; the incidence of epiglottitis due to this bacterium is decreasing. Other causal pathogens include *S. aureus, Moraxella catarrhalis,* streptococci, and pneumococci. Affected children are about 2–6 years of age. In adults, *H. influenzae* type b is also a common etiologic agent. Other implicated causes include group A streptococci and certain viruses.

HX • **Children:** acute onset of illness; rapidly progressive, with fever, sore throat, dysphagia, and drooling late in the course of illness
• **Adults:** usually less fulminant progression than in children
• **Presenting symptoms:** both children and adults can deteriorate suddenly and present with sore throat, dysphagia, "hot potato" voice, and respiratory compromise

PX • **All patients:** Often appearing ill or toxic, anxious, and sitting up with the head in a "sniffing" position; inspiratory stridor may occur. Support ABCs for any patient in extremis
• **Children:** *use caution;* allow the child to stay in the parent's arms, and examine without causing agitation
• **Adults:** may appear very ill with signs of airway compromise, similar to children

DD Pharyngitis, peritonsillar abscess, retropharyngeal abscess, diphtheria, laryngotracheobronchitis, tracheitis, uvulitis, foreign body

LB • H&P may be adequate to make diagnosis; true diagnosis takes place with direct visualization
• **Mildly ill adults** (symptom progression over several days or more with no evidence of potential airway compromise): consider direct nasopharyngoscopy with appropriate preparation in the ED (do not use intubating laryngoscope)
• **All other patients:** diagnosis and treatment in the OR

IM Portable cross-table radiograph; lateral soft tissue neck radiograph to check for thumb sign and vallecular blunting may be appropriate

TX **Supportive measures:** ABCs, including supplemental O_2 by bag-valve-mask, emergent intubation, or placement of needle cricothyrotomy if immediately necessary; otherwise intubation may take place in a more controlled manner in the OR; have all members of the surgical team assembled, including a surgeon skilled in tracheostomy, and go to the OR with the patient (and parents for children)

Antibiotics: can be started after definitive airway management
Cefuroxime: 75–100 mg/kg/day IV/IM q8hr (max 9 g/day) or
Ceftriaxone: 50–75 mg/kg/day IV/IM q12–24hr (max 4 g/day) or
Cefotaxime: 100–150 mg/kg/day IV/IM q6–8hr (max 12 g/day) or
Ampicillin: 100–200 mg/kg/day IV q6hr (max 12 g/day) and chloramphenicol: 50–75 mg/kg/day IV q6hr

DI OR or ICU

HEPATITIS

KY Generally, hepatitis is viewed as a large group of systemic infections that involve the liver with similar clinical manifestations. Although it is often caused by several different viruses, it can also be caused by nonviral infectious and toxins. Hepatitis B is a very common human carcinogen.

HX
- Malaise, low-grade fever, and other constitutional symptoms, sometimes followed by abdominal pain, pigmented urine, icterus, and jaundice
- Ascites, urticaria, arthralgias, bleeding problems, and change in mental status may subsequently develop

PX In advanced stages, change in mental status, scleral icterus, jaundice, hepatomegaly, splenomegaly, ascites, spider angiomas, gynecomastia, and testicular atrophy may be present

DD Cirrhosis, cholecystitis/cholangitis, alcoholic ketoacidosis, infectious mononucleosis, hepatic malignancy, Wilson's disease, pancreatitis

LB
- CBC, SMA-7, PT and PTT to help assess hepatic function (protein and albumin also help evaluate hepatic function and are unlikely to change ED diagnosis or management)
- LFTs, including AST (measurement of hepatocellular injury/necrosis), ALT (measurement of necrosis), alkaline phosphatase, and bilirubin (signs of cholestasis and LDH)
- Amylase, lipase, acetaminophen, and ammonia levels (may help evaluate cause and complications); alcohol level and toxicology screen; C&S
- Peritoneal paracentesis prn (to obtain ascitic fluid for analysis):
  Tube 1 (3–5 ml; red top): protein, albumin, specific gravity, glucose, bilirubin, amylase, lipase, triglyceride, LDH, fibrinogen, fibronectin
  Tube 2 (3–5 ml; purple top): cell count and differential
  Tube 3 (5–20 ml): C&S, Gram stain, AFB, fungal cultures; inject 20 ml into blood culture bottles
  Tube 4 (> 20 ml): cytology
  Syringe (2 ml): pH

IM CXR, EKG, US

TX
- **Supportive measures:** IV fluids and antiemetics for nausea, vomiting, and dehydration; give vitamin K (10 mg SQ) for patients with prolonged PT
- **Alcoholic patients:** thiamine (100 mg IM/IV), folate (2 mg IM/IV), and multivitamins (1 amp IV or 1 tab PO)
- **Signs of GI bleeding or gastritis:** IV ranitidine, famotidine, or cimetidine

- **Toxicologic causes:** general treatment recommendations for *Amanita,* acetaminophen, arsenic, and INH (see Chapter 18, Toxicologic Emergencies, General Evaluation and Treatment); stop hepatotoxic medications, including INH, acetaminophen, NSAIDs (especially diclofenac), phenytoin, α-methyldopa, lovastatin, and nitrofurantoin
- **Hepatic encephalopathy:** consider lactulose and neomycin
- **Prophylaxis:**
  HAV: hepatitis ISG (0.02 ml/kg IM) for sexual and household contacts
  HBV: hepatitis B immune globulin (0.06 mg/kg IM) for individuals without prior HBV immunization who have been exposed to a person with known active HBV via sexual contact, needlestick, or mucosal exposure and initiation of active immunization. Hepatitis B surface antigen and core antibody titer should be drawn at the time of exposure. HBV vaccine (1 ml IM; repeated in 1 and 6 weeks) is given. Previously vaccinated individuals exposed to HBV should have anti-HBs drawn (unless they are known nonresponders, in which case they should receive hepatitis B immune globulin).
  HCV: consider ISG (0.06 ml/kg IM) for parenteral exposure
  HDV: same as for HBV (see treatment)

DI Admission is not routinely required; it is necessary only in cases of severe dehydration, intractable nausea and vomiting, change in mental status, dangerous toxic etiologies, and other signs of acute or dangerous illness

HERPES SIMPLEX VIRUS (HSV) INFECTION

KY HSV disease has many manifestations. Affected patients commonly present with painful vesicles that occur in clusters on the skin, cornea, or mucous membranes. Severe forms may include pneumonia, encephalitis, or disseminated infection. Transmission occurs via contact with vesicular fluid.

- **HSV type 1:** the large majority of infections (> 80%) involve nongenital areas such as the lips, eyes (keratitis), and fingers (whitlow).
- **HSV type 2:** most infections (> 80%) affect the urogenital and anal areas.

HX Prodrome with local pain and hyperesthesias preceding vesicles; primary disease, which is more severe than recurrent infection, is usually accompanied by fever, adenopathy, and malaise

PX • Lesions, which are nondermatomal, begin as tender vesicles on red base and then ulcerate and form crusts; the lesions are contagious until after the crusts have fallen off

- Periorbital or nasal lesions: ophthalmologic evaluation is required to rule out keratitis

DD Reactivation of latent VZV (lesions appear in classic unilateral dermatomal distribution), impetigo, aphthous stomatitis, syphilitic chancre, herpangina, Stevens-Johnson syndrome

LB Culture; Tzanck smear (possible multinucleated giant cells)

TX • Primary or frequent genital infection: acyclovir
   5 mg/kg IV q8hr or 200 mg PO five times/day × 10 days (otherwise healthy patients)
   200 mg five times/day × 10 days (immunocompromised patients)
- Consider daily prophylaxis for patients with frequent recurrence
- Begin treatment with prodromal symptoms if possible
- Encephalitis: acyclovir (12.4 mg/kg IV q8hr × 10 days)
- Pregnancy: antiviral agents indicated only for encephalitis or severe pneumonitis; delivery by C-section with active lesions

DI • Outpatient follow-up for cases of localized primary or recurrent infection
- Admission for IV treatment and observation for cases of immunocompromise, encephalitis, or severe pneumonitis

INFESTATIONS (MITES, LICE, AND FLEAS)

KY Infestations with various arthropods result in skin lesions that may be difficult to differentiate. Burrowing mites, which are parasitic arachnids about 0.3 mm long, cause scabies. Lice, which are biting or sucking arthropods ≤ 3 mm long, account for pediculosis. Fleas, which are small, wingless, bloodsucking arthropods, can lead to secondary bacterial infections.

HX Close quarters, suboptimal hygiene, travel, animal contact, and indigence; pruritus is common with infestations

PX • **Mites:** small, red nodules, which become excoriated with scratching; in adults, mites are characteristically found in web spaces, flexion creases, and axillae; in children, distribution is more generalized
- **Lice:** visually resemble tiny ticks (or "crabs"), with white louse eggs and nits (larger egg cases) attached to the base of hairs
   Affected areas: pubic area (pediculosis pubis or "crabs"), scalp and eyelashes (pediculosis capitis or head lice), buttocks, shoulders, and waist (pediculosis corporis or body lice)
   Marginal blepharitis: a possible presenting condition in prepubescent children with pediculosis pubis
- **Fleas:** bites, often on legs and abdomen, perhaps in zigzag pattern

DD Other infestations, other arthropod bites, eczema, contact dermatitis

LB Examine arthropod by scraping organism or skin from affected lesion onto microscope slide

TX • **General measures:** give antipruritics and treat 2° infection prn; cut fingernails short
   • **Mites:**
      Treat family and sexual contacts, wash underclothes and bed-clothes
      Lindane 1%: apply and leave on for 8 hours or
      Crotamiton 10% (pregnant women or children < 2 years): apply for two nights and wash off 24 hours after second application or
      Permethrin 1% or 5% (pregnant women or children < 2 years): apply and leave on for 8 hours
      May repeat treatment in 1 week; lindane must be prescribed correctly because of risk of seizures
   • **Lice:** Permethrin or lindane
      Bathe, apply scabicide, leave on 1 day, bathe; repeat in 1 week
      Treat eyelash infestation with petrolatum (3–5 times per day)
      In pediculosis pubis, wash intimate clothing and bedclothes; treat sexual contacts; alert proper authorities in cases in children
   • **Fleas:** wash with soap and water; starch baths, calamine soaks, or cool soaks for comfort

DI Home

LYME DISEASE

HX The spirochete *Borrelia burgdorferi,* which is carried primarily by the tick vector *Ixodes scapularis,* causes Lyme disease. The condition most commonly occurs in northern parts of the United States, particularly in coastal areas, usually during the summer months. Lyme disease has three stages. Patients with stage I disease often present to the ED, and acute intervention is most useful at this time. Without treatment, stage I symptoms usually last for weeks. A vaccine for Lyme disease has recently been approved.

HX • **Stage I:** known tick bite in about 30% of cases (first symptoms occur about 1 week after the tick bite)
      New rash (erythema migrans) in 70% of patients
      Constitutional symptoms: possible fatigue, nausea, headache, myalgia, migratory arthralgia, low-grade fever

- **Stage II:**
    Neurologic symptoms: headache, nausea, vomiting, lethargy, cranial nerve and peripheral nerve involvement
    Ocular symptoms: eye pain, blurred vision, blindness
    Cardiac symptoms: chest pain, palpitations, syncope
- **Stage III:**
    Arthritis, most commonly monarticular, involving large joints
    Neurologic symptoms (wide ranging): AMS, severe fatigue, cranial and peripheral neuropathies, paresthesias

PX • **Stage I:** low-grade fever, erythema migrans rash usually 5–10 cm in diameter, often with target-like appearance; meningeal signs usually absent; possible lymphadenopathy and splenomegaly
- **Stage II:**
    Neurologic symptoms: cranial neuropathy, including Bells' palsy; motor or sensory neuropathy
    Ocular symptoms: blindness, conjunctivitis, keratitis, retinal detachment, papilledema
    Cardiac symptoms: bradycardia; signs of left ventricular dysfunction, including CHF
- **Stage III:**
    Arthritis
    Neurologic symptoms: AMS, dementia, cranial and peripheral neuropathies, paresthesias

DD • **Stage I:** viral syndrome or mononucleosis, erythema multiforme, meningitis
- **Stage II:** other causes of Bell's palsy, chronic fatigue syndrome, aseptic meningitis, encephalitis, MS, neuropathy, conjunctivitis, myocarditis, rheumatic fever, cardiac conduction abnormality
- **Stage III:** other causes of arthritis, Reiter's syndrome, psychosis, dementia, neuropathy

LB Provisional diagnosis must usually be made in the ED without lab testing
- CBC is usually normal
- Antibody assay may be sent if appropriate follow-up is certain; IgM titer does not peak until about 1 month after symptom onset, and false-positive and false-negative results are common

TX • Symptomatic treatment: acetaminophen or NSAIDs for fever, myalgia, and arthralgia
- Antibiotic treatment (not required emergently but may be started in the ED):
    Stage I: doxycycline (100 mg PO bid × 15–21 days); alternative treatment: amoxicillin [250–500 mg PO tid × 15–21 days (peds 25–50 mg/kg/day tid)]

Stages II and III: antibiotic regimen may depend on symptoms and systems involved; consult emergency medicine textbook

DI • Home for stage I disease unless secondary complications necessitating hospitalization exist
• Admission for patients with cardiac pathology for IV antibiotics and monitoring, those with dangerous ocular complications to ophthalmology, and those with serious neurologic sequelae who require supportive care for IV antibiotics

MENINGITIS

KY Meningitis is inflammation of the brain and spinal cord. Different pathogens cause the disease in different age groups. The incidence of *H. influenzae* type b–associated disease is decreasing as a result of the Hib vaccine. If untreated, bacterial meningitis leads to 90% mortality. Atypical presentations are common.

HX Headache, fever, nuchal rigidity, photophobia; possible prior exposure; nausea, vomiting, and change in mental status may be late findings

PX Patients often appear ill, with Kernig's and Brudzinski's signs; photophobia; nuchal rigidity; papilledema; petechiae associated with meningococcus; change in mental status, including confusion, lethargy, coma, seizure, and cranial nerve or other focal neurologic findings

DD Differential diagnosis for change in mental status (see Chapter 11, Neurologic Emergencies); viral syndromes; encephalitis or brain abscess; bacteremia; sepsis; seizures; acute narrow-angle glaucoma

LB LP (CSF analysis):
• Tube 1 (1–2 ml): cell count and differential
• Tube 2 (1–2 ml): glucose, protein
• Tube 3 (1–4 ml): Gram stain of fluid or sediment (if fluid is clear); C&S for bacteria
• Tube 4 (8–10 ml):
    Cell count and differential
    Special studies, including latex agglutination or counterimmunoelectrophoresis antigen tests for *Streptococcus pneumoniae,* *H. influenzae* type b, *Neisseria meningitidis, E. coli,* group B streptococcus, and *Cryptococcus*
    Viral cultures, VDRL
    India ink and AFB for immunocompromised or exposed patients
• **CSF findings:**
    Bacterial meningitis: glucose < 50 mg/dl or CSF:serum glucose < 0.5; elevated protein often > 100 mg/dl; WBC elevated or any granulocytes unless WBC < 5/mm³; bacterial antigens on

counterimmunoelectrophoresis; presence of organisms on Gram stain

Viral meningitis: more neutrophils in the CSF; normal glucose; and normal or only slightly elevated protein

- In addition, obtain CBC and any other studies appropriate to presentation (e.g., blood culture, UA, SMA-7)

IM CT prior to LP if papilledema or other signs of increased ICP are present, but do not delay antibiotic treatment for CT; sinus films if appropriate

TX Antibiotic treatment:

- **Neonates: < 1 month of age** (causes are B and D streptococci, *E. coli, Listeria*):

  Ampicillin: 150 mg/kg/day IV q8hr (0–7 days of age); 200 mg/kg/day IV q6hr (> 7 days) and either

  Cefotaxime: 100 mg/kg/day IV q12hr (0–7 days); 150 mg/kg/day IV q8hr (> 7 days) or

  Ceftriaxone: 50 mg/kg/day IV q24hr (0–7 days); 75 mg/kg/day IV q24hr (> 7 days)

  Alternative treatment: **ampicillin plus gentamicin** [5 mg/kg/day IM/IV over 30 minutes q12hr (0–7 days)]; [6.0 mg/kg/day IM/IV q8hr (> 7 days)]; use amikacin in place of gentamicin if gentamicin resistance is likely [10 mg/kg/day IV q12hr (0–7 days); 15 mg/kg/day IV/IM q8hr (> 7 days)]

- **Infants: 1–3 months of age** (causes are *H. influenzae, S. pneumoniae, N. meningitidis,* group B streptococci, *E. coli*):

  Ampicillin: 200 mg/kg/day IV q6hr and either

  Cefotaxime: 200 mg/kg/day IV q6hr or

  Ceftriaxone: 100 mg/kg/day IV q12hr or qd

  Alternative treatment: **chloramphenicol plus gentamicin**

  Dexamethasone (some studies recommend this agent): 0.4 mg/kg IV given 15 minutes *before* antibiotics to decrease incidence of hearing loss

- **Infants and children: 3 months–7 years of age** (causes are *H. influenzae, S. pneumoniae, N. meningitidis*):

  Cefotaxime: 200 mg/kg/day IV q6hr (max 12 g/day) or

  Ceftriaxone: 100 mg/kg/day IV q12–24hr (max 4 g/day)

  Alternative treatment: **ampicillin** [200 mg/kg/day IV q6hr (max 12 g/day)]

  Dexamethasone (some studies recommend this agent): 0.4 mg/kg IV given 15 minutes *before* antibiotic to decrease incidence of hearing loss

- **Children and adults: 7–50 years of age** (causes are *S. pneumoniae, N. meningitidis, Listeria*):

  Ampicillin: 200 mg/kg/day IV q6hr (max 12 g/day) or

Penicillin G: 20 MU/day and either

Cefotaxime: 200 mg/kg/day IV q6hr (max 12 g/day) or

Ceftriaxone: 100 mg/kg/day IV q12–24hr (max 4 g/day)

Alternative treatment: **third-generation cephalosporin** alone or **chloramphenicol plus TMP-SMX** (use ampicillin in adults when *Listeria* is high on the suspected list of causative pathogens)

Consider dexamethasone

- **Adults:** ≥ **50 years of age:** debilitated or alcoholic patients (primary cause is *S. pneumoniae*):

    Vancomycin plus third-generation cephalosporin plus rifampin

    Alternative treatment: chloramphenicol plus TMP-SMX

- **HIV-positive patients** (causes are *S. pneumoniae, Cryptococcus neoformans, Mycoplasma tuberculosis,* syphilis, *Listeria*): treat as in patients ≥ 50 years of age (see treatment):

    Amphotericin B (for *C. neoformans*): test dose [0.1 mg/kg (max 1 mg)], followed by remainder of first-day dose in 2–4 hours if tolerated at 0.25 mg/kg IV (increase to 1–1.5 mg/kg q24hr as tolerated) or

    Fluconazole (if less severe): 3–6 mg/kg/day PO qd (usually 400 mg PO qd in adults)

- **Prophylaxis**

    Health professionals and family members in household or daycare with close contact (i.e., more than being in the same room for a while): rifampin (600 mg PO q12hr × 4 doses)

    Postsplenectomy contacts: rifampin (as above)

DI Admission to ICU if necessary

OSTEOMYELITIS

KY Osteomyelitis is an acute or chronic infectious inflammation of the bones. Bacteria are usually the cause, although other microorganisms are rarely the source of infection, which is acquired by hematogenous or contiguous processes or inoculation (Table 9.1). Chronic osteomyelitis, which may result from any of these causes, is characterized by continued, indolent infection.

HX • Pain over affected bone, especially with application of resistance (e.g., standing), localized warmth, redness, swelling, and possibly fever and joint involvement

- Predisposing factors: diabetes, sickle cell disease, AIDS, alcohol, IV drug abuse, chronic steroid use, joint disease, and immunocompromise

Table 9.1   Osteomyelitis

Patient Group	Organisms	Common Routes of Infection
Children	*Staphylococcus aureus* *Streptococcus* spp. *Haemophilus influenzae* (< 5 years of age) *Enterobacter* *Pseudomonas aeruginosa*	Hematogenous
Adults	*S. aureus* *Streptococcus* spp. *Enterobacter* *P. aeruginosa*	Hematogenous
Individuals with diabetes	Polymicrobial disease	Hematogenous Direct extension from cellulitis Direct contamination from exposed bone
Individuals with sickle cell disease	*Salmonella* spp.	Hematogenous

PX • **Bone-related findings:** point tenderness, warmth, and possible joint tenderness to ROM
• **Systemic symptoms:** Possible fever, malaise, and anorexia

DD Septic joint, cellulitis, gout, fasciitis, thrombophlebitis, tumor, fracture, erythema nodosum

LB CBC and blood and urine culture are not usually helpful; ESR and serial values are obtained to follow response to treatment

IM • Possibly plain films, especially with > 7 days of symptoms (periosteal elevation, lucent lesions)
• Bone scan [accurate to within 48 hours of symptom onset ("hot spots" suggestive of blastic activity are due to destruction/reparation)]
• CT (for complex anatomy, limited to patients with > 7 days of symptoms)
• Consider MRI

TX Antibiotics and possible débridement (Table 9.2)

DI Admission for IV antibiotics

Table 9.2 Antibiotics Used in the Treatment of Osteomyelitis

Patient Age	Antibiotic Regimen*
Neonates	Penicillinase-resistant penicillin plus a cephalosporin
Children (< 3 years)	Penicillinase-resistant penicillin plus cephalosporin 3
	Cephalosporin 1 plus aminoglycoside
	Vancomycin plus cephalosporin 3 or aminoglycoside
Children (≥ 3 years)/	Penicillinase-resistant penicillin ± aminoglycoside
Adults	Penicillinase-resistant penicillin ± cephalosporin 3
	Cephalosporin 1 ± aminoglycoside
	Vancomycin plus cephalosporin 3 or aminoglycoside
	Clindamycin plus cephalosporin 3 or aminoglycoside
	Imipenem-cilastatin

*Cephalosporin 1 = cefazolin, cephalexin, or cephalothin; cephalosporin 3 = cefamandole, cefotaxime, ceftazidime, ceftizoxime, or ceftriaxone; penicillinase-resistant penicillin = methicillin, nafcillin, or oxacillin.

PARASITIC INFECTIONS

KY Primary infections with several parasites are found in both the United States and overseas travelers. *Enterobius vermicularis* and *Ascaris lumbricoides,* which are both helminthic worms, cause pinworm enterobiasis and ascariasis, respectively. Trichinosis and fluke infections represent other helminthic infections. Parasitic microorganisms include sporozoa, which cause malaria and toxoplasmosis (see AIDS, CNS toxoplasmosis); amebae, in the group Rhizopoda, which result in amebiasis; and the flagellate protozoa *Trichomonas,* which produce trichomoniasis, and *Giardia lamblia,* which causes giardiasis.

HX • **Enterobiasis:** pruritus ani or vaginalis, most commonly at night; occasional worm sighting, usually in children or familial outbreaks
  • **Malaria:** travel to an endemic area; malaise and periodic fevers and rigors followed by diaphoresis; definite periodic symptoms may not always be part of presentation
  • **Giardiasis:** crampy abdominal pain, diarrhea, pruritus ani; history of travel, camping, and day care

PX • **Enterobiasis:** presence of female worm 1-cm long (male worm, 0.3 cm); secondary infection
  • **Malaria:** fever, rigors, diaphoresis during episode; possible anemia, jaundice, and splenomegaly
  • **Giardiasis:** diffuse upper abdomen tenderness without peritoneal signs

DD • **Enterobiasis:** candidiasis, giardiasis
  • **Malaria:** other infectious causes of fever, especially associated with travel (e.g., hepatitis, dengue and typhoid fevers); other parasites

- **Giardiasis:** other causes of gastroenteritis, both viral and bacterial

LB
- **Enterobiasis:** stool sample for identification of worm or eggs (use tape to pick up)
- **Malaria:** blood smear with Wright's stain for parasites in erythrocytes; CBC, UA, C&S prn
- **Giardiasis:** stool samples for cysts or active *Giardia*

IM CXR in cases of suspected malaria

TX
- **Enterobiasis:** mebendazole [100 mg PO once, repeat in 2 weeks (peds > 2 years old: same as adult)]
- **Malaria:** chloroquine phosphate (600 mg base) [1 g PO, second dose 0.5 g PO in 6 hours, then 0.5 g PO qd × 2 days]; with suspected Plasmodium falciparum, give quinine sulfate (2 cap PO q8hr × 3–7 days) and doxycycline (100 mg PO bid × 7 days) or clindamycin (450 mg PO qid × 3 days)
- **Giardiasis:** metronidazole [250 mg PO tid × 5 days (peds 5 mg/kg tid × 5 days)]

DI Admission for patients who are dehydrated, unable to take anything by mouth, or with suspected chloroquine-resistant *P. falciparum* (generally)

PHARYNGITIS

KY Pharyngitis refers to any infection of the pharynx. Bacterial pathogens include GABHS, other streptococci, *Mycoplasma, Corynebacterium diphtheriae,* and *Neisseria.* Viral causes are EBV, adenovirus, parainfluenza, and other viruses. Pharyngitis is uncommon in children < 3 years of age, and older children should receive an antibiotic for 1 day before they return to school or day care.

HX Sore throat, fever; possible presence of other constitutional symptoms

PX Presence of fever, characteristic white plaques and/or exudate from tonsils, and cervical adenopathy all increase the probability of *Streptococcus* as the cause

DD GC, diphtheria, epiglottitis, oropharyngeal abscess

LB Controversial; laboratory studies are seldom useful; possibly culture or consider basing treatment on rapid latex agglutination assay (sensitivity ~ 85%)

TX
- **Options:** treat without culturing; treat but discontinue if culture is negative; culture and treat if positive results
- **Antibiotic treatment:**
  Penicillin VK: 250 mg tid (25–50 mg/kg/day) × 10 days or
  Erythromycin ethylsuccinate: 300–400 mg tid (30 mg/kg/day) or
  Cephalexin: 250 mg tid (30 mg/kg/day) for PO treatment or

Benzathine penicillin: 1.2 MU IM [peds 25,000 U/kg (max 1.2 MU) IM for 1 dose]

DI Home, except with complicating factors

PNEUMONIA

KY *S. pneumoniae* is responsible for 90% of all cases of pneumonia (Table 9.3).

HX • **Possible symptoms:** URI, cough, sputum, wheezing, progressive dyspnea, fever, malaise, pleuritic chest pain/abdominal pain, anorexia, nausea and vomiting, and obtundation
  • **Predisposing factors:** CHF, COPD, smoking, bronchiectasis, sickle cell disease, hypogammaglobulinemia, mental status change, seizures, aspiration, and immunocompromise

PX • **Systemic:** fever (temperature > 40°C) suggests bacterial source
  • **Chest:** congestion, tachypnea, possible retractions, sometimes splinting, cough, possible hoarseness, stridor, wheezing, rhonchi, consolidation, friction rub on auscultation, dullness to percussion, possible egophony, and sometimes obtundation (depressed gag)
  • **Skin:** perhaps exanthem

Table 9.3   Causes of Pneumonia in Patients By Age Group

Age	Etiologic Agent
Infants (neonates–12 weeks)	Group B streptococcus, coliform bacteria, *Listeria monocytogenes,* HSV, rubella, *Chlamydia,* CMV
Infants/children (1 month–4 years)	RSV (to 6 months), *Streptococcus pneumoniae, Haemophilus influenzae,* viral agents (parainfluenza, adenovirus, EBV), *Bordetella pertussis, Streptococcus pyogenes, Staphylococcus aureus,* Gram-negative bacteria, PCP
Children (5–12 years)	*S. pneumoniae, H. influenzae, Mycoplasma pneumoniae,* viral agents, TB
Older children and adults (≥ 12 years)	*S. pneumoniae, H. influenzae, M. pneumoniae,* viral agents, group A streptococcus, *Pseudomonas aeruginosa, S. aureus, Escherichia coli, Klebsiella, Legionella,* anaerobes, TB, Q fever, tularemia

DD • **Conditions to be ruled out:** CHF, tumor, pulmonary contusion, effusion (from cirrhosis, CHF, uremia, and trauma), pleural or parenchymal thickening or scarring, atelectasis
• **Etiologic agents/types of pneumonia (Table 9.4)**
• **Bacteria present in associated illnesses:** COPD and/or cigarette smoking (*H. influenzae, Klebsiella*); diabetes (*Klebsiella, E. coli,* Gram-negative species); alcohol abuse (*Klebsiella,* anaerobes, Gram-negative species, *M. tuberculosis*); sickle cell disease (*Salmonella*); IV drug abuse (*S. aureus*); cystic fibrosis (resistant *Pseudomonas aeruginosa*)

LB • CBC with differential (left shift suggests bacterial process), O_2 saturation/ABG for suspected hypoxemia, sputum Gram stain and culture, blood/urine culture for fever
• Consider analysis of thoracentesis fluid to rule out empyema and selected serologies and agglutinin studies outside of the ED based on index of suspicion

TX • **Age-related antibiotic treatment:**
0–2 weeks: ampicillin and gentamicin
> 2 weeks–2 months: erythromycin or clarithromycin
> 2 months–8 years: erythromycin
Young children and adults: erythromycin or clarithromycin
• **Certain conditions:**
AIDS: TMP-SMX, erythromycin
Diabetes or alcoholism: cefazolin and aminoglycoside
Elderly patients: erythromycin, cefuroxime, azithromycin, or clarithromycin
Aspiration pneumonia: penicillin or clindamycin and cefuroxime
Hospital-acquired pneumonia: third-generation cephalosporin and aminoglycoside

DI • Admission for patients with hypoxia, volume depletion, toxicity, serious conditions (diabetes, CAD, PVD, immunocompromise) and those who cannot receive proper care at home
• Discharge other patients only after outpatient follow-up has been arranged

SCARLET FEVER

KY Group A streptococcus–erythrogenic toxin causes scarlet fever. Without treatment, affected patients are at risk for rheumatic fever. Scarlet fever is common in school-age children in the winter and spring.

HX Pharyngitis; perhaps URI symptoms; rash after onset of pharyngitis 1–3 days' duration

Table 9.4 Types of Pneumonia

Causal Agent/Type of Pneumonia	Signs and Symptoms	Laboratory Findings	CXR Findings	Comments
Streptococcus pneumoniae	Rusty/"currant jelly" sputum	Leukocytosis Gram-positive cocci pairs and chains	Single lobular infiltrate (patchy in infants, elderly patients); ± bulging fissures, effusion (10%)	Most common causal bacterial agent in 90% of cases, especially CAP; all ages affected
Haemophilus influenzae	High fever; rigors; purulent sputum; dyspnea; pleurisy	Gram-negative, pleomorphic rods (± en-capsulated)	Patchy infiltrate, often multilobar and bilateral; no effusion	Second most common causal bacterium in patients of all ages
Mycoplasma pneumoniae	Associated symptoms: URI (50%); earache (10%); conjunctivitis; cervical nodes; pharyngitis; dry, persistent cough	Low WBC; high ESR Outside ED: cold agglutinins > 1:64; complement fixation titer > 1:64 is diagnostic	Bilateral interstitial lower lobe infiltrates; reticulo-nodular infiltrate (20%); effusion (20%)	Most common nonpyogenic pneumonitis in children and adults
Viral (e.g., RSV)	URI; sometimes with associated exanthem; 3–5 years: fever, cough, coryza, poor feeding, ± wheezing, retractions		Hyper-inflation; patchy infiltrate; superimposed bacterial pneumonia (80%); normal CXR (40%)	May be seen in infants < 1 year (e.g., RSV); less common in adults Consider in immuno-compromised hosts; bacterial super-infection common
Klebsiella pneumoniae	Toxic appearance Dark brown/ "currant jelly" sputum	Leukocytosis; Gram-encapsulated rods	Upper lobar, commonly RUL infiltrate ± AFL; classic, bulging fissure (30%); perihilar, patchy infiltrate	Rare Suspect in middle-aged and elderly patients with underlying disease (e.g., alcoholism, diabetes mellitus)

Table 9.4   *Continued*

Causal Agent/Type of Pneumonia	Signs and Symptoms	Laboratory Findings	CXR Findings	Comments
Anaerobes		Leukocytosis	Classic RLL infiltrate, but perhaps diffuse pattern; may lead to AFL	Usually results from aspiration If CAP: anaerobes most common; if nosocomial: Gram-negative aerobes
Legionella	Rapid progression of disease process Tachypnea with relative bradycardia; abdominal pain; vomiting; diarrhea; confusion or delirium common	Leukocytosis; elevated ESR; ± LFT elevation Gram stain: few polys, no preponderant bacterium Outside ED: RIA and ELISA screens have specificity but low sensitivity; elevated antibody titer of 1:128 suggests infection; 1:256, acute infection	Unilateral infiltrate (70%) to bilateral patchy infiltrate; ± consolidation, and effusion (10%)	Results from contaminated domestic water systems Occurs in summer and fall Adults, smokers, and immuno-compromised individuals at greatest risk
Aspiration	Unprotected airway leading to inflammation, infection pH < 2.5 associated with chemical and bacterial pneumonitis; particulates can lead to obstruction		Persistent hyperexpan-sion of lung; chronic granulomatous changes (particulate)	Severity based on three factors: pH and volume of aspirate Particulates (food, foreign bodies); obstruction Bacterial contamination with resulting anaerobic pneumonia

PX • **Throat:** pharyngitis, sometimes with exudate
   • **Skin:** red, blanching, papular rash with sandpaper-like texture; located in hyperpigmented areas, joint creases; flushed face, desquamation with resolution; "strawberry tongue;" circumoral pallor
   • **Complications:** same as streptococcal pharyngitis (see Pharyngitis)

DD Viral exanthem (rubeola, rubella, roseola), fifth disease, Rocky Mountain spotted fever, Kawasaki disease, *Mycoplasma pneumoniae,* adenovirus, enterovirus, meningococcemia

LB Leukocytosis, ASO serology (ASO-positive), throat culture

TX • **Supportive measures:** PO fluids
   • **Antibiotics:** penicillin G, clindamycin, erythromycin, ceftriaxone

DI • Admission for patients with complications (e.g., dehydration, pneumonia with respiratory distress, toxic appearance)
   • Outpatient follow-up for other patients

SEPSIS

KY Bacteremia is the presence of microorganisms in the blood, and sepsis is bacteremia with a systemic response to these microorganisms. The most common causal organisms include: group B streptococci and *E. coli* in neonates and *H. influenzae, N. meningitidis,* and *S. pneumoniae* in infants and adults. Infection with *S. pneumoniae* and *Salmonella* is most likely in individuals with sickle cell disease, and *S. aureus* is most probable in IV drug abusers.

HX • **Risk:**
   Highest for neonates and debilitated, immunocompromised, and elderly individuals
   The rule of 2s applies: children < 2 years of age with a rectal temperature > 102°F (38.9°C) and a WBC > 20,000/mm^3 have a 20% risk for bacteremia
   • **Symptoms:**
   Patient complaints may suggest primary focus of infection, although vague symptoms of fever, malaise, headache, and arthralgias/myalgias are quite common
   History of recent illness/infection and antibiotic use is very helpful in making the diagnosis

PX • **Course of illness:** variable, insidious to fulminant
   • **Signs** (based on studies): fever (70%, in infants < 3 months and adults > 65 years, < 60%), shock (40%), hypothermia (4%), rash [maculopapular, petechial, nodular, vesicular with central necrosis (70% with meningococcemia)], and arthritis (8%)

DD Viral exanthem, Rocky Mountain spotted fever, typhus, typhoid fever, endocarditis, vasculitis (polyarteritis nodosa, Henoch-Schönlein purpura), toxic shock, rheumatic fever, fungal septicemia; etiologic factors such as group A streptococci, *Neisseria gonorrhoeae, P. aeruginosa, E. coli*

LB CBC with differential, blood and urine culture; consider CSF analysis for suspicious symptoms; bacterial, viral, or fungal serologies based on clinical suspicion

IM CXR, CT prn

TX **Antibiotic treatment** (bacteremia or sepsis probable by clinical suspicion, perhaps with supportive laboratory data, but no identification of microorganism):

- **Neonates (birth–1 month of age):**
    Ampicillin: 200 mg/kg/day IV and cefotaxime: 50 mg/kg/day IV
    or
    Ampicillin: 200 mg/kg/day and gentamicin: 2.5 mg/kg/day IV
- **Children (1 month–15 years of age):**
    Ceftriaxone: 50–75 mg/kg/day or
    Ceftazidime: 100 mg/kg/day IV or
    Ampicillin: 200 mg/kg/day and chloramphenicol: 50–100 mg/kg/day
- **Adults (15–60 years of age):**
    Penicillin G: 6–12 MU IV qd or
    Ampicillin: 200 mg/kg/day or
    Gentamicin: 2.5 mg/kg IV q8hr and metronidazole: 7.5 mg/kg IV q6hr
- **Adults (> 60 years of age, alcoholism):**
    Ampicillin: 200 mg/kg/day and ceftriaxone: 50 mg/kg/day or
    Ampicillin: 20 mg/kg/day and gentamicin: 2.5 mg/kg IV q8hr

DI • Admission to medical floor or ICU for patients with clinical toxicity, unclear progression of symptoms, unclear follow-up, suspected meningitis and/or meningococcemia, or significant underlying medical problems
- Discharge with clear, detailed discharge instructions, follow-up arrangements, and phone accessibility for patients with minimal signs and symptoms in whom clinical suspicion is low and cultures are pending

SEPTIC ARTHRITIS

KY Septic arthritis should be considered in all cases of painful monarthritis. A hematologic source is the most common. Other sources of infection include inoculation through a laceration or bite, extension from adjacent infection, association with foreign body or surgical hardware, and indwelling central venous access. *Staphylococcus, Streptococcus* spp., and *H. influenzae* are the most common causal bacteria.

HX Fever, chills, previous infection with potential for hematogenous seeding (especially gonorrhea and meningitis), immunocompromise, IV drug abuse, trauma, and prior chronic arthritis

PX Most common in large joints, which are warm, erythematous, and tender, with decreased ROM 2° to pain; often with an effusion

DD Noninfectious arthritis, including crystalline disorders; inflammatory conditions such as SLE, polymyalgia rheumatica, and trauma

LB • Arthrocentesis, avoiding overlying cellulitis if possible (expect opaque fluid with WBC counts > 50,000/mm^3 in developed pyogenic arthritis); arthrocentesis under fluoroscopy if necessary
  • Synovial fluid for Gram stain, C&S
  • CBC, blood C&S, and search for other possibly causative, source of infection

IM Plain radiographs, which are usually normal in early infection (erosion occurs later)

TX • **Antibiotic therapy** (treatment varies according to patient age and associated conditions): β-lactamase–resistant penicillins (IV nafcillin, methicillin, or oxacillin); addition of vancomycin with history of MRSA; ceftriaxone, cefotaxime, or ceftizoxime for possible GC
    Neonates and infants (birth–3 months of age): β-lactamase–resistant penicillins and either gentamicin or cephalosporins (cefamandole, cefotaxime, ceftazidime, ceftizoxime, or ceftriaxone)
    Children (toddlers–5 years of age): β-lactamase–resistant penicillins and cephalosporins (cefamandole, cefotaxime, ceftazidime, ceftizoxime, or ceftriaxone)
    Children (> 5 years of age) and adults: β-lactamase–resistant penicillins; consider gentamicin; customize treatment for compromised adults (IV drug abuse, HIV infection, debilitated state)
  • **Surgery:** consider surgical drainage for any foreign body involvement and foot involvement

DI Admission to medical floor with orthopedic consultation; if unsure, admission and treatment pending C&S

SEXUALLY TRANSMITTED DISEASES (STDS)

Chlamydial disease

KY *Chlamydia trachomatis* is the principal causal agent. Clinical manifestations of chlamydia include nongonococcal urethritis, cervicitis, salpingitis, rectal infection, perihepatitis, and conjunctivitis. The incubation period is 2–3 weeks. At least 50% of chlamydial infections occur concomitantly with GC, and the converse is true. Patients with chlamydial infection and GC should receive treatment for both diseases.

HX Abnormal vaginal, urethral, and rectal discharge; patients may complain of painless genital or rectal vesicles and ulcers as well as inguinal adenopathy that may suppurate and form sinus tracts

PX Epididymal, prostate, or cervical tenderness is characteristic; some patients, especially infants, may also have conjunctivitis or pneumonitis.

DD GC, trichomoniasis, and bacterial vaginosis (*Gardnerella*); consider syphilis, lymphogranuloma venereum, granuloma inguinale, and chancroid for associated lymphadenopathy

LB • Discharge samples (cervical, urethral, rectal, conjunctival) to reveal associated *N. gonorrhoeae, Trichomonas,* or yeast: culture; wet mount, KOH, Gram stain
   • Screen for syphilis: RPR or VDRL

IM Consider pelvic US in women with prolonged symptoms or with adnexal tenderness or mass when TOA is suspected

TX • Doxycycline: 100 mg PO q12hr × 7–10 days (avoid in pregnancy) or
   • Tetracycline HCl: 500 mg PO q6hr × 7–10 days (avoid in pregnancy) or
   • Erythromycin base: 500 mg PO q6hr × 7–10 days
   • Amoxicillin: 500 mg PO q8hr × 7 days

DI • Outpatient follow-up in gynecologic clinic
   • Admission for IV therapy in cases of severe pain, fever, or systemic signs and symptoms

Gonorrheal infection (GC)

KY Gonorrhoea is generally considered to be an STD. Affected patients may be asymptomatic or present with penile, vaginal, cervical, rectal, pharyngeal, conjunctival, or disseminated infections.

HX The likelihood of concurrent chlamydial infection is high (50%), and patients should be treated for both GC and chlamydia. Otherwise, affected patients are healthy young individuals with a septic picture and no significant PMH.

- **Men:** infection that may be asymptomatic or involve urethral discharge and dysuria; rectal discharge, which is sometimes purulent; and pain with anal sex
- **Women:** infection that may be asymptomatic or similar to vaginitis (misdiagnosis), cervicitis with vaginal discharge, dysuria with concomitant UTI, abdominal pain with salpingitis, TOA, Fitz-Hugh–Curtis syndrome, disseminated disease, rectal discharge, and pain with anal sex
- **Both sexes:** pharyngitis, rarely symptomatic; conjunctivitis with injection and discharge (look for primary source elsewhere); contact dermatitis, with local skin inflammation; disseminated disease, which can lead to fever, rash (maculopapular with pustular, necrotic centers, and petechiae); joint disease/septic arthritis, tenosynovitis; and risk for sepsis, endocarditis, and meningitis

DD GC, trichomoniasis, and bacterial vaginosis (*Gardnerella*); consider syphilis, lymphogranuloma venereum, granuloma inguinale, and chancroid for associated lymphadenopathy

LB • Gram stain of discharge for Gram-negative intracellular diplococci
- Culture of all discharge and lesions for both *N. gonorrhoeae* and *C. trachomatis;* negative culture is common; continue culture with high suspicion, but do not wait to treat RPR/VDRL to rule out syphilis

TX **Antibiotic treatment:**

- Ceftriaxone (use in pregnant women): 125 mg IM or
- Spectinomycin (use in pregnant women): 2 g PO or
- Ciprofloxacin (contraindicated in pregnancy and in children < 17 years): 500 mg PO or
- Norfloxacin: 800 mg PO (contraindicated in pregnancy and in children < 17 years) *plus*
- Doxycycline (contraindicated in pregnancy): 100 mg PO bid × 7–10 days or
- Azithromycin (contraindicated in pregnancy and in children < 17): 500 mg PO × 1, then 250 mg PO qd × 5 days or
- Erythromycin base (pregnant women and children < 8 years): 500 mg PO qid × 7–10 days

DI • Outpatient treatment with follow-up with treatment of all sexual contacts for cases of localized or asymptomatic disease

- Admission for IV antibiotic and observation for all cases of suspected GC conjunctivitis, arthritis, or disseminated disease; many centers admit nulliparous patients with cervicitis or salpingitis for IV antibiotics to reduce risk of tubal scarring

Human papillomavirus (HPV) infection

KY Manifestations of HPV include condylomata acuminata and genital warts, and up to one-third of infected patients have concomitant GC, chlamydia, or syphilis. HPV disease, which is more common in immuno-compromised individuals, is associated with genital cancer.

HX Painless bumps, discharge, dyspareunia, symptoms of vaginitis; sexual history may be significant for other STDs and rapid growth of warts during pregnancy

PX Lesions usually exophytic, papular, verrucous; may be flat and macular; perineal, perianal, vulvar, vaginal, or cervical in location

DD Condylomata lata (caused by syphilis; smoother and moister), acrochordon (skin tag), seborrheic keratosis, nevi, fibroepithelial polyps, molluscum contagiosum, carcinoma

LB RPR/VDRL, culture for *N. gonorrhoeae and C. trachomatis,* wet mount, pregnancy test if indicated

TX
- Examination of patient and partner, and referral to primary care physician or dermatologist for treatment, which occurs outside of the ED
- Cryotherapy, laser therapy, or application of podophyllum

DI Home

Syphilis

KY Syphilis is caused by an infection caused by the spirochete *Treponema pallidum,* which may be found in semen, vaginal secretions, saliva, mucous membranes, blood from open lesions, and amniotic fluid. Syphilis may be acute, latent, or chronic, and it has three characteristic stages (Table 9.5).

HX
- Patients may present at any stage (commonly primary or secondary)
- Symptoms of another STD (GC, chlamydia, or trichomoniasis) may also be apparent; if syphilis is present, look for all other STDs

DD
- **Primary chancre:** painless, deep, ulcerated lesion with clear discharge; consider also lymphogranuloma venereum [*C. trachomatis* (painful buboes)], granuloma inguinale [*Calymmatobacterium*

Table 9.5 Stages of Syphilis

Stage	Clinical Manifestations	Occurrence	RPR/VDRL
Primary	Papule developing into painless ulceration or chancre; sometimes buboes and rubbery nontender inguinal nodes	Incubation period: 10–90 days	Often negative
Secondary	Constitutional symptoms; onset of rash with red, nonpruritic macules, papules, or plaques/warts (condylomata lata)	1–2 months after primary stage	Positive
Tertiary	Cardiovascular conditions (aortic fibrosis, dissection, rupture); skin symptoms (gummata); neurologic symptoms (tabes dorsalis)	Months to years after latent period after secondary presentation	Positive

granulomatis (painful buboes)], chancroid [*Haemopilus ducreyi* (painful lesion)]
- **Secondary rash:** condylomata acuminata (HPV); pedunculated, single or grouped warts, less plaque-like than condylomata lata; also consider Rocky Mountain spotted fever (rickettsia), pityriasis rosea (viral exanthem)

🔳 RPR, VDRL serologies in all patients and partners with STDs, pregnant patients, and patients with suggestive rash; consider CSF VDRL in change in mental status workup for neurosyphilis; darkfield microscopy of chancre fluid may reveal spirochetes

TX • **Primary, secondary, and latent (< 1 year):**
  Benzathine penicillin G: 2.4 MU IM or
  Tetracycline: 500 mg q6hr × 2 weeks or
  Doxycycline: 100 mg q12hr × 2 weeks
• **Late (> 1 year latency):**
  Benzathine penicillin G: 2.4 MU IM q7days × 3 weeks or
  Tetracycline: 500 mg q6hr × 4 weeks or
  Doxycycline: 100 mg q12hr × 4 weeks
• **Neurosyphilis:**
  Penicillin G (2–4 MU IV q4hr × 10–14 days) or
  Procaine penicillin G (2–4 MU IM qd × 10–14 days) with
    probenecid (500 mg PO q6hr × 10–14 days)
• **Suspected tertiary disease:**
  Repeat RPR or VDRL after antibiotic course to rule out treatment
    failure
  Watch for Jarisch-Herxheimer reaction (inflammatory treatment
    reaction of spirochete death from antibiotic causing fever,
    myalgias, and headache)
  IV fluids, antipyretics, and bed rest

DI • Admission to medical floor for suspected tertiary disease

SINUSITIS

KY Sinusitis is an inflammation of the paranasal sinuses. A viral URI is a precipitating factor. Gram-positive cocci and *H. influenzae* cause acute cases, and anaerobes and Gram-negative bacteria result in chronic sinusitis.

HX URI symptoms, congestion, and purulent nasal discharge

PX Fever, headache, sinus pain, possible percussion tenderness, and purulent discharge

DD Viral URI, cellulitis, erysipelas, sinus abscess, periorbital/orbital cellulitis, meningitis/abscess, Pott's puffy tumor (forehead abscess), tumor

LB Diagnosis is made clinically

IM Sinus AFL on radiograph is not reliable

TX • **Acute:** amoxicillin (500 mg PO tid) or TMP-SMX DS (PO bid)
• **Severe:** amoxicillin-clavulanate (500 mg PO tid × 21 days) or cefuroxime (500 mg PO bid × 7–21 days); addition of decongestant such as chlorpheniramine (6–8 mg PO bid), pseudoephedrine (30–60 mg PO bid), or oxymetazoline (2 sprays each nostril q4–8hr × 3 days only)

DI Admission, perhaps to the ICU, for patients with pathologic findings (see differential diagnosis)

- Toxic-appearing patients with sinusitis or those with symptoms that suggest CNS involvement warrant emergent specialty consultation either from an otolaryngologist or a neurosurgeon and immediate admission to the ICU
- Older patients, patients with diabetes, and those who are debilitated or immunocompromised, who are at risk for rhinocerebral fungal infection, should be also admitted for immediate consultation

SOFT TISSUE INFECTIONS

Cellulitis

KY Cellulitis is most commonly caused by species of *Staphylococcus or Streptococcus*. This subcutaneous infection usually involves the deeper dermal layers, down to the fascia, in contrast to erysipelas, which is restricted to the epidermis. In healthy patients, isolation of pathogens is more likely (80% to 90%) with open lesions, pustules, or broken skin; with no known source, culture of the blood or skin is less revealing (10% to 40%). In most cases of simple cellulitis, culture may be of little value.

- In otherwise healthy adults, probable causal agents are *Staphylococcus and Streptococcus*.
- In children (> 6 months of age), *Staphylococcus, Streptococcus,* and *H. influenzae* most likely account for the infection. In patients with diabetes mellitus, alcohol addiction, and immunosuppression, *Staphylococcus, Streptococcus, Enterococcus, Enterobacter,* anaerobes, *P. aeruginosa, Bacteroides, Clostridium perfringens,* and MRSA are probable etiologic agents.

HX Possibly fever; perhaps a painful, warm, red region on skin, possibly surrounding a primary lesion, sometimes with lymphangitic streaking, tender adenopathy, and induration followed by suppuration

PX Erythema, edema, and skin warmth and tenderness

DD Erysipelas, local abscess, fasciitis, myositis, thrombophlebitis, gout, foreign body, herpetic/viral exanthem

LB CBC, open wound culture, possibly skin aspirate

IM Consider radiographs of underlying bones or bone scan for deep tissue infection, prolonged course, or suspicion of concomitant osteomyelitis

TX • If possible, treatment should be guided by culture results; most patients with simple cellulitis are first treated with an antistaphylococcal–antistreptococcal antibiotic, because the culture may be of little value

- Streptococcal cause: aqueous penicillin G (600,000 U IM), then procaine penicillin (600,000 U IM q8–12hr)
- Staphylococcal cause or unknown etiology: penicillinase-resistant penicillin [oxacillin (0.5–1.0 g PO q6hr)]
- Severe infection: penicillinase-resistant penicillin [nafcillin (1.0–1.5 g IV q4hr) or vancomycin (1.0–1.5 g/day IV)]
- Gas-forming cellulitis: aqueous penicillin G (10–20 MU/day IV) or metronidazole (500 mg IV q6hr) or clindamycin (600 mg IV q8hr)
- **Bites:**
  Animal bites: penicillin or nafcillin IV × 7 days; then switch to oral antibiotics
  Human bites: amoxicillin-clavulanic acid
- Facial cellulitis (*H. influenzae* type b): cefotaxime IV
- Diabetes mellitus: clindamycin and gentamicin (cefoxitin if these drugs are toxic to the patient)
- Immunocompromise: clindamycin and gentamicin
- IV drug abuse: vancomycin and gentamicin

DI
- Outpatient treatment for healthy individuals with simple infection
- Admission for IV antibiotic and observation for signs of systemic toxicity, extension of infection, or poor host resistance

Erysipelas

KY An infection of the dermis and the subcutaneous tissues, erysipelas is most commonly seen in children and the elderly. Causal organisms include *Streptococcus* (types A, C, and D) and *S. aureus.* An unnoticed skin wound often is the source of infection. Erysipelas ranges from a localized, self-limited condition to an extensive infection with bacteremia.

HX Small wound, local infection to widespread involvement, and sometimes fever

PX Red, warm, tender skin, with no fluctuance; lesions with raised edges

DD Cellulitis, sinusitis, erysipeloid (hands), contact dermatitis, angioneurotic edema, lupus, necrotizing fasciitis

LB Examination, perhaps punch biopsy; skin aspiration is usually not helpful

TX
- **Outpatient treatment:** penicillin VK [250–500 mg/dose q6hr (peds 25–50 mg/kg/day q6h)]
- **Inpatient treatment** (for severe cases): parenteral antibiotics such as cephalosporin, penicillinase-resistant penicillin (oxacillin, nafcillin, methicillin), clindamycin, or vancomycin

DI • Outpatient PO regimen with close follow-up if patients are not toxic-appearing
 • Admission for patients with widespread infection, clinical toxicity, and failure of oral antibiotic

Myonecrosis (gas gangrene)

KY In myonecrosis, which is caused by *Clostridium* spp. (primarily *C. perfringens*), extensive tissue necrosis and edema complicate infection of muscle. As infection develops, exotoxins can lead to sepsis, diffuse edema, and RBC hemolysis. Mortality exceeds 20%.

HX • Extensive and contaminated initial wounds or surgery, compounding problems such as compartment syndrome or immunocompromise
 • Rapid onset of pain that is traditionally greater than expected for the injury, with quickly progressive edema followed by sepsis

PX Initially edema; later palpable emphysema, erythema, and bullae

DD Compartment syndrome, thrombophlebitis, cellulitis, necrotizing fasciitis

LB Gram stain for Gram-positive bacilli

IM Radiograph that shows gas along tissue planes

TX • Immediate surgical intervention with fasciotomy and débridement
 • HBO
 • Penicillin G: 5–10 MU IV q6hr (peds 0.2–0.5 MU IV q4hr); alternatives include clindamycin, cephalothin, ceftriaxone, and erythromycin

DI OR or HBO and OR

CHAPTER 10

Metabolic Emergencies

ACID–BASE DISORDERS

Metabolic acidosis

KY Metabolic acidosis occurs when pH is low (< 7.35) and plasma HCO_3 is decreased; there is a 0.15-mEq fall in pH with a 10-mEq/L decline in HCO_3 (base deficit). The decrease in $Paco_2$ is 1–1.5 times the decline in HCO_3 (see Chapter 18, Toxicologic Emergencies, Anion Gap Metabolic Acidosis).

DD • **Elevated anion gap:** the mnemonic "A MUDPILE CAT" can be used to remember the causes of anion gap acidosis (Figure 10.1)
• **Normal anion gap** (hypochloremia): causes include RTA, diarrhea, pancreatic fistula, ileostomy, ureteroenterostomy, drugs (e.g., acetazolamide, mafenide, cholestyramine, spironolactone), TPN, NH_4Cl administration, posthypocapnia

LB SMA-7, ABG

TX ABCs, IV fluids, supplemental O_2, monitoring
• 0.9% NaCl or LR (to restore BP): 20 ml/kg boluses prn; then maintenance rate to obtain urine output of 0.5–1.0 ml/kg/hr
• Specific therapy for the particular metabolic derangement or toxic ingestion
• Consider HCO_3 therapy for low pH (< 7.2); dose = base deficit (mEq/L)/4 × body weight/4

DI Admission

Alcohol
Methanol
Uremia
Diabetic ketoacidosis
Paraldehyde
Iron and Isoniazid
Lactic acidosis
Ethylene glycol
Carbon monoxide
Aspirin
Toluene

FIGURE 10.1 The mnemonic "A MUDPILE CAT," which can be used to remember the causes of anion gap metabolic acidosis.

Metabolic alkalosis

KY Metabolic alkalosis is characterized by pH > 7.35 and increased plasma HCO_3. The pH rises 0.15 for every 10-mEq/L increase in HCO_3, and the rise in $Paco_2$ is 0.25–1 times that of HCO_3.

DD Causes include:

- **NaCl-responsive conditions:** contraction alkalosis, vomiting, NG suction, villous adenoma, penicillin and carbenicillin (large doses), diuretics, rapid correction of chronic hypercapnia
- **NaCl-unresponsive conditions:** mineralocorticoid excess in primary hyperaldosteronism, hyperreninism, licorice ingestion, Cushing's syndrome, Bartter's syndrome, adrenal hyperplasia

LB ABG, SMA-7

TX
- **General measures:**
  ABCs, IV fluids, supplemental O_2, monitoring
  Give 0.9% NaCl (to stabilize BP): 20 ml/kg boluses; then adjust rate to maintain urine output of 0.5–1.0 ml/kg/hr; add 20–40 mEq/L of KCl to maintenance fluid
- **Severe cases:** consider arginine monohydrochloride and NH_4Cl
- **NaCl-resistant cases:**
  KCl infusion of 20–40 mEq/L with urine output to reduce cellular hydrogen ions and enhance HCO_3 excretion
  Spironolactone (aldosterone antagonist) and/or acetazolamide infusion to enhance HCO_3 excretion
- Dialysis is indicated in renal failure

DI Admission to medical floor

Respiratory acidosis

KY Respiratory acidosis is characterized by decreased blood pH (< 7.35), increased Pco_2, and elevated HCO_3^- (compensation). In acute cases, the expected increase in HCO_3^- ion is equivalent to the $Pco_2 \times 0.1$, and in chronic cases, the expected HCO_3^- rise is equivalent to the $Pco_2 \times 0.4$. Coincident metabolic acidosis, resulting from anaerobic metabolism, may develop.

DD Causes include acute airway obstruction (e.g., asthma, COPD), lung disease, pleural effusions, pneumothorax, thoracic cage abnormalities (e.g., flail chest, rib fractures, kyphoscoliosis, scleroderma), hypoventilation (e.g., narcotics, CVA, sedatives, tranquilizers, paralysis, neuropathy), hypokalemia, hypophosphatemia, hypomagnesemia, muscular dystrophy

LB ABG

TX • ABCs, IV fluids, supplemental O_2, monitoring; in chronic acidosis, O_2 and assisted ventilatory rates should be adjusted cautiously to avoid CO_2 retention narcosis and posthypercapneic metabolic alkalosis, respectively
• Bronchodilators, postural drainage, and antibiotics when necessary to improve alveolar ventilation and oxygenation

Respiratory alkalosis

KY Respiratory alkalosis is characterized by decreased Pco_2, increased pH (> 7.35), and decreased HCO_3 with compensation. With acute respiratory alkalosis, the expected decline in HCO_3^- is equivalent to the $Pco_2 \times 0.2$. With chronic respiratory alkalosis, the expected HCO_3^- decrease is equivalent to the $Pco_2 \times 0.5$.

DD Causes: hyperventilation, anxiety, pain, CVA, head trauma, early sepsis, fever, pulmonary embolism, CHF, pneumonia, interstitial lung disease, hepatic insufficiency, pregnancy, ASA toxicity, thyrotoxicosis, hypoxemia, mechanical ventilation

LB ABG

TX Correction of underlying condition

HYPERKALEMIA

KY Causes of hyperkalemia include acidosis, tissue necrosis, hemolysis, blood transfusion, GI bleeding, renal failure, pseudohyperkalemia (leukocytosis), thrombocytosis, spironolactone, triamterene, amiloride, excess oral potassium, RTA, high-dose penicillin, succinylcholine, β blockers, captopril, laboratory error, and decreased mineralocorticoid activity.

HX Weakness, paresthesias, confusion, and paralysis

PX Arrhythmias, cardiac ventricular fibrillation, asystole, and cardiac arrest

LB Electrolytes, glucose, Mg

IM EKG (peaked T waves, ST depression, diminished R waves, prolonged PR interval, small P waves, sine waves)

TX • Consider discontinuing the medication that may have caused the hyperkalemia
• **Therapeutic agents:**
  Calcium chloride [10% solution (13.6 mEq/10 ml)]: 5 ml; or calcium gluconate [10% solution (4.6 mEq/10 ml)]: 10 ml; given over 2 minutes via peripheral vein and repeated in 5–10 minutes if necessary; give over 30 minutes (or omit) if digitalis toxicity is suspected

NaHCO$_3$: 44–132 mEq (1–3 amp of 7.5% solution) IV over 5 minutes (give after calcium in separate IV); repeat in 10–15 minutes; then give infusion of 2–3 amp in D$_5$W titrated over 2–4 hours

Insulin (regular): 10–20 U in 500 ml D$_{10}$W IV over 1 hour or 10 U IV push with 1 amp glucose 50% (25 g) over 5 minutes; repeat prn

Sodium polystyrene sulfonate: 15–50 g in 100 ml of sorbitol 20% solution PO now and in 3–4 hours (up to 4–5 doses per day); or sodium polystyrene sulfonate retention enema: 20–50 g in 200 ml of sorbitol 20%; retained for 30–60 minutes

Furosemide: 40–80 mg IV qd

Albuterol (acute hyperkalemia): 10–20 mg in 3 ml NS neb

- **Other measures:**

   Consider emergent dialysis if cardiac complications arise or renal failure occurs

   Correction of acidosis or hypovolemia

   Continuous cardiac monitoring, frequent serial examinations, and serum electrolyte determinations q2hr for patients who are being treated emergently for severe hyperkalemia until they are out of danger

DI ICU (mandatory)

HYPERNATREMIA

KY Hypernatremia may occur in three ways.

- **Excess free H$_2$O loss** may involve renal mechanisms [diabetes insipidus, osmotic diuresis (hyperglycemia), and mannitol] as well as GI, skin, and respiratory losses.
- **Inadequate free H$_2$O intake** may result from coma, reset osmolarity, and poor oral intake.
- **Excess Na$^+$ gain** may involve iatrogenic factors (NaHCO$_3$, hypertonic saline, and exogenous steroids), hyperaldosteronism, Cushing's disease, and congenital adrenal hyperplasia.

HX Confusion, muscle irritability, and weakness

PX Flat neck veins, orthostatic hypotension, tachycardia, poor skin turgor, dry mucous membranes, seizures, coma, and respiratory paralysis

LB Hct, SMA-7, serum protein; urine osmolality, urine sodium concentration, which is useful primarily outside the ED

TX • If patients are volume depleted, give 0.5–3 L NS IV at 500 ml/hr until they are not orthostatic; then give D$_5$W (if hyperosmolar) or

D_5NS (if not hyperosmolar) IV or PO to replace one-half of body water deficit over first 24 hours (1 mEq/L/hr) and supply the remaining deficit over the next 1–2 days
- Keep urine output ≥ 0.5 ml/kg/hr
- If correction is too rapid, CNS edema and seizures may result
- Body water deficit (L) = 0.6 × (weight in kg) × ([serum Na]-140)/140

DI Admission in most cases

HYPOKALEMIA

KY Hypokalemia (K^+ concentration < 3.5 mEq/L) is the most common electrolyte abnormality. The causes of hypokalemia involve redistribution (alkalosis, insulin, vitamin B_{12} therapy, β_2-agonists, periodic paralysis); renal losses (diuretics, low magnesium, Bartter's syndrome, RTA, vomiting, glucocorticoid/mineralocorticoid excess); GI losses (gastric, diarrhea, bile, and fistula); and laboratory error.

HX Weakness, paresthesia, polyuria, and paralysis

PX Areflexia, rhabdomyolysis, orthostatic hypotension, ileus, metabolic alkalosis, glucose intolerance, and paralysis

LB SMA-7, Mg, UA

IM EKG (T-wave flattening or inversion, U-wave prominence, ST-segment depression, PVCs)

TX
- Because potassium ions can be very dangerous, overzealous administration should be avoided
- If serum potassium > 2.5 mEq/L and EKG changes are absent: KCl (20–30 mEq/hr IV with saline); may combine with KCl (30–40 mEq PO q4hr) in addition to IV [total maximal dose generally 100–200 mEq/day (3 mEq/kg/day)]
- If serum potassium < 2.5 mEq/L and EKG abnormalities are present: KCl IV (30–40 mEq/hr up to 80 mEq/L); may combine with KCl (30–40 mEq PO q4hr) [total maximum daily dose IV (3 mEq/kg/day); give one-half over 24 hours]; use supplemental potassium—phosphate preparation if phosphate is low

DI ICU with continuous monitoring for patients with any of the following conditions: malignant cardiac dysrhythmias, digitalis toxicity, profound weakness with impending respiratory insufficiency, low serum potassium concentration (< 2.0 mEq/L), and rhabdomyolysis or hepatic encephalopathy

HYPONATREMIA

KY There are three types of hyponatremia.

- **Hypovolemic hyponatremia** involves renal losses (e.g., diuretic excess, mineralocorticoid deficiency, salt-losing nephritis, and RTA with bicarbonate urea); extrarenal losses (e.g., vomiting, diarrhea); and burns, pancreatitis, and traumatized muscle.
- **Euvolemic hyponatremia** results from glucocorticoid deficiency, hypothyroidism, pain, emotion, drugs, and SIADH.
- **Hypervolemic hyponatremia** involves nephrotic syndrome, cirrhosis, cardiac failure, and acute or chronic renal failure.

HX Lethargy, apathy, disorientation, muscle cramps, anorexia, nausea, and agitation

PX Abnormal sensorium, depressed DTRs, hypothermia, pseudobulbar palsy, seizures, and Cheyne-Stokes respirations

LB Serum electrolytes, serum glucose, BUN, creatinine; urine sodium, urine osmolality

TX • **Hypervolemic hyponatremia:**
  Water restriction: 0.5–1.5 L/day
  Furosemide: 40–80 mg IV or PO qd
  For severe symptomatic hyponatremia, concurrent diuresis and sodium replacement may be necessary
- **Isovolemic hyponatremia:**
  Water restriction: 500–1500 ml/day
  Furosemide: 80 mg (1 mg/kg) IV qd—bid and 0.9% saline with 20–40 mEq KCl/L at 65–150 ml/hr (correction rate < 0.5 mEq/L/hr)
- **Hypovolemic hyponatremia:** for volume depletion, give 0.5–3 L of 0.9% saline at 500 ml/hr until the patient is no longer orthostatic; then give 125 mEq/L of 0.9% saline with 10–40 mEq of KCl/L at 65–150 ml/hr or 100 ml of 3% hypertonic saline over 5 hours

DI Medical floor or ICU as appropriate

CHAPTER 11

Neurologic Emergencies

ALTERED MENTAL STATUS (AMS) AND COMA

HX Progressive confusion, disorientation, stupor, obtundation to coma; possibly fever, and depressed mood/suicidal ideation. Search for significant PMH, including immunosuppression, endocrinopathy, CNS pathology, drug abuse, pharmacologic regimen, and trauma.

PX • The degree of AMS and coma should be assessed using the GCS (Table 11.1)
 • Certain physical conditions may indicate the cause of the AMS (Table 11.2)

DD Consider the conditions mentioned in Table 11.2; the mnemonic "TIPS AEIOU" can be used to remember the causes of AMS and coma (Figure 11.1)

LB • CBC, SMA-7, Ca, Mg, serum toxicology screen; consider urine toxicology (e.g., PCP, LSD); rectal temperature; blood, urine, and CSF culture prn
 • Consider laboratory evaluation, including CBC, LFTs, and urine protein, for preeclampsia–eclampsia in pregnant patients with change in mental status if > 20 weeks' gestation

Table 11.1   Glasgow Coma Scale

Eyes	Open spontaneously	4
	Open to verbal command	3
	Open to pain	2
	No response	1
Best Motor Response	Obeys commands	6
	Localizes painful stimulus	5
	Withdrawal from painful stimulus	4
	Flexion to pain (decorticate posturing)	3
	Extension to pain (decerebrate posturing)	2
	No response	1
Best Verbal Response	Oriented and converses	5
	Disoriented and converses	4
	Inappropriate words	3
	Incomprehensible sounds	2
	No response	1
TOTAL SCORE		3–15

Table 11.2 Physical Findings and Causes in AMS and Coma

Physical Finding	Causal Condition
Alcohol on breath	Alcohol intoxication; consider subdural hematoma
Young, healthy patient	Consider overdose
Jaundice	Hepatic failure
Petechial hemorrhage	ITP, DIC, leukemia, meningitis, hepatic/renal failure
Fecal/urinary incontinence	CVA and seizure
Barrel chest/emphysematous, pursed-lip breathing	Respiratory failure
Healthy patients with pulmonary edema on CXR	Heroin, cocaine, or salicylate overdose
Diaphoretic, cold, or hypothermic state	Consider hypoglycemia, hypothermia, adrenal crisis, sepsis
Tachypnea	Respiratory failure and acidosis [respiratory or endocrine conditions; other causes ("A MUDPILE CAT"; see Figure 10.1)]
Meningismus, Kernig's sign, Brudzinski's sign	Meningitis, sepsis, SAH
Rhinorrhea, otorrhea, Battle's sign, raccoon's eyes	Basilar skull fracture
Needle tracks	IV drug abuse/overdose
Tongue laceration	Seizure
Broken bones with petechiae, respiratory distress	Consider fat emboli

---

Trauma (hypovolemia, head injury); **T**emperature
Infection; **I**ntussusception
Psychiatric
Space-occupying lesions/conditions*

Alcohol
Endocrinopathy†
Insulin
Oxygen; **O**piates
Uremia and hypertensive crisis

*Examples include epidural and subdural hematoma; embolic or hemorrhagic CVA; subarachnoid hemorrhage; CNS tumor; cerebral edema; SAH, leading to shock.
†Disorders that involve endocrine glands, liver failure, and serum electrolytes.

FIGURE 11.1 The mnemonic "TIPS AEIOU," which can be used to remember the causes of AMS and coma.

IM Cervical spine radiographs (in-line cervical spine immobilization for suspected trauma), CXR, head CT prn, EKG

TX • ABCs, IV fluids, supplemental O_2, monitoring
• Dextrostix, D_{50} (adults 1–2 amp), D_{25} (children < 8 years 0.5–1.0 g/kg), D_{10} (neonates 0.5–1.0 mg/kg)
• Thiamine: 100 mg IV; naloxone: 0.01–0.2 mg/kg
• Gastric lavage with activated charcoal: 1.0 g/kg PO q6–8hr
• Specific antidotes to toxic drug levels found in screen or based on clinical "toxidrome"
• Consider antibiotics (ampicillin, gentamicin, metronidazole, ceftriaxone/metronidazole) for suspected sepsis/meningitis
• Trauma and/or neurosurgical consults for suspected thoraco-abdomen or CHI
• Consider benzodiazepines, phenytoin, or phenobarbital for seizures

DI Admission for suspected prolonged detoxification, infection, trauma, intractable, or first-time seizure

AMYOTROPHIC LATERAL SCLEROSIS

KY This progressive, fatal disease of unknown etiology is characterized by destruction of motor cells in the anterior gray horns of the spinal cord and degeneration of pyramidal tracts. Sensory changes are rare.

HX Weakness, atrophy, and initial muscle fasciculations of hands and arms, followed by spastic paralysis of the limbs

PX Presentation is consistent with progression of symptoms

DD Cervical spondylosis, plasma cell dyscrasias, lead intoxication, spinal muscular atrophy, primary lateral sclerosis, spinal MS, tropical spastic paraparesis

LB Muscle biopsy outside of ED

IM EMG outside of ED

TX • ABCs, IV fluids, supplemental O_2, monitoring
• Treat complications of immobility such as pneumonia, urosepsis, and respiratory problems

DI Admission to neurology or medical service

CEREBROVASCULAR ACCIDENT (CVA)

KY Cerebral ischemia/infarction is a result of occlusive syndrome from thrombi, emboli (ulcerated arterial plaques, cardiac mural thrombi, endocarditis, fat emboli of fractures, dysbaric injury), or hemorrhage (aneurysm, AVM, hypertension, blood dyscrasia, neoplasm, infection, anticoagulants). Hemorrhagic events may be either subarachnoid or intracerebral (see Intracranial Hemorrhage).

HX • Risk factors: hypertension, atherosclerosis, CAD, diabetes, hypercholesterolemia, smoking, and gout; history of previous TIAs (70% of patients who have TIAs have CVAs within 2 years)
  • Onset of symptoms: sudden with TIA or CVA
  • Clinical improvement:
    TIAs: complete improvement in hours
    Embolic/thrombotic CVAs: sometimes incomplete improvement over weeks to months
    Hemorrhagic stroke: little improvement (may see deepening picture acutely from expanding bleed or associated edema)

PX • Presence of vessel bruits suggests more than 70% stenosis and is associated with high-risk embolism (absence does not rule out ulcerated plaques)
  • Examination findings are coincident with the vascular/parenchymal distribution affected (Table 11.3)

DD Trauma [e.g., concussion, epidural or subdural hematoma, cerebral contusion (coup/contrecoup)], neoplasm, infection, abscess, metabolic abnormalities (e.g., hyponatremia), "toxidromes" (e.g., narcotics, phenothiazines, cyclic antidepressants, cholinesterase inhibitors/pesticides, pilocarpine), postictal state

LB CBC, SMA-7, Ca, Mg, ammonia, blood and urine culture, pulse oximetry or ABG, possibly CSF (negative head CT) for fever

IM • Unenhanced head CT in all patients with clinical suspicion of CVA (to rule out cerebral hemorrhage)
  • Consult with neurologist and radiologist regarding particular scanning or arteriographic techniques if further evaluation is necessary. Consider noninvasive cervical vascular Doppler US, searching for possible atherosclerotic plaques, echocardiogram (to rule out cardiac chamber mitral thrombosis), and cervical spine series for clinical suspicion of trauma.

TX • Airway (including ICP management), IV fluids, supplemental O_2, monitoring
  • Consider heparinization for patients with history and clinical evidence of TIA and for those with smaller infarcts due to embolization who have normal mental status and little deficit; consider early consultation, because the precise decision point for treatment is controversial
  • Consider antihypertensive therapy and control of ICP (see Intracranial Hemorrhage)

Table 11.3   Signs and Symptoms of CVA

Site of Occlusion/Type of Hemorrhage	Signs and Symptoms
Middle cerebral artery	Contralateral hemiplegia (upper extremity weakness greater than lower extremity weakness), hemianesthesia, homonymous hemianopsia, contralateral conjugate gaze, aphasia with dominant hemispheric involvement
Anterior cerebral artery	Contralateral extremity weakness (lower extremity weakness greater than upper extremity weakness), gait apraxia, abulia, urinary incontinence
Posterior cerebral artery	Contralateral homonymous hemianopsia, hemiparesis, hemisensory loss, ipsilateral cranial nerve III, memory loss
Vertebrobasilar artery	Ipsilateral cranial nerve deficit, cerebellar ataxia, contralateral hemiplegia, hemisensory loss; nausea, vomiting, nystagmus, vertigo, tinnitus/hearing loss
Basilar artery	Quadriplegia, upward gaze/"locked-in" syndrome
Cerebellar infarct	Ataxia (especially with vermis infarct), vertigo, tinnitus, nausea, vomiting, nystagmus (horizontal or vertical)
Lacunar infarct (lipohyalinotic, cystic infarcts off penetrating cerebral arterioles within internal capsule)	Specific syndromes: Midpons: dysarthria/clumsy hand Pons/internal capsule: ataxia, leg paresis or pure motor hemiplegia Thalamus: pure sensory syndrome
Amygdaloid/ hippocampus infarct	Transient global amnesia; common in patients > 60 years Lasts minutes to hours, with complete resolution Somatic/speech, cognition, and long-term memory are intact during and after episode, but no knowledge of event afterwards
Pontine hemorrhage	Pinpoint pupils, decerebration, coma
Thalamic hemorrhage	Contralateral hemiparesis, hemianesthesia, dysconjugate gaze
Putamen hemorrhage	Similar to middle cerebral artery syndrome but with much depressed level of consciousness
Cerebellar hemorrhage	Ataxia, dizziness, nausea and vomiting

- Urgent neurology consult for possible use of thrombolytic agents in nonhemorrhagic stroke; neurology or neurosurgery consult for possible angiography and/or surgical intervention

DI Admission to neurology or medicine (nontraumatic CVA); trauma or neurosurgery (traumatic CVA)

HEADACHE

KY Headaches result from tension, inflammation, and swelling of pain-sensitive tissues (skin, muscle, sinuses, vessels, and somatic/visceral nerves) (Table 11.4). Brain parenchymal tissue has no pain fibers.

HX Symptoms are numerous (see Table 11.4)

PX Presentation varies with type of headache (see Table 11.4)

DD Consider conditions mentioned in Table 11.4; also meningitis, encephalitis, subdural or epidural hematoma, skull fracture, sinusitis, tooth abscess, TMJ syndrome, otitis media, external otitis, parotitis, high altitude sickness

LB Customize evaluation for each presentation and include index of suspicion for a dangerous cause; consider CBC, SMA-7, Ca, Mg, ESR, septic workup for fever

IM Consider head CT, MRI, noninvasive vascular Doppler evaluation

TX • **Migraine headache:**
  Aural stage: ergotamines (PO/PR/inhaler); ergotamine–caffeine (1–2 mg PO) ASAP (max 5 mg/attack or 10 mg/week), one suppository ASAP and in 1 hour prn; *or* NSAIDs, especially naproxen (500–1000 mg PO ASAP, repeat in 12 hours prn), or isometheptene dichloralphenazone–acetaminophen [two cap PO ASAP, then one cap PO qhr (max five/day or 10/week)]
  Acute stage: metoclopramide (10 mg PO/IM/IV); chlorpromazine (0.1 mg/kg IV q15min or 25 mg IM single dose); dihydroergotamine (0.5–1.0 mg IV), perhaps with chlorpromazine; meperidine (25–50 mg IM) with hydroxyzine (25 mg PO/IM); or methylprednisolone (60–120 mg IV); or consider ketorolac (60 mg IM) [contraindications: late in pregnancy, history of PUD]
  Prevention: avoidance of alcohol, caffeine, chocolate, OCPs, tyramines, and stress; consider verapamil (80 mg PO tid/qid), amitriptyline (50–75 mg PO qd), phenytoin (200–400 mg PO qd), or ergotamine [1 mg PO bid (max 10 tab/week)]
• **Cluster headache:**
  Treatment: supplemental O_2 (7–15 L/min); ergotamines PO/PR/IV (see treatment for migraine headaches); or consider intranasal viscous lidocaine
  Prevention: avoidance of alcohol, nitrates, and histamines; verapamil (80 mg PO tid/qid), amitriptyline (50–75 mg PO qd), or lithium carbonate (300 mg PO tid)

Table 11.4   Types of Headache: Symptoms and Etiology

Type	Etiology/ Pathophysiology	Symptoms and Signs
Vascular: migraine	Environmental change, emotional stress, sleep deprivation, hunger, thirst lead to arterial vasoconstriction Hypoxia due to parenchymal distribution results in aura Vasodilation and reperfusion cause release of pain mediators [histamine, serotonin, prostaglandins, SRSA (leukotrienes)]	Severe throbbing, initially in area of hypoperfusion but may become global Associated with ocular pain, nausea, vomiting Typical patient is young woman (30s) who complains of progressively painful, unilateral to global headache associated with photophobia, nausea, vomiting Correlated with menses, family history
Vascular: cluster		Sudden onset, severe, burning, boring pain on one side of face Other symptoms: ipsilateral rhinorrhea, congestion, perhaps ipsilateral Horner's syndrome Patient is young adult (30s)
Vascular: SAH	Bleeding from leaking berry/saccular aneurysm or AVM Also commonly associated with trauma Blood tracks underneath arachnoid surrounding cerebrum cause pressure and inflammation	Pain is usually sudden ("thunder-clap") and global
Vasculitis (temporal/ cranial arteritis)	Granulomatous inflammatory changes involving carotid branches	Examination may reveal tender, pulseless temporal artery and worsened symptoms with arterial compression If temporal artery is involved, risk that retinal artery is involved as well, leading to blindness, is very high (do not misdiagnose this as migraine!)

continued

Table 11.4 *Continued*

Type	Etiology/ Pathophysiology	Symptoms and Signs
Vasculitis (temporal/ cranial arteritis) (continued)		ESR usually > 50 mm/hr Patient is usually female (> 40 years) who complains of unilateral
Tension	Muscular strain, spasm from repetitive head motion or prolonged positioning Associated with "stress"	Pain may extend globally, like a halo around the head and extend down into the neck, shoulders and back
Intraparenchymal mass (tumor, abscess)		Headache is insidious in onset Becomes progressively worse, dull, throbbing (usually unilateral), and worse on awakening Associated symptoms may include nausea and vomiting, ataxia, visual changes, LOC, tinnitus/hearing loss, unilateral/bilateral cranial nerve affects, distal somatic findings based on lesion location
Ocular	Etiology: trauma, iritis, infection, glaucoma, corneal abrasion (see Chapter 7, Head and Neck Emergencies)	Local, global pain, perhaps vision changes, retinal changes, hyphema, periorbital/conjunctival swelling, erythema, discharge

- **Arteritis:** prednisone (80–120 mg PO qd with a 2-week taper); NSAIDs for pain
- **SAH:** see Intracranial Hemorrhage
- **Tension headache:** NSAIDs, massage, stress management
- **Ocular headache:** see Chapter 7, Head and Neck Emergencies
- **Space-occupying lesion:** airway, IV fluids, supplemental O_2, monitoring, seizure prophylaxis, BP management, perhaps ICP monitoring

DI • Admission for workup for any concern of intracranial pathology or no clinical improvement from ED intervention
• With discharge: arrange appropriate follow-up and provide strict instructions to return for progressive symptoms

INTRACRANIAL HEMORRHAGE

KY Intracranial hemorrhage may be either traumatic (see Chapter 19, Trauma, Head Trauma, Acute Subdural and Epidural Hematoma) or spontaneous. Spontaneous intracranial hemorrhage causes about 10% of all CVAs (see CVA). Hypertensive hemorrhage commonly originates in small penetrating arteries that branch off the middle cerebral artery; in two-thirds of cases, the site of hemorrhage is the basal ganglia. Most often, SAH is associated with a ruptured arterial aneurysm; in some cases, AVM is the source. The 1-month mortality from a spontaneous intracranial hemorrhage is 50%.

HX • Trauma, hypertension, previous known history of aneurysm or AVM, inducing stressor; history of antithrombotic or thrombolytic medications and cocaine use
• Sudden onset of "the worst headache of my life" or previous "sentinel" headaches suggests SAH

PX • Check ABCs, determine whether gag reflex is intact
• Perform neurologic examination seeking focal deficits, change in mental status, with frequent or continuous reassessment, searching for a worsening clinical picture
• Signs of SAH (see Table 11.1)
  Grade I: no change in mental status, no focal deficits, mild headache, and meningismus
  Grade II: mild change in mental status, some focal deficit, severe headache, and meningismus
  Grade III: major change in mental status or major focal deficit
  Grade IV: semicomatose or comatose
• Other signs: BP often very high, Cheyne-Stokes respirations with elevated ICP, pinpoint pupils with pontine hemorrhage, ipsilateral third nerve palsy with posterior communicating arterial aneurysms

DD Nonhemorrhagic CVA, change in mental status, recurrence of symptoms of previous CVA prompted by a new insult (e.g., infection, metabolic abnormality), meningitis, encephalitis, metabolic derangement, brain tumor or abscess

LB Pulse oximetry or ABG, CBC, SMA-7, PT, PTT; neurosurgical consult for angiography

IM Noncontrast brain CT, CXR

TX
- **Supportive measures:** airway (including ICP management), IV fluids, supplemental O_2, monitoring (consider arterial BP monitoring)
- **BP management:** titrate to BP 160–200/100–110 mm Hg (be careful; patients with baseline hypertension who now have cerebral edema require perfusion pressure); nitroprusside (0.5 µg/kg/min up to 10 µg/kg/min), hydralazine (10–20 mg IV q30min), or labetalol (20 mg IV q10min up to 300 mg)
- **Elevated ICP or impending herniation:** RSI for intubation with care of ICP
- **Hyperventilation** (goal is P_{CO_2} of 25–30 mm Hg): elevate head of bed to 30°; consider mannitol 1 g/kg
- **Seizure control:** consider possible prophylaxis with phenytoin load: 17 mg/kg IV, no faster than 50 mg/min
- **SAH:** consider nimodipine for grades I and II (may decrease incidence of vasospasm and possible other calcium channel–mediated benefits); neurosurgical consult

DI ICU unless clearly stable

LANDRY-GUILLAIN-BARRÉ SYNDROME

KY This syndrome, an acute idiopathic polyneuritis characterized by progressive motor weakness, usually starts distally in the legs (occasionally in arms) and ascends to involve the trunk, upper extremities, and cranial and respiratory muscles. Its onset occurs over days. Recovery takes months.

HX Progressive motor weakness; some sensory loss and autonomic disturbance

PX Decreased or absent DTRs, weakness as described in history; presence of a tick

DD Tick paralysis; poliomyelitis; hypokalemia; periodic paralysis; acute transverse myelitis; radiculopathies; myopathy, including polymyositis [tender muscles (proximal muscles more affected)], elevated CK; myasthenia gravis (usually bulbar involvement); polymyalgia rheumatica (proximal muscle pain without weakness); neurotoxins, including botulism (usually bulbar involvement, with subsequent respiratory compromise as paralysis descends); tetanus; diphtheria

LB
- Acute evaluation only takes place in the ED (nerve conduction studies and other evaluation of respiratory function are inpatient concerns)

- Likely tests: CBC, SMA-7, Ca, Mg, perhaps LP (few cells with elevated protein may be found from days to weeks into the disease course)

IM Appropriate imaging (e.g., emergent MRI to rule out myelitis or extrinsic spinal cord compression)

TX ABCs, IV fluids, supplemental O_2, monitoring; plasmapheresis (inpatient)

DI
- Admission for further neurologic evaluation and treatment
- Outpatient management (should be considered only rarely) for "reliable" patients with a low suspicion of clinical deterioration who will return immediately if their condition worsens and who will seek follow-up with the primary care physician or neurologist who has been consulted and involved with their disposition

MULTIPLE SCLEROSIS (MS)

KY Scattered demyelination within the CNS characterizes MS, a progressive disease that follows a waxing and waning course. The presence of plaques is a hallmark of the disorder. Elevated body temperature, which aggravates symptoms, should be treated aggressively in the ED.

HX Usually, patients who present to the ED have previously diagnosed MS and either an exacerbation of the disease or a complication associated with impaired swallowing or airway protection, immobilization, or abnormal bladder function

PX
- Pay special attention to assessment of the airway, neurologic examination, and funduscopic examination for optic neuritis or papilledema
- Check for the potential existence of decubitus ulcers or pneumonia underlying the exacerbation

DD New, unrelated CNS lesion (e.g., CVA, meningitis, CHI), metabolic derangement, acute transverse myelitis, encephalitis

LB
- Tailor to presentation; aggressively seek insult, especially infection, that may have caused exacerbation
- Consider labs for metabolic and infectious problems: UA; blood, urine, and wound C&S as appropriate

IM CXR

TX
- Management of the airway, treatment of hyperthermia, and providing urinary drainage and skin care are initial priorities in ED management
- Antibiotics as appropriate for infection

DI Admission to neurology or medicine is frequently necessary as a result of the acute medical problem that caused the exacerbation; current management of an exacerbation of MS usually includes inpatient steroids

MYASTHENIA GRAVIS

KY Myasthenia gravis is an autoimmune condition characterized by acetylcholine receptor destruction and poor neurotransmission resulting in weakness. This disorder is classified by the extent of disease.

- **Scope of disease:**
    Localized, nonprogressive, and limited to ocular weakness (diplopia and ptosis); good prognosis

    Generalized, both cranial and skeletal muscle weakness without sensory loss; good prognosis

    Acute onset, systemic involvement with poor response to therapy; poor prognosis

    Gradual progression of symptoms several years after onset; poor prognosis

    Generalized disease with muscle atrophy beginning several months after onset; variable prognosis

- **Myasthenic crises** result from a functional lack of acetylcholine and usually occur in undiagnosed patients with severe weakness. Edrophonium (2 mg IV, then 8 mg IV slow) improves symptoms.

- **Cholinergic crises** occur in patients who are being treated for myasthenia with excess acetylcholine esterase (anticholinesterase). Severe muscle weakness is present. Edrophonium increases, not decreases, symptoms. Watch for muscarinic symptoms. The mnemonic "SLUDGE" can be used to remember the symptoms of muscarinic syndrome (Figure 11.2).

HX
- Complaints of muscle weakness, worsened by prolonged activity and improved with rest
- Most often, symptoms begin with ocular ptosis, diplopia, and blurred vision

> Salivation
> Lacrimation (tears)
> Urinary incontinence
> Diaphoresis
> Gastrointestinal symptoms (i.e., diarrhea)
> Emesis

FIGURE 11.2 The mnemonic "SLUDGE," which can be used to remember the symptoms of muscarinic syndrome.

PX Ocular weakness (ptosis, extraocular weakness, diplopia, blurred vision); facial, oral, and distal extremity weakness with depressed DTRs; and possible respiratory difficulty

DD Eaton-Lambert syndrome (symptoms improve with repetitive exercise), botulism, Guillain-Barré syndrome, tick paralysis, familial periodic paralysis (seen with normal, high, or low potassium), chronic fatigue syndrome, oculopharyngeal dystrophy, polymyositis, MS, sleep paralysis

LB Usually occurs outside ED; "double-blind" edrophonium test, which increases acetylcholine and improves symptoms; perhaps serologies for acetylcholine receptors

IM EMG (gold standard) outside ED

TX
- Edrophonium: 2 mg IV, then 8 mg IV slow
  - Clinical improvement indicates a myasthenic crisis, and worsening symptoms suggest a possible cholinergic crisis
  - Atropine [for bradycardia, low BP, wheezing/rales, or "SLUDGE" (see Figure 11.2)]: 1 mg IV prn

DI Admission to medical or neurologic ICU for monitoring

SEIZURES

KY The onset of primary epilepsy (idiopathic) occurs before the age of 20 years. Secondary epilepsy (symptomatic) caused by parenchymal abnormalities includes aneurysm, AVM, tumor cyst, abscess, contusion, hematoma, or an old scar. Although symptomatic epilepsy may develop at any age, it most commonly begins in adulthood. Status epilepticus describes seizures persisting longer than 20 minutes or repetitive events without lucid intervals; if untreated, status epilepticus is associated with 20% mortality.

HX **Types of seizures:**
- **Generalized/grand mal:** LOC (witnessed) with generalized activity
- **Petit mal (absence):** prolonged unresponsive staring without LOC, sometimes with focal muscular activity
- **Focal:** repetitive motor activity without LOC
- **Temporal lobe:** hallucinations (visual, auditory, olfactory); memory loss; and/or bizarre behavior that may progress to focal-generalized motor activity
- **Febrile:**
  Generalized activity associated with rapidly rising fever, lasting several minutes; occurs in individuals between the ages of 3 months and 5 years

Associated with no increased risk for permanent seizure disorder, mental retardation, cerebral palsy, or death

- **Infantile spasm:**
  Myoclonic jerking and spasm, especially flexion/extension of neck or back; occurs in infants who are 3–9 months old
  Associated with severe mental retardation
- **Todd's paralysis:** focal weakness or paralysis after the seizure, which lasts up to several days

PX • Check ABCs; determine seizure status and level of consciousness
- Look for trauma (head/facial abrasions, contusions, lacerations; tongue, buccal lacerations; neck deformity) and urinary or fecal incontinence
- Look for eye deviation and focal/generalized tonic-clonic activity

DD Drug intoxication/withdrawal, hypoglycemia, hyper- or hyponatremia, hypocalcemia, pyridoxine deficiency, infection, breath-holding spells, TIA/CVA, syncope, cataplexy, narcolepsy, myoclonia, pseudoseizures (watch for purposeful movement during episode)

LB O_2 saturation, Dexi-stick stat; CBC, SMA-7; consider Ca, Mg, toxicology screen (serum/urine), serum osmolality, anticonvulsant levels; serum, urine, and CSF culture for fever

IM CXR (rule out aspiration), head CT/MRI (rule out trauma as etiology or as result of episode prn with radiographic/CT evaluation), EEG

TX • Adults:
  Airway, IV fluids, supplemental O_2, monitoring, Dexi-stick or D_{50}, naloxone (2–4 mg), thiamine (100 mg IV)
  Pregnant women: begin magnesium sulfate (4–6 g IV load, then 1–2 g/hr)
  Consider pyridoxine 5%–10% solution (for suspected INH toxicity): 5 g IV
  Diazepam (to suppress activity): 5 mg/min IV q5min to 30 mg; or lorazepam: 0.1 mg/kg IV; if no response or after benzodiazepine suppression, give phenytoin: 18 mg/kg IV load at 50 mg/min
  For seizures unresponsive to benzodiazepines or phenytoin, consider phenobarbital: 10 mg/kg IV at 50 mg/min, repeated twice
  For status epilepticus unresponsive even to phenobarbital, consider lidocaine: 2–4 mg/min IV; diazepam (drip): 1 mg/kg/hr IV; pentobarbital (drip): 5 mg/kg IV load with 1–3 mg/hr; or generalized anesthesia, including halothane

- Children:

  Airway, IV fluids, supplemental O_2, monitoring, Dexi-stick or D_{25} 2–4 ml/kg, naloxone (0.01–0.1 mg/kg IV)

  Neonates: pyridoxine (50–100 mg slow infusion) and calcium gluconate (4 ml/kg IV)

  Diazepam: 0.2–0.3 mg/kg IV at 1 mg/min (10 mg max)

  If no response or after benzodiazepine suppression, give phenobarbital: 10–15 mg/kg IV at 25 mg/min

  For seizures unresponsive to phenobarbital infusion, consider phenytoin: 10–15 mg/kg IV at 50 mg/min

- **Phenytoin pearls:**

  Contraindication: second- to third-degree heart block; infuse phenytoin no faster than 50 mg/min to reduce risk of hypotension and heart block

  Drug–drug interactions: INH and chloramphenicol increase serum phenytoin levels; phenobarbital and alcohol decrease serum levels

  Phenytoin toxicity (> 20 µg/ml) (Table 11.5)

DI
- Admission to neurologic or medical ICU for all patients with status epilepticus
- Patients with possible drug intoxication/withdrawal as etiology for seizures require at least 6 hours' observation (no data to date significantly support shorter length of stay)
- Patients with first-time seizures, a negative primary workup, and no additional activity in 6 hours' observation may be discharged with neurology follow-up in 24–48 hours and instructions to return for any aura or activity
- Patients with known seizure disorders not related to drug intoxication or withdrawal may be discharged pending therapeutic anticonvulsant levels

Table 11.5 Symptoms of Phenytoin Toxicity

Drug Level	Symptoms
> 20 µg/ml	Nausea and vomiting; lateral nystagmus
> 30 µg/ml	Lateral and vertical nystagmus, ataxia
> 40 µg/ml	Lethargy, dysarthria, confusion, seizures
> 70 µg/ml	Bradycardia, heart block, idioventricular rhythm, asystole

CHAPTER 12

Obstetric Emergencies

ECTOPIC PREGNANCY

KY Ectopic pregnancy, the implantation of a fertilized ovum outside the endometrium, is most common in the lateral two-thirds of the fallopian tube. Implantation can also occur in the ovary or abdominal cavity.

HX • Amenorrhea, abdominal pain, and then vaginal bleeding occurs 6–10 weeks after the LMP
• Risk factors include tubal abnormalities, scarring from PID or tubal ligation, IUDs, recent abortion (within 2 weeks), and prior ectopic pregnancy

PX • Findings include diffuse or localized abdominal pain, pallor, and pelvic tenderness
• Shoulder pain may be present as a result of diaphragmatic irritation
• Hemorrhagic shock may be present if rupture occurs

DD PID, threatened abortion, corpus luteal cyst, dysfunctional uterine bleeding

LB • Quantitative βhCG (serial values q48hr may "plateau," with no exponential rise in value), CBC, T&C, UA, pregnancy test
• Culdocentesis (if US is not available)
   A dry tap is nondiagnostic
   Aspiration of nonclotting blood with Hct > 15% is a positive finding
   A clear tap is negative

IM Pelvic US

TX • For shock: IV fluids, supplemental O_2, monitoring, Trendelenburg's position; consider blood transfusion and stat referral for laparotomy
• For stable patients between 2 and 4–5 weeks after the LMP (when the pregnancy test may be positive but US may not yet detect an intrauterine pregnancy): consider discharge and follow-up, including serial quantitative βhCGs, within 48 hours
   If βhCG is decreasing, a D&C is indicated; the products of uterine extraction should be tested for chorionic villi
   If no villi are present, laparoscopy is indicated to locate ectopic pregnancy

If serial βhCGs "plateau" or do not increase exponentially, laparoscopy is also indicated

DI Admission to gynecologic service for patients with positive culdocentesis, shock, unreliable follow-up, or no intrauterine pregnancy with a βhCG > 6000 mIU/ml

EMERGENCY DELIVERY

HX • **True labor:** regular uterine contractions of increasing intensity that occur at decreasing intervals

First stage: results in cervical dilation and effacement; lasts 6–8 hours in multiparous women and 8–12 hours in primiparous women

Second stage: begins with complete cervical dilation and ends with the delivery of the infant; lasts several minutes to 2 hours; radiation of pain in the uterine fundus over the uterus into the lower back

• **Indications of active labor:**

"Bloody show," which consists of a bloody mucous discharge representing expulsion of the cervical mucus plug

Spontaneous rupture of membranes

PX • If vaginal bleeding (not simply "bloody show") is present, obtain a US to assess for placenta previa; avoid a pelvic examination

• Otherwise, perform a sterile speculum examination to confirm ruptured membranes by checking vaginal secretions for ferning and turning Nitrazine paper blue

• Monitor fetal heart tones and uterine contractions, if possible

• If prolonged bradycardia or tachycardia occurs after contractions, fetal distress is present

• Determine position, presentation (portion of fetus in birth canal), and lie (relation of the long axis of the fetus to that of the mother; longitudinal versus transverse) of fetus and stage of labor

• Check for cord prolapse, cervical effacement, cervical dilation (10 cm is complete), and station (relationship of fetal part to the ischial spines)

• Delivery manifests as crowning, pressure on the rectum with urge to defecate, and uncontrolled "bearing down" movements.

IM Pelvic US if vaginal bleeding is present or for help in assessing fetus

TX • **For premature delivery:** consider transfer to institution with obstetric and neonatal facilities, if possible

- **For fetal distress:** position mother on left side; IV fluids, supplemental O_2, monitoring; arrange for immediate delivery
- **For cord prolapse:**
  Exert manual pressure through vagina to lift presenting part away from the umbilical cord; place patient in knee–chest or deep Trendelenburg's position
  Use tocolytic agents to stop labor: magnesium sulfate (4–6 g IV), terbutaline (0.25 mg SQ), or ritodrine (0.1 mg/min IV)
- **Delivery:** position the mother on stretcher with thighs abducted, knees flexed, and feet on stretcher with buttocks raised on bed pan; if time permits, cleanse and drape the perineum
  Control delivery of the head with one hand on the occipital area and one hand supporting the perineum; the chin can be lifted from posterior position. After delivering the head, suction the oral cavity with a bulb syringe. If the cord is wrapped around the neck, loosen it and slip it over the head or cut it. The head will rotate to one side.
  Deliver the shoulders next. Grasp the head and exert gentle downward pressure until the anterior shoulder appears beneath the pubic symphysis, and then lift the head upward to facilitate delivery of the posterior shoulder. If the shoulders are impacted, perform an episiotomy. Anesthetize the area with lidocaine, and cut from the perineum, avoiding the anal sphincter.
  After the shoulders are delivered, support the head with one hand and prepare to catch the body and legs with other hand. Do not drop the infant! Hold the infant horizontal to the introitus and suction the mouth and nose.
  Cut the cord after clamping it twice. Send cord blood to the laboratory for infant serology and Rh determination. Place a sterile cord clamp or tie around the cord 1–3 cm distal to the navel.
  Place the neonate on warm blankets in a heated Isolette. Take Apgar scores at 1 and 5 minutes. For births with a thick meconium, intubation of the infant and suctioning under direct laryngoscopy is indicated.
  To deliver the placenta, apply pressure above the pubic symphysis, with minimal traction on the cord. A sudden gush of blood and umbilical cord protrusion signifies placental delivery. Excessive traction results in uterine inversion. Check the placenta for completeness.
  Gently massage uterus and give oxytocin (20 U IV), if needed, to control hemorrhaging.
  Inspect and repair lacerations of the cervix or vagina with 3-0 chromic catgut, and repair the episiotomy.

DI • **Infant:** admission to pediatrics or neonatal ICU
 • Mother: admission to obstetric service

HEMORRHAGING

First-trimester hemorrhage

KY First-trimester bleeding occurs as a result of ectopic pregnancy or abortion. However, bleeding from implantation may be associated with a normal pregnancy (see Ectopic Pregnancy). Abortion is defined as termination of pregnancy before 20 weeks' gestation, when the fetus weighs < 500 g. Spontaneous abortion is common, and it may be idiopathic or caused by drugs, infection, radiation, or chromosome defects.

PX **Signs of types of abortions:**
 • **Threatened:** os closed, no passage of fetal tissue, viable fetus, mild cramping and bleeding; 20% of patients eventually abort
 • **Inevitable:** os dilated and effaced, cramps and moderate bleeding
 • **Complete:** uterine contents expelled; cervix closed, little cramping or bleeding
 • **Incomplete:** clots and tissue in cervical os, os open; severe cramps and bleeding
 • **Missed:** uterus fails to expel fetus for > 2 months; os closed, fetal heart tones absent, pregnancy test negative

DD Carcinoma, polyps, cervicitis, molar pregnancy

LB CBC, T&C, SMA-7, quantitative βhCG; send products of conception to laboratory

IM Doppler US (to check for fetal heart tones), pelvic US prn

TX • **Supportive measures:** IV fluids, supplemental O_2, monitoring, positioning on left side
 • **For incomplete or inevitable abortion:** consider D&C or IV oxytocin (20 U in 1 L NS)
 • **For Rh-negative patients:** Rh immunoglobulin (50 mg)

DI • Discharge:
 Cases of threatened abortion (stable patients): instructions to avoid strenuous activity, place nothing in the vagina, and return if fever, increased bleeding, or abdominal pain occur
 Cases of missed abortion: home with close follow-up; most patients will abort spontaneously
 • Admission for patients who are hemodynamically unstable and those with incomplete abortion (OB/GYN management; usually D&C), missed abortion with coagulopathy, ectopic pregnancy, or threatened abortion with continued pain, cramps, and bleeding

Postpartum hemorrhage

KY Postpartum hemorrhage, which is defined as blood loss > 500 ml after delivery, can be immediate or delayed.

- Immediate bleeding (within 24 hours postdelivery) is caused by uterine atony and may be due to a ruptured uterus, with the potential for profound shock. Causes include prolonged or rapid labor, high parity, large or multiple fetuses, and lacerations to the vagina or cervix.
- Delayed hemorrhage (within 7–14 days postdelivery) involves retention of placental tissue or endoparametritis.

HX
- Immediate hemorrhage: steady, brisk bleeding
- Delayed hemorrhage: sudden, painless bleeding preceded by foul-smelling lochia
- Signs of vaginal hematoma: difficulties with urinating or walking

PX Perform a careful bimanual and speculum examination to look for causes; the uterus may be soft and boggy

In cases of uterine inversion, palpate or visualize the fundus near or through the os; the uterus is large, boggy, and nontender

DD Endometritis

LB CBC, PT, PTT, fibrinogen, T&C

IM Pelvic US

TX
- Supportive measures: IV fluids, supplemental O$_2$, monitoring; transfusion for shock; FFP for DIC
- For immediate hemorrhage: massage uterus and give oxytocin (20–40 U/L at 200–500 ml/hr)
- For persistent bleeding: methylergonovine (0.2 mg IM) or prostaglandin F (0.5 mg injected into uterus); repair lacerations (vaginal packing can be used for multiple small lacerations)
- For refractory immediate hemorrhage: surgery to ligate uterine artery or hysterectomy
- For delayed hemorrhage: if bleeding ceases, discharge home on ergonovine (0.2 mg PO q6–12hr)

DI Admission for D&C in cases of severe bleeding and large amounts of retained products

Third-trimester hemorrhage

HX
- **Placenta previa:**
  Placental implantation in lower uterus adjacent to or over the os

Presentation: painless, bright red vaginal bleeding after 28 weeks;

Risk factors: multiple surgeries, multiple pregnancies

- **Abruptio placentae:**

    Premature separation of the placenta from the uterine wall

    Presentation: painful, dark red bleeding (80%), and abdominal pain; DIC present in 20% of cases

    Risk factors: eclampsia, diabetes, renal disease, hypertension, abdominal trauma

PX Avoid vaginal or speculum examinations; check fundal height, contractions, or tenderness of uterus on abdominal palpation

- Placenta previa: soft and nontender uterus
- Abruptio placentae: firm and irritable uterus

DD Normal labor, uterine rupture, vasa previa, "bloody show"

LB CBC, SMA-7, T&C, PT, PTT, fibrinogen

IM Pelvic US, which can detect or rule out placenta previa but cannot reliably detect abruptio placentae; fetal monitoring using Doppler US to measure fetal heart tones

TX
- IV fluids, supplemental O_2, monitoring; positioning on left side; early transfusion, FFP (for DIC), and MAST garment
- Obstetrics consult stat

DI
- OR for unstable patients with obstetrician for examination and possible C-section; eventual admission to obstetrics
- Expectant management if bleeding is slight (bed rest and close follow-up) for stable patients with abruptio placentae who are carrying an immature fetus

GESTATIONAL HYPERTENSION

KY Gestational hypertension is BP ≥ 140/90 mm Hg during the second half of pregnancy. This BP, which is not associated with proteinuria or edema, returns to normal after delivery. Chronic hypertension is BP > 140/90 mm Hg that occurs before pregnancy and persists after delivery. Complications of hypertension in pregnancy include intracranial bleeding, papilledema, pancreatitis, renal failure, liver failure, pulmonary edema, coagulopathy, and preeclampsia–eclampsia.

- Preeclampsia is BP > 140/90 mm Hg after 20 weeks' gestation with associated edema and proteinuria
- Eclampsia, which occurs in patients with preeclampsia, involves seizures or coma in third trimester or postpartum

HX • Edema, headache, visual disturbances, mental status changes, abdominal pain, and seizures
   • Risk factors for preeclampsia, which is common in primigravidas: family history, plural gestation, diabetes, and heart or renal disease

PX • Papilledema, abdominal tenderness, and ankle clonus of hyperreflexia; tremulousness, which may indicate impending eclampsia
   • Check for cervical dilation with a bimanual examination

DD Chronic hypertension and seizures may indicate CNS pathology, meningitis, or intracranial bleeding

LB SMA-7, CBC, transaminases, T&C, UA

IM Doppler US (to check fetal heart tones)

TX • For gestational hypertension: observation for 6 hours
   • For mild hypertension without proteinuria: decreased activity recommended
   • For preeclampsia with proteinuria: hospitalization for bed rest, 24-hour urine for protein; definitive treatment of eclampsia is delivery, but seizures and BP should be controlled first
   • For severe preeclampsia (> 36 weeks' gestation):
      Position on left side, maintain urine output, use magnesium sulfate: 2–4 g IV load; 1 g/hr maintenance
      Control BP with hydralazine: 5–10 mg IV q20min with target DBP of 90 mm Hg; for refractory BP, use labetalol or nitroprusside
      Seizures: use magnesium sulfate (2–4 g IV over 5–10 minutes) [may use continuous infusion of 1 g/hr]; for resistant seizures: diazepam (5 mg IV); repeat q5min up to 15–20 mg if seizures continue or give phenobarbital (200 mg IV) and treat hypertension
   • For chronic hypertension: methyldopa, hydralazine, or labetalol
   • For conditions such as AMS, coagulopathy, increased serum CK, uncontrolled hypertension, decreased fetal movements, or fetal distress: delivery

DI • Discharge with follow-up for patients with gestational hypertension if DBP is < 90 mm Hg; limited activity and close follow-up for patients with mild preeclampsia without proteinuria
   • Admission to obstetrics for patients with preeclampsia and ICU for those with eclampsia

HYPEREMESIS GRAVIDARUM

HX Nausea and vomiting in first trimester

PX Orthostatic hypotension, decreased skin turgor, tachycardia, and thirst

DD Cholecystitis, gastroenteritis, pyelonephritis, PUD, reflux esophagitis, appendicitis

LB CBC, SMA-7, UA

TX IV fluids; prochlorperazine (both in ED and on outpatient basis); frequent small meals

DI Admission to obstetrics or medical floor for severe dehydration, acidosis, or ketosis

POSTABORTION SEPSIS

HX • Fever, excessive bleeding, uterine tenderness, and purulent bloody discharge 3–7 days postabortion
• Risk factors: advanced gestational age and untreated pelvic infections

LB SMA-7, CK, PT, T&C

TX IV fluids, supplemental O_2, monitoring, D&C, IV antibiotics:
• Clindamycin (900 mg IV q9hr) plus gentamicin (2 mg/kg IV load, then 1.5 mg/kg q8hr) or
• Cefoxitin (2 g IV q8hr) plus doxycycline (100 mg IV q12hr)

DI Admission to medical floor or ICU

PREGNANCY

HX Amenorrhea, breast fullness and tenderness, nausea, urinary frequency, fatigue, and fetal movement at 16 weeks

PX • Physical signs: darkened breast areola, blue discoloration of cervix (Chadwick's sign); fundus at pelvic brim by 12 weeks and at umbilicus by 16 weeks
• Physiologic changes: increased heart rate, decreased BP, "dilutional anemia" from increased blood volume, leukocytosis, delayed gastric emptying, cephalad displacement of abdominal organs, signs of peritoneal irritation (less reliable), decreased Pco_2 as a result of increased tidal volume and decreased residual volume

DD Amenorrhea, irregular menses, molar or ectopic pregnancy

LB βhCG:
• Level doubles every 2 days and peaks at 60 days
• May be detected 6–9 days after implantation
• βhCG > 3600–4000 mIU/ml and absence of a gestational sac signify fetal nonviability

- Quantitative βhCG by RIA (99% specific) can detect 5–40 mIU/ml
- ELISA (urine) can give a positive result (99% specific) before the first missed menses; can detect levels as low as 10–50 mIU/ml
- False-negative results are possible with dilute urine

IM • Pelvic US; transabdominal US can detect a gestational sac by 6 weeks with a corresponding βhCG level of 6500 mIU/ml; transvaginal US can detect a gestational sac at 5 weeks and show a fetal pulse and cardiac activity at 8 weeks
- Doppler at 10–12 weeks and fetoscope at 18 weeks for fetal heart tones

RETAINED PRODUCTS OF CONCEPTION

KY This condition often occurs after abortions with local anesthesia.

HX Cramping, heavy bleeding, and fever about 1 week postabortion

PX Vaginal blood, products of conception, and uterine tenderness

TX D&C, IV antibiotics:

- Clindamycin (900 mg IV q9hr) plus gentamicin (2 mg/kg IV load, then 1.5 mg/kg q8hr) or
- Cefoxitin (2 g IV q8hr) plus doxycycline (100 mg IV q12hr)

DI Admission to OB/GYN for D&C

CHAPTER 13

Orthopedic Emergencies

CARPAL TUNNEL SYNDROME

HX
- Patients, primarily women, complain of tingling, numbness, burning, cold sensitivity, and paresthesias along the distribution of the median nerve.
- Symptoms often awaken patients from sleep, and shaking or lowering the hand may lead to relief. Repetitive hand motion may aggravate symptoms.

PX
- Decreased two-point discrimination and light touch
- Positive Phalen's maneuver (reproduction of symptoms by flexing the wrist for 60 seconds)
- Positive Tinel's sign (tingling sensation in the hand resulting from tapping the wrist over the median nerve)
- Weakness of muscles innervated by the median nerve

IM Wrist radiograph to look for calcific deposits, callus, or osteophytes; cervical spine radiograph if cervical radiculopathy is considered

TX Wrist splints, NSAIDs, and discontinuation of repetitive motion

DI Discharge with referral to hand surgeon

COMPARTMENT SYNDROME

KY Increased tissue pressures in limited space lead to decreased tissue perfusion, which results in abnormal neuromuscular function.

HX Pain that is usually severe and constant; hypesthesia with tingling and numbness

PX Tenderness, swelling, increased pain with passive muscle movement, pallor, and eventually decreased or absent pulses

LB Compartment pressures (0–10 mm Hg is usually normal)
- Compromise of capillary blood flow occurs at about 20 mm Hg
- Nerves and muscles are at risk at pressures > 30–40 mm Hg

TX
- Immediate surgical consult for elevated compartment pressures
- Fasciotomy, which involves a longitudinal skin incision, should be performed in the OR

DI Admission for monitoring of compartment pressures or to OR

DISLOCATIONS

KY Rapid treatment is important to prevent injury to nerves and blood vessels as well as avascular necrosis of the bone.

- Subluxation: disruption of a joint with continued proximal and distal approximation of the articulating surfaces
- Dislocation: disruption of a joint with complete loss of articulation

HX Trauma may be major or minor; patients may complain of pain and pain with movement

PX Assessment of deformity and detailed neurovascular examination

IM Radiography

TX • **General treatment:**

Reduce after radiographic evaluation or immediately if neurovascular compromise exists, obtain postreduction films to document reduction and rule out fracture, and then splint

Referral to an orthopedic surgeon

- **Distal interphalangeal joint:** splint in full extension for 4 weeks
- **Finger or thumb proximal interphalangeal joint:** splint in 15° of flexion for 4 weeks
- **Finger and thumb metacarpophalangeal joint:** splint in 40°–50° of flexion for 4 weeks
- **Wrist:** usually requires urgent ORIF
- **Subluxation of the radial head (nursemaids' elbow),** which results when the radial head is subluxed through the annular ligament with sudden traction and generally affects children 1–4 years of age: apply simultaneous traction and supination; a "click" confirms reduction. Do not splint.
- **Elbow** (associated with median nerve, ulnar nerve, and brachial artery injury): treat with reduction and then splint posterior dislocation in 120° of flexion and anterior dislocation in 90° of flexion
- **Shoulder** (in anterior dislocation, the most common type; the risk for axillary nerve injury is high; posterior dislocations are rare): reduce and apply a sling for 2–3 weeks with initial gentle ROM out of sling in 2–3 days
- **Hip** (occurs with large forces; high incidence of avascular necrosis of the femoral head): often requires operative reduction; then treat with traction
- **Knee** (associated with popliteal artery and peroneal nerve injury): if suspicion of arterial injury, obtain arteriography; reduce and then splint in 20° of flexion
- **Patella** (associated with osteochondral fracture): after reduction, splint in a knee immobilizer for 3–4 weeks
- **Ankle** (almost always associated with fracture): ORIF is usually necessary. A cast should be worn for 6 weeks.

DI Admission for most patients with hip, knee, and ankle dislocations after consultation to orthopedic service

FRACTURES

HX Patient age (e.g., Salter-Harris fractures in young children; hip fractures in the elderly), mechanism of injury, pain site and character, and changes in sensation

PX • Examine for edema, skin integrity, tenderness, deformity, and distal neurovascular and motor function
  • Several complications may result (Table 13.1)

Table 13.1   Complications of Fractures and Other Orthopedic Injuries

Complication	Resulting Condition
Hemorrhage	Blood volume lost: radius and ulna, 150–250 ml; humerus, 250 ml; tibia and fibula, 500 ml; femur, 1 L; pelvis, 1.5–3 L
Nerve problems (type of injury/nerve)	Shoulder dislocation/axillary; elbow/medial (supracondylar) and ulnar; sacral/cauda equina; hip dislocation/femoral; acetabulum/sciatic; femoral shaft/peroneal; knee dislocation/peroneal or tibial; lateral tibial plateau/peroneal
Compartment syndrome	Pain with passive stretching, active flexing against resistance, or with pressure applied to compartment
Vascular injury	First rib and clavicle fractures: associated with vascular bleeding
	Knee fractures and dislocation: associated with popliteal artery injury
Avascular necrosis	Tends to occur in comminuted fractures of bones with poor blood supply such as capitate, scaphoid, and femoral head
Fat embolism	Commonly follows long bone fractures (e.g., tibia, fibula, hip)
	Symptoms: tachypnea, dyspnea, tachycardia, pulmonary edema, restlessness, confusion, petechial rash, fever, jaundice, retinal changes, renal involvement
	Fat may be found in the urine
Immobilization complications	Pneumonia, UTI, ulcers, muscle atrophy, GI hemorrhage, DVT, pulmonary embolism, joint immobility, and psychological disorders
Cast problems	Pain, local irritation, swelling, and numbness "Bivalve" cast and inspect the area; if this cast does not relieve symptoms, consider compartment syndrome

- **Terms used to describe fractures:**
  - Anatomic location: proximal, middle, and distal
  - Position: valgus, in which the fractured part is angled away from midline; or varus, in which the fractured part is angled toward the midline
  - Apposition: contact between fracture surfaces (i.e., apposed, displaced, or distracted)
  - Angulation: degree of the angle formed by the bone segments in relation to the longitudinal bone
  - Fracture line direction: transverse, spiral, or oblique
- **Types of fractures:**
  - Open: skin integrity is compromised (e.g., lacerated or abraded) near the fracture or bone is protruding
  - Closed: skin is intact
  - Comminuted: bone is broken into more than two fragments
  - Avulsion: bone fragment pulled away from its normal position by ligament or muscle
  - Articular: involvement of joint surfaces; the percentage of articular surface involvement should be given
  - Pathologic: break that occurs in bone that is not normal
  - Stress: caused by repeated low-intensity trauma
  - Impaction: bone is driven into adjacent bone at fracture site
- **Types of fractures common in children:**
  - Complete versus incomplete: a complete fracture involves disruption of both cortices, whereas an incomplete fracture involves disruption of one cortex
  - Greenstick: an incomplete fracture of long bones with angulation
  - Torus: buckling or wrinkling of the cortex
- **Classification of fractures in children** (Figure 13.1)

IM
- Plain films of pain site as well as joint above and below
- CT, which may confirm suspicious fractures and define alignment, fragmentation, or displacement

TX
- **Open fractures:**
  - Obtain culture and start antibiotics [cefazolin (1 g IV)]
  - Irrigate with saline solution and cover with Betadine (concentration < 5%)-soaked sponges
  - Tetanus immunoglobulin if indicated
  - Obtain immediate orthopedic consult
- **Closed fractures:**
  - Splint or immobilize all fractures or suspected fractures
  - Obtain orthopedic consult
- **Nondisplaced fractures:**
  - May not be apparent on initial radiographs

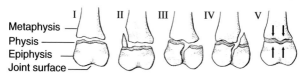

FIGURE 13.1 Salter-Harris classification of physeal fractures. Type I injuries involve slip of the zone of provisional calcification. Type II injuries are similar to type I, with fracture extension into metaphysis. Type III injuries involve slip of the growth plate plus fracture through the epiphysis and the articular surface. Type IV injuries are similar to type III, with involvement of a metaphyseal fracture. Type V injuries are crush injuries of the metaphyseal plate. Type III, IV, and V injuries may result in growth problems.

     If fracture is clinically suspected, splint and repeat films in 7 days
     or perform a more definitive test (i.e., CT or bone scan)

DI Admission for patients with open fractures, fractures that require surgery (e.g., hip fractures, trimalleolar fractures), or fractures with neurovascular compromise; discharge for all other patients

HAND INFECTIONS

KY The risk of morbidity and mortality is high with soft tissue infections. Examples of such infections include: necrotizing fasciitis, which spreads very quickly and is typically caused by *Escherichia coli*; and cat and dog bites, which often become infected with *Pasteurella multocida*. Fungal hand infections occur among gardeners who become infected with *Sporothrix schenckii*. Wounds are especially dangerous in immunosuppressed patients.

HX Trauma; usually a puncture, cut, bite, or crush injury

PX Possible crepitus, erythema, vesicle formation, change in skin color, pain with passive or active movement, and pus

LB Consider CBC, blood culture, culture of pus from wound

IM Radiograph to rule out foreign body, air in tissue or joint, or associated fracture

TX • Irrigate with high-pressure saline, leave wound open
    • Dress wound, splint in position of function, and start appropriate antibiotics

DI Admission for patients with signs of serious hand infection; immediate consult with hand surgeon

HAND INJURIES

HX • Patient age, occupation, and dominant hand, mechanism of injury, and clean or contaminated environment

PX Location; amount of bone exposure; neurovascular status, including color, pallor, cyanosis, and capillary refill (Figure 13.2)
  • Allen test for radial and ulnar artery evaluation
  • Nerve (motor and sensory) and tendon evaluation

IM Plain films

TX Treatment of selected hand injuries is given in Table 13.2

HIP FRACTURES AND DISLOCATIONS

HX Falls and MVAs

PX • **Physical examination:**
      Gentle palpation; dullness on auscultation of symphysis pubis while tapping patella suggests fracture (Wood's sign)
  • Evaluation of distal neurovascular status
  • **Types of hip injuries:**
      Femoral neck fracture: extremity is slightly shortened, externally rotated, and abducted
      Intertrochanteric fracture: extremity is shortened and markedly externally rotated
      Anterior dislocation: extremity is abducted and externally rotated
      Posterior dislocation: extremity is shortened, internally rotated, and adducted

LB CBC, T&C, labs as indicated for associated trauma

IM Plain films of the pelvis and hips, CT, bone scan

TX Treat hemorrhage; obtain immediate orthopedic surgical consult

DI Admission to orthopedic service

KNEE SOFT TISSUE INJURIES

HX Mechanism of injury, position of injury, abnormal bending, force applied, and audible sounds (e.g., popping suggests anterior cruciate tear, ripping or click indicates meniscus tear)

PX • Edema and effusion suggest fracture or ligament disruption
  • Varus and valgus stress are associated with collateral ligament tears

A

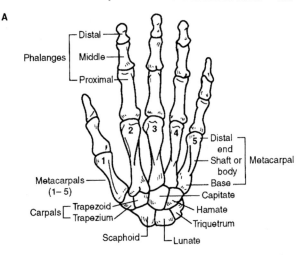

B

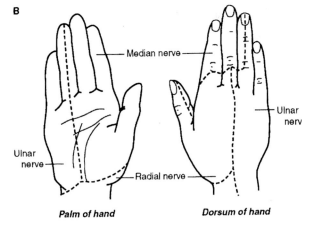

FIGURE 13.2 *(A)* Bones of the hand. *(B)* Sensory nerve distribution in the hand.

Table 13.2   Emergency Treatment of Selected Hand Injuries

Type of Injury	Emergency Treatment
Flexor tendon injury	Referral to a hand surgeon
Extensor tendon injury	Repair by trained emergency physician with close follow-up
Amputation	Cleaning of amputated part to remove gross debris, wrapping in a moist saline towel or sponge, and placement in a plastic container on ice
	Immediate referral to a hand surgeon
Boutonnière deformity (sudden forced flexion of the proximal interphalangeal joint, disrupting the central slip of the extensor tendon)	Splinting of the proximal interphalangeal joint in extension for 6–8 weeks
Mallet finger (flexion of the distal interphalangeal joint, which ruptures the extensor tendon at the base of the distal phalanx)	Splinting of the distal interphalangeal and proximal interphalangeal joints in extension for 6 weeks; if avulsion of the bone occurs, splinting in hyperextension
	Immediate consult with hand surgeon if a bony avulsion involves one-third or more of the joint
Subungual hematoma	Drainage of blood by making a hole over the center of the hematoma using either electric cautery or heated paper clip
Ganglion cyst (benign tumor-like swelling, which generally occurs on the volar-radial aspect of the wrist and dorsum of the wrist; lesions are filled with a jelly-like substance)	Surgical removal may be required if pain, tenderness, or weakness is present (outpatient surgery)
De Quervain's tenosynovitis (occurs in the abductor pollicis longus and extensor pollicis brevis; usually seen with repetitive motion; the Finkelstein test, placing the thumb in the palm and then deviating the wrist radially, produces pain)	Rest and splinting; hand surgeons may inject steroids or perform a release

- Anterior drawer test for anterior cruciate tears consists of gentle forward traction of the flexed knee, looking for laxity
- Apley and McMurray's tests for meniscal tears

    Apley compression test: the patient lies prone with the knee flexed 90°. The examiner holds the thigh while applying downward pressure on the plantar surface of the foot and rotating the lower leg. Pain is elicited on the affected side, or crepitance may be felt.

    McMurray test: the patient lies supine, hyperflexing the knee. One hand applies pressure on the distal anterior thigh while the other applies caudal pressure on the plantar surface of the foot and rotates the lower leg. Pain or clicking is a positive result.

LB Consider arthrocentesis for large effusions

IM Plain films to evaluate for fracture

TX After fracture and dislocation are ruled out, treat with ice applied for 20 minutes several times a day, elevation, crutches, avoidance of weight-bearing activities, and knee immobilization

DI Discharge, with referral to an orthopedic surgeon for further evaluation

LOW BACK COMPLAINTS

KY Causes of this very common problem may include trauma, neoplasms, congenital disorders, degenerative disease, metabolic disorders, infections, inflammatory disorders, vascular disorders, psychosocial disorders, and visceral inflammation.

HX
- Location, duration, frequency, and radiation of pain; neurologic symptoms and weakness
- Ask about any changes in bowel or bladder function and "saddle anesthesia"; such symptoms may indicate spinal cord suppression

PX
- Evaluate neurologic function, extent of deformity, tenderness, ROM, straight-leg raises, gait, reflexes, muscle strength, and rectal tone or sensation

IM Plain films; consider CT, MRI, or bone scan to rule out focal lesions or unexplained symptoms; myelogram or MRI for cord compression

TX
- Fractures: bed rest on firm surface without movement; orthopedic or neurosurgical referral
- Disk herniation, rupture, extrusion without neurologic involvement: analgesics, NSAIDs, muscle relaxants, perhaps bed rest, physical therapy, and orthopedic referral

- Disk herniation, rupture, extrusion with neurologic involvement or acute cauda equina syndrome, and presence of bladder or rectal dysfunction: bed rest, immediate neurology/neurosurgery/orthopedic surgery referral
- Osteomyelitis, diskitis, paraspinal abscess (disk space narrowing usually present 10–14 days after symptoms): admission, immediate consult, and IV antibiotics
- Neoplasia: bone scan, myelogram (usually inpatient); immediate oncology/radiology and neurosurgical referral

DI Admission to orthopedics for patients with disk herniation with neurologic compromise, infectious spinal cord/paraspinal process, neoplasm, or intractable pain

PELVIC FRACTURES

KY Pelvic fractures usually occur as a result of falls or high-speed blunt trauma and may cause severe hemorrhage. High mortality is associated with severe fractures, and immediate intervention is required. Pelvic fractures are associated with injury to the pelvic organs, especially the bladder. These fractures can be classified into four groups:

- I: fracture of individual bones without break in continuity of the ring; stable
- II: single break in the pelvic ring; stable. Twenty-five percent of these fractures are associated with tissue, visceral, and GU injuries and bleeding.
- III: double break in pelvic ring; unstable. These fractures are associated with soft tissue, visceral, and GU injuries and major hemorrhage.
- IV: fracture of the acetabulum, which is associated with nerve injury

HX Trauma and pelvic pain

PX • Evaluate for shock
- Gently palpate pelvis for pain sites; perform pelvic and rectal examinations if they are not contraindicated
- Evaluate neurovascular status

LB • CBC, T&C, PT, other labs as indicated for associated trauma
- If urethral bleeding, a high-riding or boggy prostate, or scrotal hematoma is present, check urethrogram before inserting Foley catheter

IM • Radiography; consider CT; urethrogram, cystogram to evaluate bladder integrity

TX • Treat for hemorrhage and shock; consider MAST garment

- Consult trauma, orthopedic, and urologic surgeons; placement of external fixator or other operative management may be required

DI ICU for patients with hemodynamic compromise or directly to OR for repair

SPRAINS

HX
- Abnormal or exaggerated force on joint; often a pop or a snap is audible
- History should include position and forces applied

PX
- Evaluate for swelling, hemorrhage, point tenderness, function, and joint stability
- Classification:
  First degree: minor tear ligamentous fibers with mild hemorrhage and swelling; stress joint produces pain but no abnormal joint motion
  Second degree: partial ligament tear; moderate hemorrhage, swelling, tenderness, pain, and loss of function
  Third degree: complete ligament tear with loss of joint stability

IM Plain films to rule out fracture (in most cases)

TX Ice, elevation, analgesia, avoidance of weight bearing, and immobilization; orthopedic referral prn

DI Home

STRAINS

KY A strain is a pulled muscle that usually results from rapid acceleration or use of excessive force.

PX
- Local tenderness, swelling, spasm, ecchymosis, and loss of function
- Classification:
  First degree: minor tearing of musculotendinous unit with spasm, swelling, tenderness, and mild loss of function
  Second degree: more tearing without complete disruption; swelling, muscle spasm, ecchymosis, and loss of strength
  Third degree: complete disruption of muscle or tendon; often accompanies avulsion fracture

TX
- Rest, ice, elevation, NSAIDs, immobilization, and orthopedic consult
- Passive stretching soon after the injury may impede healing and result in calcium or fibrosis in the injured muscle

DI Home

CHAPTER 14

Pediatric Emergencies

RESUSCITATION

KY Hypoxia is the cause of cardiorespiratory compromise in the vast majority of cases in which resuscitation is necessary. Bradycardia that results in asystole from hypoxia constitutes the majority of cardiac dysrhythmias. VT and VF, which are actually rare, are also associated with cardiac anomalies, and PSVT commonly results from Wolff-Parkinson-White syndrome. Other conditions that may necessitate resuscitation include prematurity, birth trauma, congenital disorders and other medical problems, trauma, environmental injury, acute infection, toxic ingestion, and seizures.

HX Try to obtain from EMS or caregiver while initiating ABCs

PX Assess ABCs

LB • Appropriate laboratory evaluation after stabilization (e.g., CBC, chemistry profile, UA); pulse oximetry or ABG may be useful during resuscitation
• Refer to the algorithms and instructions in Appendices A and B as well

IM Appropriate radiographic evaluation for index of suspicion (e.g., CXR, cervical spine series, "baby-gram")

TX • **Newborn resuscitation:**
On presentation of the head, suction the mouth and nares. At delivery, hold the neonate in a slight Trendelenburg's position, and suction the nares and oropharynx. Clamp and cut the cord, move to a radiant warmer, dry and stimulate the neonate, and suction again. If spontaneous respirations are present, but hypoxia persists via O_2 saturation monitor, provide 100% O_2.
Assist ventilation with bag-valve-mask (rate, 40–60/min) for a pulse < 100 bpm or the presence of persistent apnea and/or cyanosis
Suction the pharynx with a De Lee trap for suspicion of meconium aspiration. Intubate for persistent apnea, cyanosis, hypoxia, or difficulty with bag-valve-mask ventilation (see Airway)
Initiate chest compressions for pulse < 60 bpm or persistent pulse < 80 bpm after taking the preceding steps (CPR rate, 120/min with depth of 1/2–3/4)

Table 14.1 Equipment Sizes Used in Pediatric Resuscitation

Patient Characteristics		Equipment Used		
Age/ Weight (kg)	Pulse (bpm)/ SBP (mm Hg)	ET Tube Size/ Length (cm)	Laryngo- scope Blade	NG Tube
Premature infant/< 2	140/55	3.0/6 + weight	0	5F
Full-term infant/3	125/65	3.5/6 + weight	1	6F
6 months/7	120/90	3.5/11	1	8F
1 year/10	120/96	4.0/11	1	10F
3 years/15	110/100	4.5/13	2	10F
5 years/18	100/100	5.0/14	2	12F
6 years/20	100/100	5.5/15	2	12F
8 years/25	90/105	6.0/17*	2	14F
12 years/40	85–90/115	6.5/19*	3	18F

*Cuffed ET.

Begin pharmacologic intervention for a pulse < 80 bpm after taking the preceding steps: epinephrine 1:10,000 (0.1 mg/ml) [0.01–0.1 mg/kg]; $NaHCO_3$ (1 mEq/ml) [1 mEq/kg]; consider naloxone (0.01 mg/kg); consider dextrose 10% (1 mEq/kg) and obtain access via the umbilical vein using a 5F umbilical venous catheter.

- **Airway** (Table 14.1)

  ET tube size: use the formula [16 + age (years)/4] or see Table 14.1; use uncuffed tube in children < 6 years of age

  Foreign body removal: back blows, chest thrusts, and the Heimlich maneuver (avoid Heimlich maneuver in children < 1 year of age) [see Chapter 7, Head and Neck Emergencies, Foreign Bodies]

  Intubation: increase succinylcholine to 2 mg/kg in children < 6 years of age; consider atropine (0.01 mg/kg) if using succinylcholine, especially in children < 3 years of age

- **Basic measures:** ABCs, including intubation; CPR as appropriate; supplemental O_2; reassessment after each step; IV or IO access; see Table 14.2 for information concerning drug dosing

- **Asystole:**

  Institute basic measures (see treatment)

  Hyperventilate

  Check two leads for cardiac activity

  Epinephrine 1:10,000: 0.01 mg/kg IV/IO q3–5min

  Epinephrine 1:1000: 0.1 mg/kg IV/IO q3–5min

Table 14.2   Drug Doses Commonly Used in Pediatric Resuscitation

Drug Name	Dose
Atropine*	0.02 mg/kg
	(min 0.1 mg; max 0.5 mg children, 1.0 mg adolescents)
Bretylium	5 mg/kg; repeat at 10 mg/kg to 30 mg/kg total
Diazepam*	0.3 mg/kg q2–5min (max 10 mg)
	(titrate 0.5 mg units)
	0.5 mg/kg rectal dose
Dobutamine	5–15 µg/kg/min
Dopamine	2–20 µg/kg/min for pressor
	(0.5–2 µg/kg/min increases renal and splanchnic blood flow)
Epinephrine 1:1000*	0.1 mg/kg ET tube
Epinephrine 1:10,000*	0.01 mg/kg IV/IO
	0.1–1.0 µg/kg/min
Isoproterenol	0.1–1.0 µg/kg/min
Lidocaine*	1 mg/kg, repeat up to 3 mg/kg
	20–50 µg/kg/min
NaHCO$_3$ 8.4%*	1 mEq/kg IV/IO
NaHCO$_3$ for neonates*	0.5 mEq/ml
Naloxone	0.01 mg/kg
Phenobarbital	10–15 mg/kg slow IV or IM; may repeat q20min (max 30 mg/kg)

*The mnemonic "NAVEL" can be used to remember the drugs that can be administered via the ET tube [**N**aloxone, **A**tropine, **V**alium (trade name for diazepam), **E**pinephrine, **L**idocaine].

- **Bradycardia:**
  Institute basic measures (see treatment)
  Epinephrine 1:10,000: 0.01 mg/kg IV/IO q3–5min [epinephrine 1:1000 (0.1 mg/kg via ET tube if IV/IO access is not available)]
  Atropine: 0.02 mg/kg [min 0.1 mg; max 0.5 mg (child), 1.0 mg (adolescent)]; repeat once
  Consider pacing
- **PEA:**
  Institute basic measures (see treatment)
  Hyperventilate
  Seek and treat cause (hypoxia, hypovolemia, tension pneumothorax, cardiac tamponade, hypothermia, acidosis)
  Epinephrine 1:10,000: 0.01 mg/kg IV/IO q3–5min [epinephrine 1:1000 (0.1 mg/kg via ET tube if IV/IO access not available)]
  Epinephrine 1:1000: 0.1 mg/kg IV/IO/ET tube q3–5min

- **Supraventricular VT (unstable):**
  Institute basic measures (see treatment)
  Cardioversion: synchronized shock (0.5–1 J/kg, 2 J/kg, 4 J/kg;
    repeat 4-J/kg shock after each drug treatment)
  Adenosine: 0.1 mg/kg rapid IV; double dose and try again up to
    two more times
  Verapamil: 0.1–0.3 mg/kg up to 5 mg (do not use in children
    < 1–2 years of age)
- **Supraventricular VT (stable):**
  Institute basic measures (see treatment)
  Vagal maneuvers (ice on face, simulated dive reflex)
  Adenosine: 0.1 mg/kg rapid IV; double dose and try again up to
    two more times
  Digoxin or β-blocking agent
  Verapamil: 0.1–0.3 mg/kg up to 5 mg (do not use in children
    < 1–2 years of age)
- **VF/pulseless VT:**
  Institute basic measures (see treatment)
  Cardioversion: shock (2 J/kg, 4 J/kg, 4 J/kg; repeat 4-J/kg shock
    30–60 sec after each drug treatment)
  Epinephrine 1:10,000: 0.01 mg/kg IV/IO [epinephrine 1:1000
    (0.1 mg/kg via ET tube if IV/IO access is not available)]
  Lidocaine: 1 mg/kg IV/IO
  Epinephrine 1:1000: 0.1 mg/kg IV/IO/ET tube q3–5min
  Lidocaine: 1 mg/kg IV/IO
  Bretylium: 5 mg/kg IV/IO (first dose); 10 mg/kg IV/IO (second
    dose)
- **VT (stable):**
  Institute basic measures (see treatment)
  Lidocaine: 1 mg/kg IV
  Phenytoin: 2–4 mg/kg IV over 5 minutes or
  Procainamide: 2–6 mg/kg slowly or
  Bretylium (children > 12 years of age): 5 mg/kg IV slowly

DI ICU

ANALGESIA/SEDATION

KY Use of medications for pain management and/or sedation carries an inherent risk that should be understood and considered when selecting the proper regimen. Adequate patient monitoring as well as the equipment and personnel necessary for airway management should be in place as appropriate for each situation. Some of the pharmacologic agents that are used in clinical practice are listed in Table 14.3; check contraindications before use.

Table 14.3   Dosing Information for Sedatives and Analgesics

Drug	Route of Administration	Dose (mg/kg)/ Maximum Dose (mg)	Contra-indication(s)
Analgesics			
Ibuprofen	PO/PR	10–15/975	PUD
Acetaminophen	PO/PR	5–10/800	
Sedative– analgesics			Respiratory depression
Morphine	IV/IM/PO	0.1–0.2/10	
Meperidine	IV/IM	1.0–2.0/100	
Fentanyl	IV/IM	0.001–0.005/0.05	
Codeine	PO	1.0/60	
Hydrocodone	PO	0.2/7.5	
Sedatives			Respiratory depression
Midazolam	IV/IM	0.01–0.08/4	
	PR/intranasal	0.3–0.7/4	
Diazepam	IV	0.05–0.2/10	
	PR	0.5/10	
Chloral hydrate	PO	50–100/1000	Liver disease
Pentobarbital	IV/IM	2.0–5.0/200	
Thiopental	IV	3.0–5.0/500	Hypotension
Etomidate	IV	0.2–0.5	Nausea, vomiting
Other agents			
Ketamine	IV	1.0/100	Laryngospasm
	IM	3.0–5.0/50	Vomiting, dysphoric reactions
	PO	6.0–10.0/50	
Nitrous oxide	Inhaled	30%–50%/50%	

Adapted from *Ann Emerg Med* 23(2):241, 1994.

APNEA

KY Apnea means no spontaneous respirations for > 20 sec.

- **SIDS,** the leading cause of death in infants in the first year of life, is more common in males (male:female incidence, 2:1). Risk factors include prematurity, low birth weight, intrauterine growth retardation, bronchopulmonary dysplasia, and maternal smoking or IV drug abuse. It occurs more often during the winter months and in the early morning hours.

- **ALTE,** or near-miss SIDS, is associated with brief periods of apnea, cyanosis, listlessness, or LOC with complete resolution.

HX Infants are found unconscious, unresponsive, apneic, and sometimes cyanotic. Associated factors include gastroenteritis, possible recent URI, and absence of trauma.

- **SIDS:** infants remain unresponsive despite CPR
- **ALTE:** infants are aroused spontaneously via tactile stimulation

PX Unconsciousness, unresponsiveness, apnea, sometimes cyanosis; in SIDS, no vital signs or asystole on monitor

DD Seizures, hypoglycemia, sepsis/meningitis, cardiomyopathy, botulism

LB O_2 saturation or ABG, CBC, SMA-7; septic workup, including blood, urine, CSF, and stool culture

IM EKG, head CT with and without contrast, inpatient Holter, pneumogram, and possibly a swallowing study

TX ABCs, including IV fluids, supplemental O_2, and monitoring

DI Admission for monitoring and workup for any apneic episode if there is any question of ALTE

BRONCHIOLITIS

KY Most cases of bronchiolitis occur within the first 2 years of life, and the vast majority of deaths occur in infants < 6 months of age. RSV is the most common cause of the disease in infants, followed by parainfluenzavirus; epidemics usually result from infection with RSV. *Mycoplasma pneumoniae* occurs most frequently in school-aged children with bronchiolitis.

HX Poor feeding, apparent dyspnea, coryza, and rhinitis; symptoms most evident at night

PX Tachypnea, chest hyperexpansion, nasal flaring, wheezing, and anxiety; retractions and grunting (late signs)

DD Asthma, pneumonia, other debilitating respiratory or cardiac illness, cystic fibrosis, foreign body aspiration

LB Pulse oximetry; consider ABG

IM CXR

- Peribronchiolar cuffing visible as small white circles of edematous tissue around airways, especially near the periphery
- Flattened diaphragms associated with air
- Trapping/hyperinflation; rib-angle flattening also associated with trapping

TX • Antibiotics are not useful unless secondary pneumonitis is present
- Bronchodilators are likely to be helpful; consider ribavirin for RSV when verified or if patient is very ill
- IV hydration prn

DI • Admission (generally) for patients who are younger, have other underlying disease or immunocompromise, or are more ill appearing
- Discharge, with follow-up within 1 day

CELLULITIS (ORBITAL AND PERIORBITAL)

KY Infection of orbital and/or periorbital structures is more common in children than adults. The common cause is extension of sinusitis (ethmoid). Other etiologic factors are URI and otitis media with effusion. *Haemophilus influenzae* and *Streptococcus pneumoniae* are found in 90% of blood cultures (*H. influenzae* occurs more often in children). (See Chapter 9, Infectious Disease Emergencies, Soft Tissue Infections, Cellulitis.)

HX • Lid swelling and pain, usually in one eye, occurring over a day or two; no direct ocular symptoms
- Symptoms are often accompanied by a history of URI and/or sinus infection

PX Fever is not uncommon; other findings include:
- Periorbital cellulitis: erythema, edema, warmth, tenderness of one or both lids, and closure of the palpebral fissure; mucopurulent discharge
- **Orbital cellulitus:** chemosis, proptosis, tenderness, ophthalmoplegia, pupillary sluggishness or paralysis, and decreased visual acuity; tenderness or pain with extraocular movements

DD • Orbital cellulitis (more serious condition) must be distinguished from periorbital cellulitis
- Other conditions include allergy, trauma, orbital abscess, subperiosteal abscess, cavernous sinus thrombosis, neoplasm, thyrotoxicosis

LB CBC, chemistries, blood cultures (mostly negative)

IM CT of orbit (used to distinguish orbital from periorbital cellulitus)

TX • Children > 5 years (adults as well): nafcillin (150 mg/kg/day q6hr); penicillin-allergic patients: vancomycin (40 mg/kg/day q6hr)
- Children ≤ 5 years: cefuroxime 75 mg/kg/day q8hr
- Immediate ophthalmologic consult

DI Admission is necessary for all children (all but the mildest cases in adults)

Table 14.4 Physical Findings in Children Who are Dehydrated

Clinical Finding	Degree of Dehydration (%)		
	5	10	15
Tachycardia	−	+	+
Orthostatic hypotension	−	±	+
Dry mucous membranes	±	+	+
Poor skin turgor	−	±	+
Increasing BUN	−	+	+
Decreasing urinary output	±	+	+
Urine specific gravity	1.020	1.030	1.035

DEHYDRATION

HX Associated conditions: fever, nausea, vomiting, diarrhea, and decreased oral intake from any cause

PX Various physical findings, depending on degree of dehydration (Table 14.4)

LB CBC, SMA-7, UA, and other appropriate evaluations for underlying problem

TX NS (for severe dehydration): 20 mg/kg IV bolus, repeat prn for pulse and BP; then give maintenance fluids using 1/4 to 1/2 NS. Give 100 ml/kg/24 hr for the first 10 kg of body weight plus 50 ml/kg/24 hr for each kg body weight from 11–20 kg plus 10 ml/kg/24 hr for each kg body weight over 20 kg; consider adding 20–40 mEq KCl/L when patient is urinating

DI Admission in severe cases

FEVER

KY Fever (temperature > 38.0°C rectal) sometimes has no evident source in patients < 3 years of age, and management is both challenging and controversial. Optimal management is unknown. A thorough search should always be made to discover the source of the fever, using information from the patient history; physical examination; and laboratory evaluation, especially UA (see Chapter 9, Infectious Disease Emergencies, Sepsis). In children < 90 days of age, the risk for serious bacterial infection is:

- 17.3% for those who meet toxic criteria (decreased level of consciousness, poor or absent eye contact, no interaction with environment, septic or cyanotic appearance, decreased perfusion or ventilation).
- 1.4% for those who meet low-risk criteria [previously healthy; bacterial source found on examination; WBC of 5000–15,000/mm³

(bands < 1500/mm³); UA normal; WBC < 5/HPF in diarrhea (if present)]; (in children < 28 days of age who meet these criteria, the risk for serious bacterial infection is ±1%).

HX • **Symptoms and signs:** fever with or without vomiting and diarrhea, and signs of toxicity
  • **Historical evidence:** duration and magnitude of fever; presence of any other symptoms; and recent oral intake and urinary output or number of diaper changes (both determined as accurately as possible)

PX • Perform a thorough examination to determine the source of the fever and gauge the degree of dehydration (see Table 14.4)
  • Examine the skin for signs of rash or petechiae that might be associated with meningococcal sepsis

DD Causes of septic appearance:
  • **Infectious:** bacterial sepsis, meningitis, UTI, congenital syphilis, viral infection
  • **Noninfectious:** gastroenteritis with dehydration, congenital heart disease, paroxysmal atrial tachycardia, MI, pericarditis and myocarditis, congenital adrenal hyperplasia, hypoglycemia, Reye's syndrome, anemia or methemoglobinemia, pyloric stenosis, intussusception, child abuse, other metabolic derangement

LB Controversial; consider CBC, SMA-7, LP, UA, blood and urine culture. The conservative approach is presented in Table 14.5.

IM CXR if appropriate (see Table 14.5)

TX • ABCs, IV fluids, supplemental O_2, monitoring if appropriate
  • Specific management as appropriate (see Table 14.5)
  • NS: 20 mg/kg IV for dehydration, repeat prn (see Dehydration)
  • Antipyretics for children > 1 year: acetaminophen (15 mg/kg); if no response to acetaminophen, give ibuprofen (10 mg/kg)

DI Admission, unless patients appear nontoxic and close follow-up is arranged (see Table 14.5)

IMMUNIZATION

KY Check the patient's vaccination history. The usual vaccination schedule is presented in Table 14.6. Lack of appropriate vaccinations may indicate poverty, isolation, cultural differences, or neglect.

Table 14.5 Conservative Approach to the Management of Fever in Young Children

Age	Laboratory/Imaging	Treatment/Disposition
0–28 days	Complete workup (see Fever)/± CXR	Perhaps parenteral antibiotic [usually if patient does not meet low-risk criteria (see Fever)], pending culture results/ Admit
29–90 days (toxic appearance)	UA, blood and urine culture, LP	Parenteral antibiotic/ Admit
29–90 days (nontoxic appearance)	Two options: • UA, blood and urine culture, LP • Urine culture	• Ceftriaxone (50 mg/kg IM up to 1 g)/ Discharge home with follow-up in 1 day • No ceftriaxone/ Discharge home with close observation and follow-up within 1 day
3 months–3 years (toxic appearance)	Sepsis workup	Parenteral antibiotic/ Admission
3 months–3 years (nontoxic appearance; temperature > 39.0°C)	Urine culture in males < 6 months and females < 2 years; stool culture if blood or mucus in stool or 35 WBC/HPF; blood culture (some recommend only if WBC > 15,000/mm^3)/ CXR for respiratory symptoms or findings	Empiric antibiotic (some recommend only if WBC > 15,000/mm^3)/ Discharge with follow-up in 1–2 days
3 months–3 years (nontoxic appearance; temperature < 39.0°C)	No laboratory workup	Discharge with acetaminophen, with instructions to return for worsening or if fever persists > 2 days; follow-up in 1–2 days

Table 14.6 Immunization Schedule*

Age	Vaccination(s)
2 months	DTP, polio, Hib
4 months	DTP, polio, Hib
6 months	DTP, polio,† Hib
15 months	DTP/DTaP, polio, Hib, MMR
4–6 years	DTP/DTaP, polio, MMR
14–16 years	Td

*Variation exists in the timing of doses of Hib; alternate regimen provides for Hib at 2, 4, and 12 months. DTaP is approved only for infants ≥ 15 months of age; it is not a substitute for those children with contraindication to pertussis vaccine.
†In endemic areas.

LARYNGOTRACHEOBRONCHITIS (CROUP)

KY The incidence of croup peaks at the age of 2 years. Etiologic factors include parainfluenzavirus types 1, 2, and 3; RSV; influenza A; and rhinovirus. Spasmodic croup is associated with personal or family history of allergies and multiple bouts of croup.

HX • A few days of viral prodrome often precedes the gradual onset of the characteristic barking, seal-like cough
• Inspiratory stridor can progress to respiratory distress
• Fever is variable; severe symptoms occur most commonly at night

PX Barking cough; patients may not appear toxic

DD Epiglottitis (slightly higher age; rapid onset; absence of cough; muffled, "hot potato" voice; ill or toxic appearance; anxiety; sitting up and drooling), tracheitis, foreign body, tracheal stenosis, diphtheria

LB Consider CBC, ABG, blood C&S; UA, urine C&S, urine antigen screen; nasopharyngeal washings for direct fluorescent antibody (RSV, adenovirus, parainfluenzavirus, influenza virus, *Chlamydia*) and viral cultures

IM CXR; AP neck radiograph to check for "steeple sign," lateral radiograph if there is concern about possible epiglottitis and "thumb sign"

TX • Use a nonthreatening approach (leave the child in the parent's arms)
• Oropharyngeal and surgical airway materials must be placed at the bedside at all times in the event of acute respiratory failure
• For symptomatic patients, use humidified O_2 by blow-by or 40%–60% by mask; maintain O_2 saturation > 92%. For many patients, particularly those with spasmodic croup, changes in temperature or breathing humidified air can cause significant, rapid improvement.

- For stridor at rest, retractions, and tachypnea, initiate treatment with racemic epinephrine 2.25% solution [0.05 ml/kg/dose (or 0.5 ml/dose) nebulized in 4 ml NS, repeat q1–6hr]; some authors recommend dexamethasone (0.25–0.5 mg/kg IV/IM q6hr)
- Patients with serious respiratory compromise should be intubated using an ET tube 0.5–1.0 mm smaller than usual size [16 + age (years)/4]

DI • Admission to pediatric ICU for all patients requiring treatment with racemic epinephrine or steroid (except for patients observed in the ED who still appear well > 6 hours after such treatment; they can probably be safely discharged)
- Consider admission for patients who do not have a pediatrician or quick access to an ED
- Discharge for patients who respond well to conservative treatment in the ED, with instructions for using a vaporizer or a shower to make steam in a closed bathroom and to return for any worsening

RETROPHARYNGEAL ABSCESS

KY This condition is most common in children < 3 years of age. Abscess formation occurs between retropharyngeal fascial planes (alar fascia), prevertebral fascia, and vertebral bodies. Usual causes include mixed mouth flora, anaerobic infection, *Staphylococcus aureus,* and *H. influenzae.* Tissue inoculation may occur via retropharyngeal trauma (e.g., surgery, dental work, fall onto popsicle or lollipop stick). Other etiologic factors include otitis media, parotitis, and retropharyngeal adenopathy from nasopharyngitis. If a retropharyngeal abscess goes untreated, morbidity or mortality is high. The potential exists for mechanical airway obstruction and abscess extension inferiorly to the mediastinum and/or pericardium.

HX • Sore throat; progressive sensation of mass in throat; dysphagia, and pleuritic chest pain; sometimes breathing difficulty, fever, toxic appearance, and cough
- Recent trauma to mouth or pharynx (ask about this)

PX Hyponasal voice, muffled voice, noisy breathing, toxic appearance, dehydration, stiff and painful neck, redness or swelling to the neck with tenderness to palpation; pharyngeal wall may appear erythematous and boggy, with displacement toward the uvula

DD Pharyngitis, foreign body, epiglottitis, croup, tonsillar abscess, submandibular abscess, Ludwig's angina, diphtheria, vascular anomaly

LB CBC, SMA-7; throat, blood, and urine culture for fever

IM Soft tissue neck films may reveal prevertebral soft tissue swelling, perhaps AFL, normal trachea and epiglottis; CT if necessary

TX • ABCs, careful monitoring for respiratory distress (equipment for emergency management of the airway, including a cricothyrotomy set, must be available)
 • Otolaryngologic consult for surgical I&D
 • IV antibiotics:
   Nafcillin (100–150 mg/kg/day divided q4hr IV) with metronidazole (35–50 mg/kg/day divided q8hr IV) or
   Clindamycin (15–40 mg/kg/day divided q6–8hr IV) with cefoxitin (80–160 mg/kg/day divided q6hr)

DI Admission, usually either to ICU or directly to OR

CHAPTER 15

Psychiatric Emergencies

ANOREXIA NERVOSA

HX Refusal to maintain body weight more than the minimum normal level, profound weight loss, disturbed body image, preoccupation with weight loss, excessive dieting and exercise, and amenorrhea

PX Bradycardia, hypothermia, pedal or pretibial edema, brittle hair and nails, petechiae or purpura, peripheral neuropathy, paresthesias of the fingers and toes, diminished DTRs, and possible impairment of gross motor coordination

DD Schizophrenia, depressive illness, hysteria, borderline personality disorders, superior mesenteric artery syndrome, inflammatory bowel disease, chronic hepatitis, Addison's disease, diabetes, hyperthyroidism, hyperemesis gravidarum, tuberculosis, malignancy

LB Consider CBC, electrolytes, BUN, creatinine, LFTs, glucose, Mg, lipase

IM Consider EKG

TX • Aggressive replacement with isotonic saline, thiamine, multivitamins, and magnesium
• Consider admission with psychiatric and internal medicine consults

DI Admission is suggested in the following circumstances: weight loss > 30% in 3 months, significant dehydration, severe metabolic disturbance, depression that is sufficiently severe to put patients at risk for suicide, severe binging and purging, failure to maintain outpatient weight contract, psychosis, family crisis, need to confront patient and family denial, need for initiation of therapy (individual, family, and pharmacotherapy), or complex differential diagnosis

BULIMIA NERVOSA

HX Eating binges, self-induced vomiting, diarrhea secondary to laxative abuse, preoccupation with diet and exercise, and disturbed body image; symptoms of esophagitis

PX Normal weight, parotid and submandibular swelling, scars and abrasions on the knuckles and hands, and unexplained amenorrhea

DD Primary affective or schizophrenic disorder

LB Electrolytes, CBC, Mg, lipase, LFTs, BUN and creatinine, glucose

TX Aggressive replacement with isotonic saline, thiamine, multivitamins, and magnesium; determination of the extent and severity of illness and its complications may require admission

DI Admission (an eating disorders unit is best) is suggested in the following circumstances: weight loss > 30% in 3 months, severe metabolic disturbance, depression that is sufficiently severe to put patients at risk for suicide, severe binging and purging, failure to maintain outpatient weight contract, psychosis, family crisis, need to confront patient and family denial, need for initiation of therapy (individual, family, and pharmacotherapy), or complex differential diagnosis

CONVERSION DISORDER

HX Conversion symptoms typically involve loss of neurologic function and include blindness, aphonia, seizures, paralysis, hemianesthesia, tunnel vision, unresponsiveness, and amnesia. Vomiting and symptoms of pregnancy may also occur. An attitude of relative unconcern may exist despite the seriousness of the symptoms that may be present (la belle indifférence).

PX • Inconsistent and incomplete sensory loss in one leg, with preservation of DTRs and antigravity muscle activity
  • Slowness of motion, inconsistencies in physical signs during unresponsiveness
      Nystagmus on oculovestibular stimulation in some nonorganically unresponsive patients
      Inconsistencies in blindness
  • "Cogwheel" response on manual muscle testing

DD Organic illness, malingering, Munchausen syndrome, somatization disorders, hypochondriasis

TX • Patients with conversion disorders must be handled delicately, deftly, and with a great deal of respect. They should be told that although the symptoms are bothersome, they do not appear to be manifestations of a serious illness. In many cases it often helps to suggest that such symptoms may resolve quickly.
  • Simultaneously, the physician can probe for underlying psychosocial conflicts that may be associated with symptoms. Consider a neurologic consult.

DI • Many patients with conversion disorders experience resolution of their physical symptoms during their ED stay, but some require admission

- If the diagnosis of conversion disorder is uncertain and if presenting symptoms may signify dangerous illness, admission is warranted
- Even when the diagnosis of conversion disorder is clear, patients whose manifestation persists and who cannot manage on their own require inpatient care

DEPRESSION AND SUICIDE

HX
- Vague, ill-defined somatic symptoms; self-inflicted wounds; drug overdose; fall from heights; previous suicide attempts; active suicidal or homicidal ideation
- Diminished sense of self-esteem and general physical and mental well-being; loss of interest in pleasurable activities; loss of energy; poor appetite; sleep disturbances, including insomnia or hypersomnia; decreased attention span and concentration ability; nervous symptoms such as increased tension and feelings of anxiety; decreased effectiveness at school, work, or home; episodes of tearfulness; irritability or excessive anger; pessimistic attitude toward the future; and recurrent thoughts of death or suicide

PX Neurologic evaluation, including an MSE

LB Consider CBC, Chem-7, LFTs; ammonia levels where indicated

TX
- Chemical and mechanical restraint where indicated
- Provide as supportive an environment as possible

DI Admission is indicated for patients who are a threat to themselves or others (e.g., active suicidal ideation) or for those who cannot care for themselves

MANAGEMENT OF DIFFICULT PATIENTS

KY In difficult-to-manage patients, a high index of suspicion for an organic cause must be maintained to reach an accurate diagnosis. Acutely psychotic patients may harm themselves or others out of confusion or in an effort to avoid imagined threats. *Security personnel should be on hand to prevent the outbreak of any physical violence.*

HX
- Determine the onset of abnormal behavior, psychiatric history, and history of violent behavior or assault
- Ask about medications and any drugs or alcohol that may have been used recently

PX If patients are confused, their wallets, purses, or pockets should be searched for medication, identification, or physician appointment cards

Muscle tone and overall state of attention may indicate a readiness for fight or flight. Speech may be loud or profane, indicating impending loss of control. Motor activity such as restlessness or pacing, especially if it is escalating, is a concern.

DD Drug or alcohol withdrawal, hypoglycemia, meningitis or encephalitis, hypertensive encephalopathy, intracranial hemorrhage, subdural or epidural hematoma, thyrotoxicosis, porphyria, hemorrhagic shock

LB CBC, electrolytes, blood cultures, BUN, creatinine, glucose; consider LFTs with ammonia, alcohol level, screen for drugs of abuse

IM CT scan, EKG, CXR (as indicated)

TX • Physical restraints may be required for protection of the patient and staff
   • Chemical restraints such as neuroleptic drugs may be required to reduce agitation; these agents may be titrated to effect
      Haloperidol: 5–10 mg IV/IM q30min (max 40 mg) or
      Droperidol: 2.5–5.0 mg IV/IM q3–6hr or
      Lorazepam: 0.5–2 mg IV/IM/PO q6–8hr
   • Consider prophylactic administration of an antiparkinsonian drug such as benztropine (2 mg IM) when administering a phenothiazine
   • When using physical restraint, each staff member is responsible for controlling movement in one extremity. The patient is brought to the ground backwards, protecting the head. The legs are restrained at the knees and feet. Once physical control is established, the patient is physically restrained on a gurney.

DI Admission should be considered for psychiatric evaluation of agitated or violent patients for whom the use of restraints or medication is necessary

PANIC DISORDER

HX Sudden extreme surge of anxiety, dread, palpitations, tachycardia, shortness of breath, chest tightness, dizziness, sweating, and tremulousness

PX Typically, there are no specific physical findings other than tachycardia and tachypnea

DD Thyrotoxicosis, carcinoid syndrome, hypoglycemia, pheochromocytoma, migraine, MI, cardiac arrhythmia, schizophrenia, depressive disorders, somatoform disorders, phobic disorders, post-traumatic stress disorder, drug withdrawal, complex-partial seizures, alcohol withdrawal

LB CBC, electrolytes, BUN, creatinine, glucose

IM Consider EKG, CXR

TX • Benzodiazepines are generally considered the first line of treatment because they are safe and have a relatively rapid onset of action; antihistamines, diphenhydramine, and hydroxyzine are other helpful sedating drugs

• When diagnosis is certain, outpatient psychiatric consultation is indicated

DI • Consider inpatient care for all patients who do not respond to supportive measures in the ED

CHAPTER 16

Pulmonary Emergencies

AIRWAY MANAGEMENT AND INTUBATION

KY There is no single guideline for airway management. Differences in clinical presentation and condition, patient anatomy, and physician and institution practices mandate that airway management be individually customized. Airway management should be performed by medical students and house officers only under the supervision of the ED attending physician. Consultation should be obtained with appropriate specialists where clinically indicated.

TX • **Orotracheal intubation:**

Prepare all equipment (e.g., suction device, supplemental O_2, bag-valve-mask device, ET tubes, cricothyrotomy or needle-jet equipment, CO_2 indicator, laryngoscope, pulse oximeter)

Use the proper ET tube size (interior diameter): women, 7.0–9.0 mm; men, 7.5–10.0 mm; children, (age + 16)/4 mm

If sedation and/or paralysis is required, prepare all medications, including those necessary if a rapid-sequence induction is planned (Table 16.1).

Refer to Table 16.2 for guidelines for orotracheal intubation.

• **Nasotracheal intubation:**

Nasotracheal intubation may be preferred <u>if prolonged</u> intubation is anticipated (increased patient comfort).

Intubation is easier if the patient is awake and breathing spontaneously. ET tube sizes are usually 0.5–1.0 mm smaller than orotracheal tube sizes to allow passage and reduce trauma to the nasopharynx.

Use of a tube with directional tip control ("ringed," Endotrol) may also facilitate the procedure.

Proper ET tube sizes: women, 6.0–7.0 mm; men, 6.0–8.0 mm; children: (age + 16)/4 mm

Refer to Table 16.3 for guidelines for nasotracheal intubation.

ASTHMA

HX Previous history, recent exposure to trigger, and worsening wheezing and dyspnea

PX Findings include anxiety, tachypnea, wheezing, accessory muscle use, cough, and cyanosis

Table 16.1   Medications Used for Rapid-Sequence Induction*

Pharmacologic Agent	Dose (IV)
Fentanyl	50-μg increments (max ≈ 4–6 μg/kg)
Midazolam	1 mg IV q2–3min (max 0.1–0.15 mg/kg)
Vercuronium	0.015 mg/kg (priming dose) (≈ 1 mg adult dose); 0.15 mg/kg (paralytic dose) (≈ 7–10 mg adult dose)
Atropine	0.01 mg/kg (children < 3 years)
Lidocaine	1.5 mg/kg
Thiopental	3–5 mg/kg
Succinylcholine†	1–1.5 mg/kg (increase to 2 mg/kg in infants and small children)

*Considerable expertise is required for use of paralyzing agents and RSI.
†Relative contraindications include prolonged seizures, rhabdomyolysis, suspected hyperkalemia, or globe injury. Because of the risk for vomiting and aspiration, cricoid cartilage pressure should be applied as soon as the patient may be unable to protect the airway (Sellick maneuver).

Table 16.2   Guidelines for Performing Orotracheal Intubation

1. **Position the patient.** Put the patient's head in the "sniffing" position (i.e., with the head flexed at the neck and extended). If necessary, elevate the head with a small pillow or towel.
2. **Preoxygenate the patient.** Allow the patient to breathe 100% oxygen. Avoid unnecessary gastric filling by minimizing assisted bag-valve-mask ventilation.
3. **Position the laryngoscope.** Holding the laryngoscope handle with left hand, insert the laryngoscope along the right side of the mouth to the base of tongue, and push the tongue to the left. If using a curved blade, advance to the vallecula (superior to the epiglottis) and lift anteriorly. If using a straight blade, place the laryngoscope beneath the epiglottis and lift anteriorly.
4. **Intubate the patient.** Stop just after the cuff disappears behind the vocal cords. If intubation is unsuccessful after 30 seconds, stop and resume bag-valve-mask ventilation before reattempting.
5. **Inflate the cuff** with a syringe and attach the tube to an Ambu bag or a ventilator.
6. **Confirm the location of the ET tube** by checking for equal bilateral breath sounds, absence of gastric air, CO_2 monitoring, a syringe test, or CXR. If there are any questions concerning proper ET tube location, repeat laryngoscopy with the tube in place to be sure it is in the trachea.
7. **Secure the tube** with tape, and note the centimeter mark at the mouth. Suction the oropharynx and trachea.

Table 16.3   Guidelines for Performing Nasotracheal Intubation

1. **Administer necessary medications.** Spray the nasal passage with vasoconstrictor spray: cocaine 4% (4 ml) or phenylephrine 0.25% (2 ml) unless contraindicated. Apply topical anesthesia with viscous lidocaine 2% or topical spray. If sedation is required, administer fentanyl (1 µg/kg) or midazolam 0.05–0.1 mg/kg (titrate).
2. **Position the patient.** The procedure may be performed with the patient in the sitting position.
3. **Intubate the patient.** Place the tube into the nasal passage, and guide it into the nasopharynx. Monitor progress by listening for air movement and observing fogging of the tube. As the tube enters the oropharynx, gradually guide it downward. If the sounds stop, withdraw the tube 1–2 cm until breath sounds are heard again. Reposition the tube, and if necessary, extend the head and advance the tube. If difficulty is encountered, perform laryngoscopy under direct visualization or use Magill forceps. Successful intubation occurs when the tube passes through the cords; a cough may occur and breath sounds will reach maximum intensity if the tube is correctly positioned.
4. **Confirm the location of the ET tube** by checking for equal bilateral breath sounds, absence of gastric air, CO_2 monitoring, a syringe test, or CXR. If there is any doubt concerning proper ET tube location, repeat laryngoscopy with the tube in place to be sure it is in the trachea.

Be alert for patients who "move" so little air that they are not wheezing and those who tire from respiratory effort

DD Pneumonia, bronchitis, croup, bronchiolitis, COPD, CHF, pulmonary embolism, allergic reaction, upper airway obstruction

LB Peak flow measurement is mandatory; pulse oximetry or ABG may be useful in patients with severe symptoms; consider other lab tests such as CBC, chemistry profile, UA

IM CXR prn

TX • Supplemental O_2 (maintain O_2 saturation > 90%); monitor peak flow rates before and after bronchodilator treatments
• Pharmacologic agents:
   Albuterol or metaproterenol nebulized: 0.2–0.5 ml (2.5 mg) in 3 ml NS q20min
   Epinephrine 1:1000: 0.3–0.5 ml SQ q20min × 3; relative contraindications include age > 40 years (epinephrine is virtually never used in patients with known CAD)
   Terbutaline: 0.25 mg SQ q30min × up to 3 (preferred over epinephrine for pregnant women)
   Steroids such as methylprednisolone (60–120 mg IV) [optimal dosing unknown] or prednisone (40–60 mg PO); recent

research suggests that glucocorticoid effectiveness may be just as rapid with the PO route as with the IV route

Magnesium sulfate: 2 g IV over 20 minutes (may be useful transiently)

DI • No asthmatic patient need stay in the ED > 4 hours; during that time, a decision to admit or discharge can be made based primarily on clinical impression and peak flow measurements

• Admission for patients who are not improving who:

Are tiring from work of breathing (objectively measured by rising CO_2)

Have low peak flows, especially without improvement

Have complications such as pneumonia or ischemia

Are returning to an ED after a recent previous visit

Are pregnant (low threshold for admission of pregnant women with asthma)

• All patients with asthma who are discharged from the ED should have their medications carefully checked, provided with adequate prescriptions, and advised to seek appointments for an outpatient visit within 1 week

CHRONIC OBSTRUCTIVE PULMONARY DISEASE (COPD)/BRONCHITIS

KY The treatable component of COPD is caused by tracheobronchial inflammation and mucus production, leading to chronic, productive cough. The pathology of this condition, which is implicated in its etiology, includes previous infection, cigarettes, and environmental pollutants, which increase secretions and impair mucociliary response. Although most episodes of COPD are associated with viral etiology, superimposed and chronic bacterial infections contribute to inflammation and chronic obstruction.

HX The various stages of COPD (early to late):

• Morning cough or smoker's cough, with no respiratory difficulty

• Periodic exacerbations of copious, purulent sputum; chest "cold," with little dyspnea or disability

• Chronic cough, DOE, and disability; worsened symptoms with "colds;" clinical evidence suggestive of central cyanosis, chronic hypoxia/hypercarbia, and early right-sided heart failure

• Progressive disability; DOE with minimal exertion; chronic respiratory difficulties of cough paroxysms and wheezing; cor pulmonale

• End stage: incapacitation, O_2 dependence, chronic dyspnea at rest and respiratory failure, refractory cor pulmonale

PX • Physical findings sometimes include obesity and possible central cyanosis, with pursed-lip breathing, loose rales, rhonchi, and diffuse wheezing
  • Cor pulmonale may produce JVD, peripheral edema
  • S_4 suggests low right ventricular compliance; S_3, right ventricular failure; and systolic murmur, tricuspid insufficiency
  • Polymicrobial sputum

DD Congestive heart disease, pneumonia, atelectasis, asthma, cardiogenic shock, ARDS, pulmonary embolism, foreign body, aspiration pneumonitis, tumor

LB • ABG; PCO_2 (adequacy of ventilation); PO_2 (degree of hypoxia: e.g., stage A, 80–100 mm Hg; stage B, 60–80 mm Hg; stage C, < 60 mm Hg); pH and HCO_3 values (degree of respiratory and renal compensation); FEV_1 (establish < 60 to > 300 ml) [useful for comparison of patient's baseline value (if available) as well as an indicator of clinical response to treatment]

IM CXR (possible atelectasis, edema, infiltrate; rarely hyperexpansion; perhaps cardiomegaly)

TX • Airway, IV fluids, supplemental O_2 (increase O_2 by 1–2 L/min prn), monitoring
  • Bronchodilators:
      ß-Adrenergics: albuterol 0.5% (0.5 ml); metaproterenol 0.5% (0.3 ml)
      Anticholinergics (glycopyrrolate in nebulized form or ipratropium bromide via metered-dose inhaler) may play a role in acute ED management
  • Steroids:
      Prednisone: 40–60 mg PO initial dose or
      Methylprednisolone [60–125 mg IV (or equivalent) q6hr for acute flare; taper doses of outpatient prednisone over 5–7 days, beginning at 40–60 mg]
  • Antibiotics (data concerning efficacy are unclear):
      Inpatient: ampicillin (1 g IV q6hr or 250–500 mg PO q6–8hr), TMP-SMX (160/800 mg PO bid), ampicillin–sulbactam (1.5 g IV q6hr), or cefuroxime (1.5 g IV q8hr)
      Outpatient: doxycycline (100 mg PO q12hr × 10 days); erythromycin (333 mg PO q8hr ×10 days); TMP-SMX DS (PO q12hr × 10 days); either azithromycin (500 mg PO initial dose, followed by 250 mg daily × 4 days); cefazolin, cephalexin, or cephalothin; ciprofloxacin; or amoxicillin– clavulanate may be used, but they are no more effective)

DI • Admission for acute exacerbation; little clinical improvement with treatment
 • Consider outpatient follow-up if respiratory status has improved, FEV_1 has improved, the patient "road tests" well, or the patient returns to baseline

HEMOPTYSIS

HX Possible cough, sputum, wheezing, congestion, chest pain, dyspnea, fever, chills, night sweats, weight loss, tobacco abuse, or previous episodes of mild hemoptysis

PX • Quantify the bleeding as massive (600 ml in 24–48 hours or a rate of > 100 ml/hr) or submassive
 • Seek a history of pulmonary embolism associated with coagulopathy

DD Causes may be inflammatory (bronchitis, bronchiectasis, lung abscess, pneumonia, TB), neoplastic, cardiovascular (AVM, CHF, pulmonary embolism, pulmonary hypertension, mitral stenosis), congenital (cystic fibrosis), immunologic, or even extrapulmonary (thrombocytopenia, coagulopathy, trauma)

LB Pulse oximetry, ABG, CBC, platelets, SMA-7, PT, PTT, T&C 4–6 U packed RBCs, sputum Gram stain, C&S, AFB, parasites and fungi, cytology; consider nasopharyngoscopy to rule out upper airway source

IM CXR, EKG; consider $\dot{V}/\dot{Q}$ scan and contrast CT scan

TX • Manage airway
 • Keep patient in lateral decubitus and Trendelenburg's positions
 • Obtain immediate thoracic surgical consult for massive hemoptysis
 • Quantify amounts of all sputum and blood; suction prn
 • Transfuse and manage coagulopathy as indicated
 • Consider empiric antibiotics if an infection may be contributing to the hemoptysis

DI • ICU for massive bleeding with immediate surgery consult
 • Discharge only those patients who are reliable and stable, with appropriate follow-up in < 24 hours

PLEURAL EFFUSION

KY The many causes of pleural effusions include CHF, pulmonary infection, tumor, cirrhosis, pancreatitis, nephrotic syndrome, acute aortic dissection, esophageal rupture, and myxedema.

HX • Occasionally asymptomatic

- If symptomatic: weight loss, fever, orthopnea, edema, cough, dyspnea, and chest pain

PX Decreased breath sounds with dullness to percussion

DD Pneumonia or other infiltrate, tumor, widened mediastinum, herniated diaphragm with viscera in thorax

LB • Pulse oximetry, ABG, CBC, SMA-7, PT, LFTs, amylase, lipase, protein
- Thoracentesis (for sample of pleural fluid):
    Tube 1 (10 ml): LDH, protein, amylase, lipase triglyceride, glucose
    Tube 2 (20–60 mg heparinized): Gram stain, C&S, AFB, fungal C&S, wet mount
    Tube 3 (5–10 ml EDTA): cell count and differential

IM CXR, EKG

TX Manage airway and maintain adequate oxygenation with supplemental O_2; consider thoracentesis for diagnostic or therapeutic purposes

DI • Consider admission, especially if thoracentesis performed in ED
- Patients with an effusion not evacuated may require admission depending on the severity of symptoms, underlying diagnosis, and response to treatment

RESPIRATORY FAILURE AND VENTILATOR MANAGEMENT

KY Potential indications for ventilatory support include: severe respiratory distress, inability to state name due to respiratory distress, impending respiratory failure, and uncorrectable hypoxia by ABG or pulse oximetry. The decision to initiate treatment in the ED is based primarily on clinical impression.

- Sample initial orders: FIO_2 = 100%; PEEP = 3–5 cm H_2O; assist control 8–14 bpm; tidal volume = 800 ml (10–15 ml/kg ideal body weight); set rate so that minute ventilation is approximately 10 L/min
- If the patient is "fighting" the ventilator, despite appropriate sensitivity, flow rate settings, and tidal volume:
    Consider IMV or SIMV or
    Add sedation with or without paralysis (exclude complications or other causes of agitation); never use paralytic agents without concurrent analgesia/sedation

RHINITIS

KY There are two major types of chronic rhinitis: allergic and nonallergic. Allergic rhinitis (hay fever) is an immunologic disease triggered by repeated exposure to allergens in predisposed individuals. Nonallergic rhinitis is a group of heterogeneous diseases that results from the use of sympatholytic medicines, aspirin, pregnancy, hypothyroidism, nasal polyps, nasal tumors, or vasomotor rhinitis.

HX Nasal discharge, difficult nasal breathing, cough, and symptoms of URI

PX Use a nasal speculum and adequate light to focus on the nasal mucosa

DD Sinusitis, sinus fracture, sinus squeeze, nasal tumors, conjunctivitis

LB Nasal secretion smear for eosinophilia; (other tests are not helpful unless a complication such as bacteremia or drug abuse is suspected)

IM Consider sinus radiographs

TX • Allergic rhinitis: antihistamines are the treatment of choice
  OTC preparations, including triprolidine or pseudoephedrine (Actifed), chlorpheniramine (Chlor-Trimeton), or diphenhydramine (Benadryl)
  Prescription medications such as fexofenadine (60 mg PO bid) or terfenadine (60 mg PO bid)
• Nonallergic rhinitis: referral to an otolaryngologist for rhinitis from mucosal damage from intranasal drug use

DI Home; patients should be referred to a specialist if they fail to improve with the usual symptomatic therapy

CHAPTER 17

Rheumatologic/Allergic Emergencies

ANAPHYLAXIS

KY Anaphylaxis is a life-threatening allergic reaction that occurs in sensitized individuals, leading to the release of histamine, prostaglandins, and kallikrein from mast cells and basophils. These mediators cause massive vasodilation and capillary leakage that results in hypotension, urticaria, and angioedema of the skin, upper airway, and GI tract. Penicillin and bee and wasp stings are the most common antigens. Death usually results from laryngeal edema, causing acute upper airway obstruction and hypotension with poor cerebral and coronary perfusion.

- **Urticaria,** which is edema of the superficial dermis, is marked by red wheals.
- **Angioedema** is edema of the deep dermis. It appears as swelling of mucous membranes, which are prominent in the face, lips, and pharynx.

HX
- Antibiotics, NSAIDs, aspirin, iodinated contrast media, bee and wasp stings, seafood
- Onset occurs < 1 hour after exposure
    Early symptoms: itching, a warm feeling, chest tightness, and a throat lump
    Later symptoms: dizziness secondary to hypotension

PX Tachycardia, arrhythmia, and hypotension angioedema, stridor, wheezing, decreased breath sounds, and urticaria

DD Hereditary angioedema, viral or bacterial infection, scombroid fish poisoning, reaction to monosodium glutamate, carcinoid syndrome

TX **Mild anaphylaxis:** diphenhydramine (50 mg PO) [IV if severe]
- **Severe anaphylaxis:** methylprednisolone [60–125 mg IV push (peds 1 mg/kg)]; ranitidine (50 mg IV); epinephrine 1:1000 [0.3 ml SQ (peds 0.01 ml/kg) q15min or 0.5 ml SL]
    Life-threatening situations: epinephrine 1:10,000 (0.3–0.5 mg IV)
    Persistent shock: epinephrine 1:10,000 (1 mg in 250 ml D_5W; infuse at 2 µg/min IV LR wide open)
    Persistent hypotension: MAST suit and dopamine infusion

DI
- ICU for all unstable patients
- Admission for observation for moderate-to-severe cases (usually)

- Observation in ED for 3 hours and discharge for patients with mild allergic reaction who respond rapidly and completely; stable patients who are discharged must continue diphenhydramine (25 mg PO q6hr × 72 hours) to reduce the risk for symptom reexacerbation due to systemic leukotrienes

MONARTICULAR ARTHRITIS ("HOT JOINT")

KY Causes of monarticular arthritis include trauma; inflammation, both crystal-induced and non–crystal-induced; immunologic disorders; degenerative joint disease; and infection (Table 17.1). The timely diagnosis of septic arthritis is the most important consideration in the ED.

HX Viral syndrome, pharyngitis, trauma, fever, vaginal or urethral discharge, rash, alcohol or IV drug abuse, previous episodes, major diseases, and medications

Table 17.1 Etiologic Agents and Antibiotic Regimens in Septic Arthritis

Patient Age/ Condition	Organism(s)	Antibiotics
Infant (< 3 months)	*Staphylococcus aureus* Enterobacteriaceae Group B streptococcus	PRSP + third-generation cephalosporin
Child (3 months–6 years)	*Haemophilus influenzae* S. aureus Streptococcus Enterobacteriaceae	PRSP + third-generation cephalosporin
Adult	S. aureus Group A streptococcus Enterobacteriaceae	PRSP + aminoglycoside
Adult with possible STD contact	*Neisseria gonorrhoeae*	Ceftriaxone or cefotaxime
IV drug abuse	S. aureus Pseudomonas	PRSP + aminoglycoside
Sickle cell disease	*Salmonella*	Ampicillin, TMP-SMX, ciprofloxacin
Prosthetic joint, postoperative or postintra-articular injection	S. aureus Enterobacteriaceae Pseudomonas Staphylococcus epidermidis	Vancomycin + ciprofloxacin

PRSP = penicillinase-resistant synthetic penicillin.

Table 17.2 Synovial Fluid Characteristics

Cause/Diagnosis	Appearance	Viscosity	WBC/mm³	Glucose (% of serum glucose)
Normal	Clear	High (viscous)	< 200	100
Hemorrhagic (trauma, coagulopathy)	Bloody	Low	Approaching peripheral	Approaching peripheral
Inflammatory (osteo-arthritis, rheumatoid arthritis, psoriatic arthritis)	Cloudy, yellow	Low	2000–50,000	90–100; (75 in rheumatoid arthritis)
Crystal-induced (gout, pseudogout)	Turbid, with urate crystals (gout) or positively birefringent calcium pyrophosphate crystals (pseudogout)		5000–50,000	90
Infectious	Opaque, turbid	Low	> 50,000	> 40

PX • Fever, tachycardia, tophi, pharyngitis, rales, murmur, and abdominal organomegaly or tenderness
- Affected joint: hot, edematous, red, tender, with decreased ROM
- Joint involvement: first metatarsophalangeal joint or ankle (gout); knee (pseudogout, infectious); and sternoclavicular joint (IV drug abuse)

DD Cellulitis, bursitis, gout, pseudogout, septic arthritis, trauma, osteoarthritis, rheumatoid arthritis, collagen vascular disease, coagulopathy

LB • CBC, SMA-7, ESR; blood C&S, PT, PTT prn
- Arthrocentesis to obtain synovial fluid for analysis to check appearance, viscosity, cell count with differential, glucose level, presence of crystals, Gram stain, and C&S (Table 17.2)

IM Joint radiograph

TX • **Tense joint effusion:** therapeutic arthrocentesis
- **Hemorrhagic arthritis:** splinting, elevation, protection from weight bearing, analgesia, and appropriate therapy for bleeding disorder
- **Inflammation:** indomethacin (25 mg q6hr prn) or aspirin
- **Crystal-induced arthritis:** indomethacin (50 mg qid x 2 days, then 25 mg qid prn) or colchicine [either 2 mg IV (diluted in 20 ml NS injected slowly) or 0.6 mg PO q2hr] until symptoms subside or nausea or diarrhea occurs
- **Infectious arthritis** (see Table 17.1)

DI • Admission for patients with infectious causes
- Outpatient management for all other patients (see Table 17.1)

CHAPTER 18

Toxicologic Emergencies

GENERAL EVALUATION AND TREATMENT

KY Toxicity results from ingestion of or exposure to a toxic substance or overdose of a prescription or nonprescription drug.

HX History is extremely important
- Obtain information from the patient, friends, relatives, and EMS personnel
- Find out about the time and amount of ingestion and whether vomiting has occurred as well as any psychiatric history, previous similar episodes, drug and alcohol abuse, and change in mental status before and after ingestion
- Drug bottles should be brought to the ED

PX • Vital sign—related symptoms: possible hyperthermia, tachycardia or bradycardia, hyperventilation or bradypnea
- Skin: redness, track marks, diaphoresis
- HEENT: signs of trauma; pupil size and light reaction; fundi, visual acuity, nystagmus
- Neurologic symptoms: change in mental status, including level of consciousness (GCS) [see Table 11.1], confusion/delirium, mania
- Neuromuscular symptoms: dystonic reaction (phenothiazines)

LB Depends on presentation; CBC, SMA-7, toxicology screen, or levels of ASA, acetaminophen, or alcohol; specific drug levels, ABG, osmolality, CO, and UA may be useful

IM Consider CXR, KUB

TX • ABCs, IV fluids, supplemental O_2, monitoring
- Reduced level of consciousness: opioid antagonist [naloxone (2 mg IV)], thiamine (100 mg IV), glucose (1 amp 50% dextrose IV)
- Prevention of absorption:
  Activated charcoal (1 g/kg PO or NG tube) [do not use if toxicity is due to caustics, hydrocarbons, lithium, or Fe]; repeat doses q2–4hr in some cases
  Gastric lavage may be performed if within 1 hour of ingestion or when otherwise indicated (if decreased level of consciousness and no gag reflex, intubate the patient first)
- Dialysis (e.g., methanol, ethylene glycol, salicylates, lithium)

DI Admission for all patients, except those with benign ingestions; psychiatric consultation as indicated

ACETAMINOPHEN TOXICITY

KY Most acetaminophen is metabolized in the liver, but a small portion is metabolized via the cytochrome P450 oxidase system to a toxic metabolite that is detoxified by glutathione and excreted in urine. In acetaminophen overdose, glutathione is depleted, and the toxic metabolite accumulates in the liver, causing hepatic necrosis. Acetaminophen toxicity occurs in stages:

- Phase I (0–24 hours): anorexia, nausea, and vomiting
- Phase II (24–72 hours): abdominal pain
- Phase III (3–5 days): jaundice, hypoglycemia, coagulopathy, and encephalopathy
- Phase IV (1 week): resolution of hepatic dysfunction (if phase III is not lethal)

HX
- Identification of drug, time of ingestion, medical and psychiatric illnesses, and current medications
- Nausea, vomiting, abdominal pain, diaphoresis, malaise, and jaundice; sometimes asymptomatic

PX Change in mental status, scleral icterus, hepatomegaly, RUQ tenderness, pallor, diaphoresis, and jaundice

DD Liver disease, including alcoholic and viral hepatitis, gallbladder and biliary tract disease; *Amanita* mushroom poisoning

LB CBC, SMA-7, PT, LFTs, toxicology screen, serum acetaminophen level (at 4 hours) (Figure 18.1)

IM Consider CXR

TX
- Airway, IV fluids, supplemental O_2, monitoring
- Naloxone; thiamine; glucose if indicated for decreased mental status; charcoal; consider gastric lavage if presentation within 1 hour of ingestion (see General Evaluation and Treatment)
- Toxicity (> 150 µg/ml at 4 hours) [see Figure 18.1] requires administration of glutathione-substitute NAC

    Standard loading dose: 140 mg/kg diluted with soda or juice, then 70 mg/kg q4hr × 17 doses

    Increased loading dose if administering charcoal: 235 mg/kg PO

    Consider IV NAC (not yet FDA approved): 140 mg/kg IV load, increase over 1 hour

DI Admission for all patients who require NAC

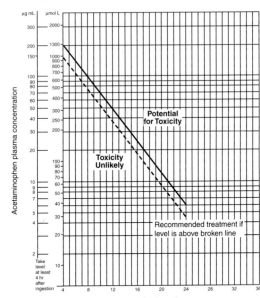

How to use this graph:

1. **Determine serum acetaminophen level.** Serum levels drawn within 4 hours of ingestion may not represent peak levels; therefore, the acetaminophen level should be determined **at least 4 hours after the overdose.**

2. **Plot coordinate.**
   a. If the point falls **above the broken line,** treatment is required and the entire course of **acetylcysteine should be administered.**
   b. If the point falls **below the broken line,** acetylcysteine treatment is not necessary, or, if already instituted, may be discontinued.

FIGURE 18.1 Acetaminophen poisoning nomogram. This nomogram has been developed to estimate the probability that plasma levels (in relation to the time after ingestion) will result in hepatotoxicity. The *broken line*, which represents a 25% allowance below the solid line, is included to allow for possible error in acetaminophen plasma assays and estimated time from ingestion of an overdose. This graph relates only to plasma levels following a single, acute overdose ingestion. (Redrawn with permission from Rumack BH, Matthew H: Acetaminophen poisoning and toxicity. *Pediatrics* 55:871, 1975.)

ALCOHOL POISONING

KY Toxic alcohols cause morbidity and mortality. Ethanol is discussed elsewhere (see Chapter 3, Endocrinologic Emergencies, Alcoholic Ketoacidosis). Ethylene glycol, which is found in detergents, paints, antifreeze and coolants, is metabolized to glycolic and oxalic acids. Methanol (wood alcohol), which is found in antifreeze, paint solvents, canned fuels (e.g., Sterno), gasoline additives, and home heating fuels, is metabolized in the liver to formic acid. Both of these alcohols are severely toxic and cause profound anion gap acidosis. Isopropyl alcohol (rubbing alcohol), which is metabolized to acetone, does not cause acidosis.

HX • **Ethylene glycol toxicity:**

> 1–12 hours after ingestion: slurred speech, lethargy
>
> About 12 hours: cardiac and respiratory symptoms, including palpitations and shortness of breath
>
> About 48 hours: renal failure occurs because of intratubular deposition of oxalate crystals

• **Methanol toxicity:** symptoms occur 1–2 days after ingestion and include nausea, vomiting, abdominal pain, and change in vision

• **Isopropyl alcohol ingestion:** symptoms, which are similar to those of acute ethanol intoxication, include CNS depression, nausea, and vomiting

PX General: decreased level of consciousness

• Vital sign–related symptoms: tachycardia, hypertension (ethylene glycol), hyperventilation (compensatory, from metabolic acidosis; ethylene glycol or methanol)

• Photophobia, mydriasis, hyperemia of optic disk, papilledema (methanol), nystagmus (ethylene glycol)

• Rales, arrhythmias (ethylene glycol)

• Abdominal: diffuse tenderness (methanol, isopropyl alcohol)

• Neurologic: ataxia, myoclonus (ethylene glycol), confusion, and seizures (ethylene glycol or methanol)

DD Differential diagnosis for change in mental status; the "A MUDPILE CAT" (see Figure 10.1) and "TIPS AEIOU" mnemonics (see Figure 11.1) may be useful (see Anion Gap Metabolic Acidosis)

LB CBC, SMA-7, ABG, UA, serum osmolality, toxicology screen, serum methanol and ethylene glycol (see Anion Gap Metabolic Acidosis)

IM CXR, EKG (as needed)

TX • Airway, IV fluid, supplemental O_2, monitoring; naloxone, thiamine, and glucose (see General Evaluation and Treatment)

• **Ethylene glycol/methanol:**

> If ingestion occurred within 1 hour, gastric lavage (minimal absorption to charcoal)

NaHCO$_3$ (to correct acidosis): 1–2 amp IV (up to 400 mEq may be required)

Ethanol 10% (competitively blocks conversion to toxic metabolites): IV loading dose of 10 ml/kg, followed by maintenance infusion of 1.5 ml/kg/hr to achieve level of 100 mg/dl

Consider fomepizole if available

Hemodialysis if (1) no improvement with NaHCO$_3$, ethanol, or fomepizole; (2) serum level of either substance > 50 mg/dl; or (3) visual impairment is present (methanol)

- **Isopropyl alcohol:** symptomatic treatment
- Psychiatric consult as appropriate

DI
- Admission for cases of ethylene glycol/methanol toxicity; ICU as needed, plus renal and ophthalmologic consults as necessary
- Observation and discharge for cases of ethanol and isopropyl alcohol toxicity when patients are no longer clinically intoxicated, unless they exhibit respiratory depression or decreased level of consciousness

ANION GAP METABOLIC ACIDOSIS

KY The anion gap may be calculated as follows: anion gap = [Na+] - ([HCO$_3$] + [Cl$^-$]). The normal range is 8–12 mEq/L. Anion gap metabolic acidosis has several causes; the mnemonic "A MUDPILE CAT" can be used to remember these etiologic factors (see Figure 10.1).

- **Clinical information** (based on history and physical examination):
    Alcoholic ketoacidosis: affected patients often have lower blood sugar and mild or absent glucosuria

    Methanol: common symptoms include visual disturbances and headache; anion and osmolar gaps are high

    Uremia: condition becomes advanced before it causes an anion gap

    DKA: usually results in both hyperglycemia and glucosuria

    Lactic acidosis (check serum level): has a broad differential diagnosis itself

    Ethylene glycol: causes calcium oxalate or hippurate crystals in urine; anion and osmolar gaps are high

    Salicylates: high levels are required to contribute to the anion gap
- **Size of the anion gap:**
    > 35 mEq/L: usually caused by ethylene glycol, methanol, or lactic acidosis

    16–22 mEq/L: may be due to uremia, which must be quite advanced before it causes an increase

Table 18.1   Effect of Various Substances on the Osmolar Gap in Anion Gap Metabolic Acidosis

Substance	Amount (mg/dl) Needed to Increase Serum Osmolarity by 1 mOsm/L	Increase in mOsm/L due to Each mg/dl
Methanol	2.6	0.38
Ethanol	4.3	0.23
Ethylene glycol	5.0	0.20
Acetone	5.5	0.18
Isopropyl alcohol	5.9	0.17
Salicylate	14.0	0.07

- **Osmolar gap,** which is the difference between the measured osmolality and the calculated osmolarity

  Osmolar gap = measured osmolality − calculated osmolarity

  Calculated osmolality = 2(Na) + (glucose/18) + (BUN/2.8)

  Normal osmolality = 275 mOsm/L − 285 mOsm/L (normal gap < 10 mOsm/L)

  Different substances contribute to the osmolar gap to various extents (Table 18.1). Small amounts of methanol lead to greater increases in osmolality, and large amounts of salicylate eventually increase the osmolar gap. Note also that the contribution to an osmolar gap due to alcohol may be calculated; this can be useful when a mixed alcohol ingestion is suspected.

  For more information, see Chapter 10, Metabolic Emergencies, Acid–Base Disorders, Metabolic Acidosis

ANTICHOLINERGIC TOXICITY

KY A wide variety of prescription and nonprescription drugs have anticholinergic properties: antidepressants, antiemetics, antihistamines, antiparkinsonian medications, major tranquilizers, antispasmodics, ophthalmoplegics, OTC cough and cold medications, and sleep aids. Parasympathetic blockade leads to the anticholinergic clinical picture: "hot as a hare, blind as a bat, dry as a bone, red as a beet, mad as a hatter."

HX • Identification of drug, time of ingestion, medical and psychiatric illnesses, and current medications

  • Dry mouth, fever, blurred vision, and confusion

PX • Altered level of consciousness or AMS

- Look for hyperthermia, tachycardia, hypertension, mydriasis, poor visual acuity, flushed and dry face, decreased bowel sounds, disorientation, and confusion

DD CNS infection, dehydration, psychiatric disorder, sepsis

LB CBC, SMA-7; consider toxicology screen

IM CXR, EKG

TX
- Airway, IV fluids, supplemental O_2, monitoring
- Naloxone, thiamine, glucose, charcoal (see General Evaluation and Treatment); conservative and supportive therapy in ED
- Psychiatric consult as appropriate

DI
- Admission, usually to the ICU, for severe symptoms or complications
- Observation in ED until condition resolves

ANTIPSYCHOTIC TOXICITY

KY Antipsychotic (neuroleptic) drugs block dopaminergic, adrenergic, and muscarinic and histaminic receptors. Dopamine blockade modifies behavior and can result in dystonic reactions. Alpha-adrenergic blockade causes vasodilation (orthostatic hypotension). Antipsychotics have anticholinergic properties (see Anticholinergic Toxicity). Common phenothiazines include chlorpromazine, fluphenazine, prochlorperazine, thioridazine, and trifluoperazine. Common butyrophenones are haloperidol and droperidol.

HX
- Dosage of antipsychotic and other medications, psychiatric history
- Nervousness, stiff neck, and pacing

PX
- Level of consciousness is usually not affected, except with severe overdoses
- Other findings: hyperthermia; tachycardia; orthostatic hypotension; dystonias, including torticollis, involuntary movements, spasms; akathisia

DD Malignant hyperthermia, heatstroke, extrapyramidal reaction, hyperthyroidism, infectious disease

LB CBC, SMA-7; consider toxicology screen

IM EKG; consider CXR

TX
- Airway, IV fluids, supplemental O_2, monitoring
- Naloxone, thiamine, glucose, charcoal (see General Evaluation and Treatment)
- Hypotension: LR or NS IV

- Dystonias: diphenhydramine (50 mg IV or IM) or benztropine (2 mg IM, repeat prn)

DI Discharge with psychiatric follow-up unless otherwise indicated

β BLOCKERS/CALCIUM CHANNEL BLOCKER OVERDOSE

KY β Blockers block adrenergic receptors and can cause hypoglycemia. Calcium channel blockers prevent movement of calcium in slow channels of the myocardium, depress SA and AV nodes, and inhibit calcium-dependent insulin release, causing hyperglycemia. Toxicities of both agents are similar; symptoms include bradycardia, depressed myocardial contractility, and hypotension. CNS effects occur secondary to hypoperfusion. Common β blockers include metoprolol and atenolol (both agents are cardioselective), labetalol, nadolol, propranolol, and esmolol and timolol. Frequently used calcium channel blockers are diltiazem, nifedipine, verapamil, and nicardipine.

HX
- Identification of drug, time of ingestion, medical and psychiatric illnesses, and current medications
- Chest pain, lethargy, nausea, and vomiting

PX
- Mental status is usually not decreased
- Bradycardia, hypotension, bradyarrhythmias, and rales (pulmonary edema)

DD Digoxin toxicity, cholinergic agents (organophosphate insecticides), cyclic antidepressant toxicity, α-methyldopa, anaphylaxis, cardiogenic shock, sepsis

LB CBC, SMA-7; consider toxicology screen

IM CXR, EKG

TX
- ABCs, IV fluids, supplemental O_2, monitoring
- Naloxone, thiamine, glucose, charcoal (see General Evaluation and Treatment)
- Bradycardia or hypotension:
   From β blockers: LR or NS IV; atropine (0.5–1 mg IV), glucagon (stimulates membrane receptors, cardiac contractility, heart rate, BP) [5 mg IV, followed by infusion of 1 mg/hr]
   From calcium channel blockers: LR or NS IV; calcium gluconate (3 g slow IV push, up to 5 g); glucagon as in β blocker overdose; pacemaker as needed

DI
- Discharge after 4–6 hours in cases of mild toxicity, with possible psychiatric consult
- ICU as needed in all other cases

CARBON MONOXIDE POISONING

KY CO is a colorless, odorless gas, with an affinity for hemoglobin 240 times that of O_2. Toxic exposure occurs as a result of smoke inhalation during fire and from improperly vented exhausts of stoves, furnaces, and automobiles. Hypoxia results from toxic exposure because of the decrease in O_2 carrying capacity. The half-life of CO in the human body after breathing room air is about 6 hours; on 100% O_2, it is only about 1.5 hours, and on 100% O_2 HBO, about 0.5 hours.

HX • Occupational exposure, use of home and business heaters, operation of automobiles, and attempted suicide
• Symptoms:
  Early symptoms (CoHb level, 10%–20%): mild headache, dyspnea on exertion, angina
  20%–30%: moderate headache, dyspnea, nausea, dizziness
  30%–40%: severe headache, vomiting, fatigue, poor judgment
  40%–50%: confusion, syncope, tachypnea, tachycardia
  50%–60%: syncope, seizures, coma
  > 60%: convulsions, respiratory failure, arrhythmias, death

PX • Decreased level of consciousness; tachycardia, tachypnea, cyanosis versus red color (rare)
• Soot around nose, lips, mouth, and stridor if involved in a fire (see Chapter 4, Environmental Emergencies, Smoke Inhalation)
• Lungs: rales or rhonchi
• MSE: confusion, poor judgment

DD Differential diagnosis for change in mental status; "TIPS AEIOU" mnemonic (see Figure 11.1)

LB CBC, CoHb level

IM CXR, EKG

TX • Airway, IV fluids, supplemental O_2, monitoring; *all* patients should receive 100% oxygen via tight-fitting nonrebreather mask or ET tube
• Psychiatric consult as appropriate

DI • Admission for all patients with CoHb level of 25%–30%; LOC; those with cardiac, pulmonary, or neurologic disease; and those with anemia
• Treatment with HBO is indicated for any period of unconsciousness, seizure activity, or a CoHb level > 35%, as well as in respiratory failure, in pregnant women who have any of the previously mentioned conditions or a CoHb level > 15%, and in infants

CAUSTIC INGESTIONS

KY The major types of caustic agents (corrosives) are acids and alkalis.

- **Acids** such as hydrochloric, sulfuric, and nitric acids are found in toilet bowel cleaners, battery acid, drain cleaners, and industrial cleaners. The result of ingestion is coagulation necrosis and burns to the distal stomach, duodenum, and jejunum.
- **Alkalis** (lye) such as sodium, potassium, and ammonium hydroxide are found in paint removers; drain and pipe cleaners; toilet bowl cleaners; dishwashing liquids; bleaches; laundry detergents; disinfectants; oven cleaners; and tile, wall, and floor cleaners. Ingestion causes liquefaction necrosis and burns with tissue penetration as well as high risk for perforation in esophagus and stomach. Household ammonia or bleach (sodium hypochlorite) is usually *not* caustic, except in large amounts.

HX
- Time, type, concentration, and amount of corrosive is important
- Symptoms include drooling, throat pain, chest pain, vomiting, abdominal pain, hematemesis, hoarseness, and shortness of breath

PX Vital sign–related symptoms: fever (alkali), hypotension (perforation)

- HEENT: soapy mucosal lesions (alkali), white/gray-white necrotic areas (acid), dysphagia, aphonia, stridor, dyspnea
- Abdominal: rigidity (perforation and peritonitis)
- Rectal: Hemoccult-positive stool

DD Foreign body ingestion, iron ingestion, esophagitis, gastritis, PUD, esophageal varices, Mallory-Weiss syndrome, Boerhaave's syndrome, perforated viscus, epiglottitis, croup, retropharyngeal abscess, malignancy

LB CBC, SMA-7, coagulation studies, UA, T&C; consider toxicology screen

IM CXR, abdominal series, lateral soft tissue radiograph of neck

TX
- Airway, IV fluids, supplemental O_2, monitoring
- Naloxone, thiamine, glucose (see General Evaluation and Treatment); charcoal is *not* indicated
- Large ingestions of acidic liquids may benefit from NG aspiration
- Analgesia (NPO) for pain control
- Emergency endoscopy for significant ingestions; immediate surgical intervention if GI hemorrhage or perforation
- Use of steroids for alkali ingestions is controversial
- Psychiatric consult as appropriate

DI ICU, immediate gastroenterology, and otolaryngology consult

COCAINE TOXICITY

KY Cocaine can be ingested, inhaled, or injected. IV use of heroin and cocaine ("speedballing") is common. This drug causes central and peripheral sympathetic stimulation, which primarily affects the CNS and cardiovascular systems. Hyperthermia results from the combined effects of increased motor and metabolic activity, vasoconstriction, and hypothalamic stimulation.

HX • Route of administration, amount ingested, time of ingestion, medical and psychiatric illnesses, and current medications; history of IV drug use, complications, and hospitalizations
  • Palpitations, chest pain, and nervousness

PX • Agitation and altered level of consciousness
  • Look for hyperthermia, tachycardia, tachypnea, hypertension, dilated pupils, rales, track marks, restlessness, paranoia, and hallucinations

DD • Toxicity due to anticholinergic agents, sympathomimetics, or hallucinogens; pheochromocytoma, hypoglycemia, drug withdrawal, thyrotoxicosis, malignant hypertension, MAO reaction, serotonin syndrome, psychiatric illness
  • Differential diagnosis for change in mental status; "TIPS AEIOU" mnemonic (see Figure 11.1)

LB CBC, SMA-7; consider toxicology screen

IM EKG

TX • Airway, IV fluids, supplemental O₂, monitoring
  • Naloxone, thiamine, glucose, charcoal for oral ingestions (see General Evaluation and Treatment)
  • Diazepam (to reduce agitation and help resolve chest pain and hypertension): 2.5–5 mg IV prn; avoid β blockers alone (for treatment of chest pain and indications of occurrence of an AMI, see Chapter 1, Cardiovascular Emergencies, Acute Myocardial Infarction)
  • Psychiatric consult as appropriate

DI • Usually discharge after 3–6 hours ED observation
  • Admission to medical floor or ICU for patients with sustained chest pain, altered vital signs, EKG changes, or AMI

CYCLIC ANTIDEPRESSANT OVERDOSE

KY Cyclic antidepressants are the leading cause of ingestion-related deaths and account for one-half of ICU admissions for drug toxicity. The major mechanisms of toxicity are blockade of sodium channels, resulting in myocardial depression, quinidine-like effects, and alpha-adrenergic blockade effects that primarily involve the cardiovascular system and the

CNS. Common cyclic antidepressants are imipramine, amitriptyline, nor-triptyline, and doxepin. Newer unicyclic and bicyclic agents such as flu-oxetine, trazodone, and bupropion block serotonin and dopamine reup-take and have fewer CNS and cardiovascular effects.

- The three primary toxic effects of cyclic antidepressant overdose are (1) hypotension, (2) cardiac arrhythmias or heart blocks, and (3) decreased level of consciousness
- Of all the patients who die from cyclic antidepressant overdose, 25% are responsive on initial presentation

HX • Identification of drug, time of ingestion, medical and psychiatric illnesses, and current medications
- Palpitations, dry mouth, slurred speech, and drowsiness

PX General: decreased level of consciousness (monitor very frequently or constantly), presentation with anticholinergic signs (see Anticholinergic Toxicity)

- Vital sign–related symptoms: hyperthermia; hypotension (monitor every 15 minutes); tachycardia; bradycardia; irregular rhythms, including unstable wide complex tachycardias
- HEENT: mydriasis, dry mouth, flushed face
- Heart: abnormal rate and rhythm
- Abdomen: decreased bowel sounds
- Neurologic symptoms: hyperreflexia, myoclonus, seizure activity
- MSE: disorientation to unresponsiveness

DD • Hypoxia; metabolic abnormalities; cardiac disease; toxicity (β blockers, propoxyphene, quinidine, procainamide, pheno-thiazines, cocaine, amphetamines, anticholinergics); withdrawal from sedative–hypnotic drugs
- Differential diagnosis of change in mental status; "TIPS AEIOU" mnemonic (see Figure 11.1)

LB CBC, SMA-7, ABG, toxicology screen

IM EKG [arrhythmias, blocks, widened QRS (QRS > 100 msec has a specificity of 75% and a sensitivity of 60% for serious complications)]; a normal EKG does *not* rule out a serious overdose

TX • Aggressive airway management with very low threshold for intu-bation; IV fluids, supplemental O_2, monitoring
- Naloxone, thiamine, glucose, charcoal (see General Evaluation and Treatment)
- For paralysis, a nondepolarizing agent such as vecuronium is pre-ferred; succinylcholine (a depolarizing agent), with more vagal effects, should be avoided
- Basis of treatment: serum alkalinization to reduce sodium channel blockade and increase plasma protein binding and excretion; either

hyperventilate the patient and/or provide $NaHCO_3$ (2 mEq/kg IV initially, then mix 3 amp in 1 L of D_5W, run at 250 ml/hr, and titrate) to maintain arterial pH of 7.5

- Hypotension: NS, $NaHCO_3$, epinephrine, norepinephrine, and phenylephrine (all IV) may be tried; dopamine and dobutamine are not usually helpful
- Seizures:

    Alkalize with $NaHCO_3$ (1–5 mEq/kg IV)

    Diazepam (5–10 mg IV)

    Phenobarbital

    Thiopental

    Consider paralysis (will not stop seizures but will halt increasing acidosis resulting from seizure activity)

    Phenytoin (has decreased efficacy in treatment of seizure caused by cyclic antidepressant toxicity; used to treat conduction defects but does not treat myoclonic jerks)

- Arrhythmias: alkalization as in seizures, with usual treatment thereafter

DI ICU for all but the most benign ingestions

- Discharge for all asymptomatic patients after 6 hours observation

DIGOXIN TOXICITY

KY The therapeutic serum digoxin level is 0.5–2.0 ng/ml. Toxicity usually results from dosing anomalies and exaggerating therapeutic effect (e.g., bradycardia, AV blocks).

HX • Time and amount of ingestion, frequency and dosage of chronic therapy; other medications and illnesses
- Acute toxicity: weakness and slow heart rate with skipped beats
- Chronic toxicity: confusion, depression, fatigue, headache, weakness, disturbances of color vision, and skipped beats

PX • General: decreased level of consciousness or confusion
- Vital sign–related symptoms: bradycardia, hypotension
- HEENT: scotoma, white colors appear yellow
- Heart: bradyarrhythmias
- Neurologic symptoms: confusion, muscle weakness, paresthesias

DD MI; cardiac disease with arrhythmia; hyperkalemia; hypokalemia; glaucoma; toxicity due to cyclic antidepressant, β blocker, or calcium channel blocker

LB CBC, SMA-7 (hyperkalemia represents acute form; hypokalemia, chronic form), serum digoxin level

IM EKG (most common arrhythmia is PVC; PSVT with block is pathognomonic)

TX
• ABCs, IV fluids, supplemental O_2, monitoring; naloxone, thiamine, glucose, charcoal (see General Evaluation and Treatment)
• Bradyarrhythmias (see Chapter 1, Cardiovascular Emergencies, Bradyarrhythmias)
• Acute ingestion, life-threatening dysrhythmias, coma, or hyperkalemia:
  Digoxin-specific Fab fragments, 10 vials IV over 30 minutes
  For chronic toxicity: body load = serum concentration × 5.6 × patient's weight (kg)/1000. Example: 4 ng/ml × 5.6 × 70 (kg)/1000 = 1.57 mg. For the number of vials required for neutralization, this figure (1.57) is divided by 0.6; the result is 3 (vials).

DI Admission to monitored bed if patient is symptomatic; ICU if unstable

HALLUCINOGEN USE

KY Common hallucinogens are PCP ("angel dust"), LSD ("acid"), peyote, mescaline, and marijuana. These substances cause sensory misperceptions and mood changes from stimulation or distortion of multiple receptor sites in the CNS. In addition, PCP results in dissociative anesthesia.

HX
• Identification of drug, time of ingestion, medical and psychiatric illnesses, and current medications
• Mood swings and bizarre behavior

PX
• Level of consciousness is not usually affected
• Vital sign–related symptoms: hyperthermia, tachycardia, tachypnea, hypertension
• HEENT: pupil size and reactivity, vertical nystagmus (PCP)
• Skin: diaphoresis (PCP) and track marks
• Neurologic symptoms: sensory loss, hyperreflexia, dystonia, ataxia, analgesia (PCP); mental status: hallucinations and/or delusions, agitation

DD Differential diagnosis for change in mental status; "TIPS AEIOU" mnemonic (see Figure 11.1); cocaine use

LB CBC, SMA-7, oximetry or ABG, UA (including myoglobin for PCP); consider toxicology screen

TX
• Airway, IV fluids, supplemental O_2, monitoring; naloxone, thiamine, glucose, charcoal (see General Evaluation and Treatment)

- Reduce environmental stimulation (e.g., dim lights, quiet room); restrain using physical and pharmacologic measures, including haloperidol (5–10 mg IV or IM q30min prn)
- For hypertension: sedate with haloperidol (5–10 mg IM q30min prn), or diazepam (5 mg IV prn)
- For rhabdomyolysis: vigorous crystalloid hydration
- Psychiatric consultation as appropriate

DI
- ICU as indicated for patients with unstable vital signs or mental status and medical floor for those with rhabdomyolysis
- Observation for several hours with discharge for mild cases

IRON (FE) TOXICITY

KY Fe is present in three major forms: ferrous compounds, vitamins with Fe, and prenatal vitamins.

- The overuse of multivitamins with Fe is the most common cause of pediatric poisoning.
    First stage (first few hours): GI symptoms, although hypotension and CNS symptoms may occur
    Second stage (up to 12 hours): asymptomatic (iron is being absorbed)
    Third stage (several hours later): impaired oxidative phosphorylation, hepatic dysfunction, obtundation, hypovolemia with hypotension, metabolic acidosis, and shock
    Fourth stage (days to weeks): gastric outlet or small bowel obstruction
- Symptoms may also follow ingestion of 20 mg/kg of elemental Fe; serious poisoning occurs at 40 mg/kg. Amounts of elemental Fe in selected Fe-containing compounds are: ferrous gluconate, 11%; ferrous sulfate, 20%; and ferrous fumarate, 33%.

HX Time and amount are important; early symptoms include abdominal pain, nausea, vomiting (occasionally hematemesis), diarrhea (sometimes black and tarry stools), weakness, lethargy, later obtundation, and seizures

PX Change in mental status, tachycardia, tachypnea, hypotension, pallor, diffuse abdominal tenderness, and increased bowel sounds

DD Aspirin and other NSAIDs, theophylline, caustics, isopropyl and ethyl alcohol (see Anion Gap Metabolic Acidosis, clinical information)

LB CBC, SMA-7, ABG, clotting studies, serum Fe (reliable if within 6 hours), TIBC (see Anion Gap Metabolic Acidosis)

IM KUB (may show radiopaque tablets)

TX • Airway, IV fluids, supplemental O_2, monitoring; consider naloxone, thiamine, glucose, gastric lavage (charcoal does not bind Fe)
   • Indications for chelation therapy (severe symptoms, serum Fe > TIBC, serum Fe > 350 µg/dl): treat with deferoxamine mesylate (15 mg/kg/hr IV infusion); do not delay treatment in symptomatic patients to wait for Fe levels

DI Admission if chelation therapy is required; ICU as necessary

NARCOTIC OVERDOSE

KY Narcotics (opioids) include morphine, codeine, heroin, propoxy-phene, meperidine, and fentanyl. They stimulate opiate receptors in the CNS, causing analgesia, euphoria, miosis, and respiratory depression.

HX • Method of administration, frequency, and other drugs
   • Previous complications such as hepatitis, pneumonia, AIDS, endo-carditis, and hospitalizations
   • Drowsiness and slurred speech

PX • Decreased level of consciousness (GCS [see Table 11.1])
   • Vital sign–related symptoms: hypothermia, bradycardia, brady-pnea, hypotension
   • Seek fever, track marks, pupillary miosis (midrange or mydriasis with diphenoxylate, meperidine, and other drugs), rales, murmurs, and other stigmata of endocarditis

DD Differential diagnosis for change in mental status ("TIPS AEIOU" mnemonic; see Figure 11.1) [see Chapter 11, Neurologic Emergencies, Altered Mental Status and Coma]; see also Sedative–Hypnotic Overdose

LB CBC, SMA-7; consider toxicology screens (serum and urine) and ABG

IM CXR and EKG prn

TX • Airway, IV fluids, supplemental O_2, monitoring; activated charcoal for oral ingestion
   • Decreased level of consciousness: after placement of restraints, administer naloxone (initial dose, 0.4–2.0 mg IV; then titrate to effect) [larger doses may be required for diphenoxylate, propoxyphene, pentazocine, and fentanyl]; give naloxone infusion (1 mg/hr) prn; thiamine (100 mg IV), 50% dextrose (1 amp IV)

DI Admission for all patients with coma and respiratory depression unre-sponsive to naloxone, persistent naloxone requirement, unstable vital signs, or fever

PETROLEUM DISTILLATES

KY Petroleum distillates (hydrocarbons) include gasoline, kerosene, lighter fluid, and mineral oil. Other less frequently ingested hydrocarbons are turpentine, diesel fuel, motor oil, toluene, xylene, benzene, and carbon tetrachloride. GI symptoms are almost always present. The most frequent adverse effect is chemical pneumonitis from aspiration. The lower the viscosity (higher volatility/gasoline, kerosene), the more likely the occurrence of aspiration. Some individuals, primarily children, experience a change in mental status or LOC.

HX • Identity, amount, and concentration of distillate, time of ingestion, symptoms present at time of ingestion, other medications, as well as past and present medical and psychiatric history
  • Vomiting almost always follows ingestion and increases likelihood of aspiration; coughing and gagging are common

PX Change in mental status, tachycardia, tachypnea, dusky appearance, oral tenderness, dysphagia, drooling, nasal flaring, stridor, coughing, wheezes, and rales

DD Corrosive ingestion, infectious gastroenteritis, food poisoning, asthma, allergic reaction, pulmonary infection, noxious gas inhalation

LB CBC, SMA-7; consider ABG and toxicology screen

IM CXR, EKG

TX • Airway management, which may need to include early intubation and PEEP, IV fluids, supplemental O_2, monitoring; naloxone, thiamine, glucose; the efficacy of charcoal is unknown
  • Gastric lavage if hydrocarbon ingestion > 2 ml/kg or toxic hydrocarbon
  • Treat bronchospasm
  • Psychiatric consult as appropriate

DI • Home if patients are asymptomatic for 6 hours and second CXR (taken after 2 hours) is normal
  • Admission for symptomatic patients; ICU as needed

PHENYTOIN TOXICITY

KY Phenytoin is an anticonvulsant and type Ib antiarrhythmic that prevents spread of abnormal electrical discharges by stabilizing neuronal membranes, inhibiting sodium channels, and decreasing the effective refractory period of myocardium. The majority of toxic cases arise from patient or caregiver dosing errors. Cardiac arrhythmias occur virtually only after IV (iatrogenic) administration.

- 20–40 µg/ml (serum): dizziness, ataxia, tremors, lethargy, nausea, vomiting, slurred speech, diplopia, blurred vision, and nystagmus
- 40–90 µg/ml (serum): confusion, psychosis, hallucinations, and decreased level of consciousness
- > 90 µg/ml: coma and respiratory depression

HX Time, amount, and preparation taken; onset of symptoms; other medications; and present and past illnesses

- Early symptoms: dizziness, nausea, vomiting, diplopia, blurred vision
- Later symptoms: confusion, psychotic behavior

PX Bradycardia, hypotension, mydriasis, nystagmus, bradyarrhythmia, ataxia, tremor, slurred speech, confusion, and hallucinations

DD Other anticonvulsive medications, sedative–hypnotic overdose, alcohol, DKA, hypoglycemia, Wernicke's encephalopathy, postictal state, cerebellar lesion or bleed

LB CBC, SMA-7, serum phenytoin level; consider toxicology screen

IM EKG

TX
- Airway, IV fluids, supplemental O_2, monitoring; naloxone, thiamine, glucose, charcoal (see General Evaluation and Treatment)
- Arrhythmias (see Chapter 1, Cardiovascular Emergencies, Arrhythmias)
- Seizures: phenobarbital (20 mg/kg IV), repeat as needed

DI Admission for all symptomatic patients, with monitoring for those whose symptoms are a result of IV phenytoin; psychiatric consultation as appropriate

SALICYLATE/NONSTEROIDAL ANTI-INFLAMMATORY DRUG (NSAID) TOXICITY

KY Aspirin (acetylsalicylic acid, ASA) and NSAIDs inhibit prostaglandin synthesis. Repeated administration of charcoal, alkaline diuresis, and hemodialysis enhance ASA elimination. Toxicity with NSAIDs is rare even with massive doses, and treatment consists of supportive care.

- **Acute aspirin poisoning** causes gastric irritation; stimulates the respiratory center, leading to hyperventilation and respiratory alkalosis; uncouples oxidative phosphorylation, resulting in fever and anion gap metabolic acidosis; and mobilizes glycogen stores, leading to hyperglycemia (*hypoglycemia* is common in children).
- **Chronic aspirin poisoning** causes lethargy, disorientation, and sometimes ARDS. The PT is elevated, but the salicylate level is usually normal.

HX • Drug identification, time of ingestion, medical and psychiatric illnesses, current medications
   • Symptoms of early toxicity: nausea, vomiting, abdominal pain, vertigo, and tinnitus
   • 12–24 hours: fever, diaphoresis, pallor, confusion, disorientation, tachycardia, and tachypnea
   • > 24 hours: cerebral edema, coma, seizures, pulmonary edema, arrhythmias, and bleeding may develop

PX • Confusion, lethargy, unresponsiveness
   • Seek fever, tachycardia, hyperpnea, hypotension, flushing or pallor, rales, stool for blood, disorientation, and presence of hallucinations

DD Theophylline toxicity, acute Fe poisoning, DKA, anxiety, cardiopulmonary disease, cerebrovascular disease, sepsis, alcohol withdrawal, meningitis, COPD; factors cited in the mnemonic "A MUDPILE CAT" (see Figure 11.1)

LB CBC, SMA-7 and ABG (to check for anion gap metabolic acidosis), PT, PTT, UA, toxicology screen, salicylate level (Done nomogram valid at 6 hours in acute ingestion of non–enteric-coated tablets/capsules)

IM EKG, CXR

TX • Airway, IV fluids, supplemental O_2, close monitoring; naloxone, thiamine, glucose, charcoal (see General Evaluation and Treatment)
   • Rehydration: 1–2 L D_5NS ± $NaHCO_3$ (1–2 amp/L) and potassium (10–20 mEq/L) over first 1–2 hours to make up preexisting deficit; then slow IV to < 500 ml/hr
   • Alkaline diuresis
      Indicated for signs of significant toxicity and acid–base abnormalities; contraindicated for cerebral or pulmonary edema, pH > 7.55, and oliguric renal failure
      $NaHCO_3$ (1–2 amp/L initially; then about 2 mEq/kg in 500 ml sterile H_2O over 2 hours); add to IV or provide separately; titrate to urine pH > 7.5
      Aggressive repletion of potassium will probably be required to achieve alkaline diuresis
   • Hemodialysis: necessary if salicylate level > 100 mg/dl, coma, seizures, cerebral/pulmonary edema, and renal failure
   • Psychiatric consultation for acute ingestions
   • Chronic poisoning:
      For prolonged PT, phytonadione (10 mg IM) [consider test dose]; can provide IV at 1 mg/min with likely higher risk of anaphylaxis (peds 0.4 mg/kg); repeat q6hr as needed
      FFP is not indicated

DI Admission for all symptomatic patients (ICU as necessary)

SEDATIVE–HYPNOTIC OVERDOSE

KY Sedative–hypnotics act by stimulating GABA synaptic inhibition in the CNS. Common benzodiazepines are diazepam, lorazepam, chlordiazepoxide, alprazolam, flurazepam, temazepam, and triazolam. Short-acting barbiturates are amobarbital, pentobarbital, and secobarbital. Long-acting barbiturates are anticonvulsants such as phenobarbital and primidone.

HX
- Identification of drug, time of ingestion, medical and psychiatric illnesses, and current medications
- Drowsiness and slurred speech

PX
- General: decreased level of consciousness (GCS)
- Vital sign–related symptoms: hypothermia (barbiturates), bradycardia, bradypnea, and hypotension
- HEENT: miosis, corneal reflex, and neck suppleness
- Lungs: rales [aspiration pneumonia (barbiturates)]
- Neurologic symptoms: serial coma scale assessments (GCS) [(see Table 11.1]

DD See mnemonic "TIPS AEIOU" for causes of coma or decreased level of consciousness (see Figure 11.1) [see also Chapter 11, Neurologic Emergencies, Altered Mental Status and Coma]

LB CBC, SMA-7; consider toxicology screen and ABG

IM CXR, EKG

TX
- Airway, IV fluids, supplemental O_2, monitoring; naloxone, thiamine, glucose, charcoal (see General Evaluation and Treatment); supportive care
- Benzodiazepine toxicity
    Consider flumazenil (antidote), a competitive inhibitor of the benzodiazepine receptor site (may induce seizure and use is controversial)
    Dose: 0.2 mg IV over 30 seconds; may repeat at 1-minute intervals (0.5 mg) to total dose of 3 mg
- Phenobarbital poisoning
    Activated charcoal q6hr × 6 doses
    Excretion enhanced by urinary alkalization (2 mEq/kg) to maintain urine pH ≥ 7.5
    Severe cases: hemodialysis or charcoal hemoperfusion

DI ICU for patients with unstable vital signs or decreased level of consciousness; psychiatric consult

CHAPTER 19

Trauma

GENERAL EVALUATION

The evaluation and management of trauma patients consists of a primary survey that involves identification and treatment of life-threatening conditions followed by a detailed secondary survey.

Primary survey (ABCs)

PX • **A (airway and cervical spine control):** perform a chin lift or jaw-thrust maneuver, and remove foreign debris; assume that a cervical spine fracture is present; maintain in-line immobilization
  • **B (breathing and ventilation):** evaluate oxygenation; supplement with bag-valve-mask ventilation or intubation as necessary; insert a chest tube prn (Table 19.1)
  • **C (circulation and hemorrhage control):** check pulses, skin color, capillary refill, and level of consciousness
  • **D (disability):** perform a neurologic assessment; use the AVPU scale (Alert, responsive to Vocal or Painful stimuli, or Unresponsive)
  • **E (exposure):** patients should be undressed completely

LB CBC, chemistry profile, UA, T&C, toxicology and alcohol screen; ABG, pregnancy test, cardiac enzymes prn

IM EKG monitoring; CXR; cervical spine and pelvic radiographs

TX **Primary management:**
  • Airway, supplemental O_2, two large-caliber IV lines, urinary and gastric catheters (contraindications to placement of urinary catheter are blood at meatus, scrotal hematoma, and high-riding or "boggy" prostate)
  • Immediate administration of thiamine, 50% dextrose, and naloxone immediately if a change in mental status occurs; reassess AVPU

Secondary survey

PX • **Eyes:** check pupil size, fundi for hemorrhage and papilledema, lens for dislocation, conjunctiva for hemorrhage, and penetration
  • **Ears:** evaluate tenderness, CSF leak, hemotympanum, and perforation

Table 19.1   Instructions for Chest Tube Insertion

1. Place the patient in a supine position, with the arm abducted > 90°. The usual insertion site is the fourth or fifth intercostal space, between the midaxillary and anterior axillary line (drainage of air or free fluid). The point at which the anterior axillary fold meets the chest wall is a useful guide. Alternatively, the second or third intercostal space, in the midclavicular line, may be used for pneumothorax drainage alone.

2. Clean the skin with iodine solution and drape. Determine the intrathoracic tube distance (lateral chest wall to the apices), and mark the tube length with a clamp.

3. Infiltrate lidocaine 1% generously into the skin, subcutaneous tissues, intercostal muscles, periosteum, and pleura using a 25-gauge needle. Use a scalpel to make a transverse 2- to 3-cm skin incision over the rib just inferior to the interspace where the tube will penetrate the chest wall.

4. Bluntly dissect a subcutaneous tunnel from the skin incision extending just over the superior margin of the lower rib using a Kelly clamp. Avoid the neurovascular bundle located at the upper margin of the intercostal space.

5. Bluntly dissect over the rib, penetrate the pleura with the clamp, and open the pleura 1 cm.

6. With a gloved finger, explore the subcutaneous tunnel and palpate the lung medially. Exclude possible abdominal penetration, and ensure correct location within the pleural space; use a finger to disrupt any local pleural adhesions.

7. Use the Kelly clamp to grasp the tip of the thoracostomy tube (36F; internal diameter, 12 mm), and direct it into the pleural space in a posterior, superior direction. Guide the tube into the pleural space until the last hole is inside the pleural space.

8. Attach the tube to an underwater seal apparatus containing sterile NS, and adjust to 20 cm H_2O of negative pressure. Suture the skin of the chest wall using 0–0 silk and tie to the tube. Apply gauze impregnated with petroleum jelly, 4 × 4-gauze sponges, and elastic tape. Obtain a CXR to verify correct placement and reexpansion of the lung.

- **Maxillofacial trauma:** stabilize the patient, and then evaluate and treat
- **Cervical/neck:** maintain in-line immobilization; evaluate for tenderness, deformity, penetrating wounds, JVD, and bruits
- **Chest:** assess breath sounds and look for deformities and penetrating wounds; insert a chest tube if necessary (see Table 19.1); check heart rate, rhythm, and tones
- **Abdomen:** inspect, auscultate, and palpate for bowel sounds, tenderness, masses, guarding, and rebound; consider DPL
- **Pelvis:** inspect and palpate for fractures; perform a genital examination
- **Rectum:** check sphincter tone; look for blood in lumen, fractures, and a high-riding prostate

- **Extremities:** inspect and palpate for fractures and penetrating trauma; evaluate pulses
- **Integument:** check for lacerations, warmth, diaphoresis, and edema
- **Back:** inspect and palpate for tenderness, fractures, and penetrating trauma
- **Neurologic status:** check for focal or lateralizing signs, assess the cranial nerves, perform a muscular and sensory examination, use the GCS to assess the level of consciousness (see Table 11.1)

IM Bedside US if available, extremity radiographs as indicated; consider CT of head, chest, abdomen, or pelvis; IVP, retrograde urethrogram, angiography as indicated

TX **Secondary management:**

- DPL
- Crystalloid: 1–2 L (peds 20 ml/kg bolus), followed by PRBCs

Airway management:

- Prevent hypercarbia, especially in patients with head injuries
- Manage the airway, deliver oxygen, and support ventilation
- Look for agitation and cyanosis, which may suggest hypoxia
- Auscultate breath sounds bilaterally; gurgling and snoring indicate occlusion of the pharynx, and hoarseness suggests laryngeal obstruction; a verbal response suggests a patent airway, intact ventilation, and adequate brain perfusion

Specific management techniques:

- **Chin lift:** place the fingers of one hand under the mandible, gently lift the chin anteriorly, and use the thumb to depress the lower lip to open the mouth; avoid hyperextension of the neck
- **Jaw thrust:** grasp the angles of the lower jaw, with one hand on each side, and displace the mandible forward
- **Suction:** use a rigid suction catheter to clear the airway
- **Nasopharyngeal airway:** insert the device into one nostril to provide passage into the hypopharynx; this prevents the tongue from falling posteriorly
- **Oropharyngeal airway:** insert the device into the mouth behind the tongue
- **ET intubation:**
    Orotracheal intubation (see Table 16.2: RSI may be required; if there is any risk of injury to the cervical spine, in-line manual cervical immobilization is necessary
    Nasotracheal intubation (see Table 16.3): commonly used with suspected cervical fractures

Table 19.2   ATLS System for the Classification of Hemorrhagic Shock

	Class			
	I	II	III	IV
Blood loss (% blood volume)	< 15	15–30	30–40	> 40
Blood loss (ml)	< 750	750–1500	1500–2000	> 2000
Pulse (bpm)	< 100	> 100	> 120	> 140
BP	Normal	Normal, with narrowed pulse pressure	Hypotensive	Hypotensive
Urinary output (ml/hr)	> 30	20–30	5–15	< 5
Mental status	Slight anxiety	Some anxiety (more than in class I)	Anxiety, confusion	Confusion, lethargy
Treatment	Crystalloid	Crystalloid	Crystalloid, blood*	Crystalloid, blood*

*Transfuse either type-specific blood (preparation time, 10 minutes) or crossmatched blood (preparation time, 60 minutes). Use type O-negative PRBCs for acute class III and IV shock.
(Adapted from American College of Surgeons: *Advanced Trauma Life Support Course for Physicians*, 5th ed. 1993, p. 86.)

- **Cricothyrotomy:** incise skin through the cricothyroid membrane, dilate with a hemostat, and insert a small ET tube or tracheostomy tube (avoid in children under the age of 12 years)
- **Jet insufflation (needle cricothyrotomy):** insert a large-caliber (12- or 14-gauge) plastic cannula into the trachea through the cricothyroid membrane below the level of the obstruction

Hemorrhagic shock: refer to Table 19.2 for the ATLS system for classification of shock.

ABDOMINAL TRAUMA

Abdominal injuries

KY Blunt trauma typically produces spleen and liver injury. Both penetrating and blunt wounds to the lower chest (nipple line anteriorly and the tip of the scapulae posteriorly) often involve the abdomen.

HX • **Blunt trauma** (e.g., from MVA): knowledge of direction and amount of forces applied; position at impact; location; seat belt type and use; damage to windshield and steering column; extrication requirements; and status of other victims
  • **Penetrating trauma:** size and length of knife; number of shots fired, type of weapon

PX • Expose and visualize entire body, perform log-roll, inspect abdomen for distention, contusions, abrasions, lacerations; auscultate for bowel sounds; palpate for signs of peritoneal irritation and focal tenderness
  • Physical examination may be unreliable; despite absence of clinical signs, dangerous pathology may be present
  • Appropriate diagnostic options such as bedside US, CT, DPL, and immediate laparotomy should be considered depending on clinical circumstances and availability of personnel, and a Foley catheter and an NG tube should be placed if no contraindications are present

LB CBC, SMA-7, amylase, lipase, T&C, UA, toxicology screen

IM • **Plain films** may detect retroperitoneal or free air, fractures, and abnormal fluid collections
  • **Contrast gastroduodenography** may be indicated in stable patients with suspected pancreaticoduodenal injury
  • **ERCP** may be indicated if pancreatic ductal injury is suspected in a patient who does not require laparotomy
  • **Contrast enemas** may be used to diagnose colorectal perforations

TX • **Stabilization:**
    Control bleeding by using direct pressure and large-bore IV lines
    Give hypotensive patients 2 L LR (peds 20 ml/kg); if no response, give O-negative blood and obtain immediate surgical intervention
    Coagulopathy should be treated with FFP (1 U) for every 4 U PRBCs, with calcium chloride (0.2 g IV) [2 ml of 10% solution] when PRBCs are transfused at a rate > 100 ml/min (max 1 g)
  • **Surgery:**
    Consult a trauma surgeon when trauma patients are anticipated in the ED or on the arrival of multiply-injured patients
    Patients in profound shock who are unresponsive to initial fluid resuscitation may require transthoracic aortic clamping followed by laparotomy
  • **Antibiotic treatment:** consider cefazolin 1 g IV or tobramycin or gentamicin (1.5 mg/kg IV) plus clindamycin (600 mg IV) or cefoxitin (1 g IV)

- **Td prophylaxis**
- **Blunt trauma–related conditions:**
  - **Acute abdomen or pneumoperitoneum:** exploratory laparotomy
  - **Nonacute abdomen:** consider bedside US, DPL, or CT (positive: consider laparotomy; negative: observation)
  - **Criteria for positive peritoneal lavage in blunt trauma:** 5 ml gross blood; RBC > 100,000 cells/mm^3; WBC > 500 cells/mm^3; food particles, bile, feces, or bacteria on Gram stain; exit of lavage fluid via a chest tube or bladder catheter
- **Penetrating trauma–related conditions:**
  - **GSW wounds to abdomen:** require exploratory laparotomy; tangential wounds may be assessed by DPL
  - **Stab wounds (unstable patients):** laparotomy for acute abdomen, signs of peritoneal injury, shock, hypotension, upper or lower GI bleeding, evisceration or pneumoperitoneum
  - **Stab wounds (stable patients):** DPL should be performed or abdominal CT obtained (see Chest Trauma) if the wound is between the fourth intercostal space and the costal margin or fasciae are involved or penetrated on local exploration; 24 hours of observation after local wound care and antibiotic treatment may be clinically appropriate if no fascial penetration is apparent on wound exploration. Laparoscopy may be considered to evaluate for diaphragmatic injury.

DI • Admission for observation and treatment; victims of multisystem trauma should remain in the hospital for 12–24 hours despite normal diagnostic studies
- After initial stabilization, transfer to a trauma center should be considered

Trauma in pregnancy

KY Abruptio placentae is the number one cause of fetal death after blunt trauma. The fetus may be in shock before the mother shows signs of shock, so adequate resuscitation is important. Treatment priorities in pregnant patients are identical to those in nonpregnant individuals. However, some important factors should be considered in the evaluation and treatment of trauma in pregnant women, including:

- **Anatomic changes:** after the 12th week of gestation, the pelvis no longer protects the uterus
- **Hemodynamic changes:** gravid patients normally have elevated cardiac output and heart rate; decreased systolic and diastolic blood pressure (5–15 mm Hg); increased plasma volume and WBC count

- **Pulmonary changes:** increased tidal volume, but no change in respiratory rate

HX See Abdominal Trauma, Abdominal Injuries

PX
- Expose and visualize entire body; perform log-roll; inspect abdomen for contusion, distention, abrasion, and laceration; auscultate for bowel sounds; and palpate for signs of peritoneal irritation and focal tenderness
- Perform a complete pelvic examination *unless* blood is present at the introitus or pelvic fracture is obvious

LB
- Kleihauer-Betke test to assess amount of fetomaternal hemorrhage and appropriate dose of Rh immune globulin for an Rh-negative mother; trauma labs as usual
- For DPL (if indicated), the open technique above the uterus should be used

IM
- Bedside US if available, pelvic US if blood at the introitus, radiographs are indicated (as usually performed)
- Fetal heart tones, tocographic monitoring

TX Unless spinal trauma is suspected, tilt the patient to her left side to prevent uterine compression of the vena cava

- Trauma workup and evaluation as previously discussed (see General Evaluation)
- Obstetric consult

DI OR or ICU admission to trauma or obstetric service as indicated; consider admission with observation with cardiotocodynamometry for 4 hours

BURNS

KY Burn management involves airway maintenance, assessment of breathing, restoration of intravascular volume, pain control, prevention of infection, evaluation of extent of injury, and appropriate referral.

HX Time and duration of contact, heat source, closed or open space, associated trauma or toxic inhalation

PX
- **Classification of burns (including depth):**
  First-degree burn (epidermis only [e.g., sunburn], with no inclusion in estimate of extent of burn injury): painful, edematous, and indurated blanching erythema
  Second-degree burn: superficial and deep partial-thickness burn, with destruction of epidermis extending to the dermis; red or mottled appearance, with swelling, blister formation, and pain

Third-degree burn: full-thickness burn, with destruction of the epidermis and dermis, extension into subcutaneous tissues, muscle, fascia, or bone; involvement of nerve fibers; translucent, waxy, mottled, leathery, charred, painless, insensate, pale or white appearance; and no blanching with pressure. Constricting full-thickness burns should be identified

- **Size of burn:** the "rule of nines" divides the adult body surface area into areas of approximately 9% each. In children, the head accounts for a larger proportion of the body surface area (Figure 19.1). (A modified Lund-Browder chart may also be used for children.)
- **Other signs:** evidence of inhalation injury (i.e., carbon deposits on the nasal and oral mucosa, carbonaceous sputum); depressed consciousness, which suggests toxic inhalation

LB CBC, SMA-7, T&C for FFP or shelf-stored plasma, CO, cyanide, PT/PTT, UA, myoglobin as indicated

IM EKG, CXR; other imaging as indicated for associated trauma

TX
- **Supportive measures:** airway, IV fluids, supplemental O_2, monitoring
- **Fluid resuscitation:** fluids are necessary for ≥ 20% TBSA; LR should be infused through an IV line (≥ 16-gauge)

  The Parkland formula may be used as a guide: 4 (ml) × body weight (kg) × area of second- or third-degree burn (%) ÷ 24 (hr) = hourly fluid requirement for the first 24 hours. One-half of the total 24-hour requirement should be administered during the first 8 hours after the injury, with the remainder given over the next 16 hours

  Vital signs and urine output should be monitored (30–50 ml/hr in adults; 1 ml/kg/hr in children who weigh < 30 kg)
- **Pain:** IV narcotics: diazepam (5–10 mg IV) [for anxiety], after circulation is stabilized
- **Airway burns:** maintain airway; give stable patients humidified, 100% high-flow oxygen by mask; intubate patients with possible unstable airway early and provide mechanical ventilation; bronchoscopy should be considered, with HBO prn
- **Tar:** cool immediately, remove with anti-infective ointments (Neosporin, Polysporin) and silver sulfadiazine ointments
- **Burn care:**

  General measures: clean with sterile saline (avoid vigorous scrubbing); remove charred epithelium and surface debris; excise ruptured blisters; apply silver sulfadiazine or gauze impregnated with antibiotic ointment

  Other measures: perform immediate escharotomy for circumferential full-thickness burns that threaten extremity circula-

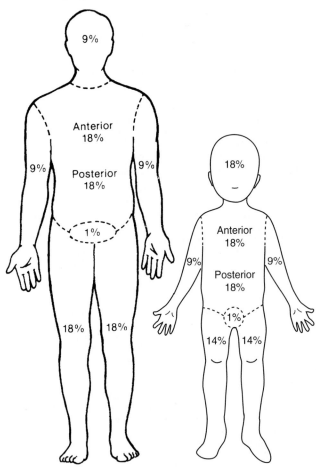

FIGURE 19.1 "Rule of nines" for estimating percent of body area burned. The area covered by a person's palm is approximately 1% of the body surface area. (Reprinted with permission from Plantz SH, Adler JN: *NMS Emergency Medicine.* Baltimore, Williams & Wilkins, 1998, p. 557.)

tion or for similar chest burns with severely decreased compliance; administer Td toxoid, place NG tube, and give antacids and IV H$_2$ blockers

DI • Outpatient care for individuals with partial-thickness burns < 15% of TBSA in adults (< 10% in children)
  • Admission to burn service for patients with full-thickness burns > 10% TBSA who are of extreme age, with involvement of face, hands, feet, or perineum or a complicating medical illness
  • Transfer to burn unit for patients with:
      Burns that involve > 25% TBSA or > 20% in children under 10 and adults over 40
      Third-degree burns that involve > 10% of TBSA and second-degree burns > 20% of TBSA
      Burns that involve the eyes, face, ears, hands, feet, or perineum, and those associated with traumatic injury

CHEST TRAUMA

Aortic disruption

KY Traumatic rupture of the aorta tends to occur at the level of the ligamentum arteriosum. This condition is associated with a 90% mortality rate at the scene of the accident; survivors usually have a contained hematoma.

HX Rapid deceleration injuries warrant a very high index of suspicion

PX Palpable first or second rib fractures, chest wall tenderness or bruises, pneumothorax or flail chest

LB CBC, SMA-7, T&C 10 U, PT

IM • CXR
      Fractures of the first or second ribs
      Tracheal deviation to the right; widened mediastinum; obliteration of the aortic knob; presence of a pleural cap; depression of the left main stem bronchus; obliteration of the space between the pulmonary artery and the aorta, elevation and rightward shift of the right main stem bronchus; deviation of the esophagus to the right as seen with NG tube
  • Chest CT, transesophageal echocardiography, or arteriogram (with surgical consult)

TX • ABCs, IV fluids, supplemental O$_2$, monitoring
  • Stat cardiothoracic surgery consult; thoracotomy prn

DI OR

Esophageal injury

KY After injury, the esophageal contents leak into the mediastinum. Immediate or delayed rupture into the pleural space (usually on left) follows, with resulting empyema.

HX
- Associated conditions (usually) include penetrating injuries to the chest, severe blunt trauma to the abdomen, or instrumentation of the esophagus with NG tube or endoscopy
- Patients may complain of chest pain or shortness of breath
- High index of suspicion is required

PX Look for signs of severe blows to the abdomen associated with pleural effusion, subcutaneous or mediastinal emphysema, and shock

LB CBC, SMA-7, T&C, PT, amylase, lipase, LFTs

IM CXR (left or sometimes right pleural effusion), Gastrogaffin swallow or endoscopic examination

TX
- **Surgical treatment,** which consists of primary repair, if feasible, or esophageal diversion in the neck and a gastrostomy
- **Empiric broad-spectrum antibiotic therapy** should be started ASAP

DI OR or ICU

Flail chest

KY Uncomplicated flail chest is usually well tolerated with no secondary hypoxia. However, major secondary dysfunction may result from disrupted mechanical chest function and possible injuries to the underlying lung parenchyma (contusion or laceration).

HX Usually secondary to severe, blunt chest injury, with multiple rib fractures

PX Freely moving rib segment without bony continuity with the rest of the chest wall; the segment moves in a paradoxical fashion with respect to the chest as a whole

LB ABG

IM CXR

TX
- Aggressive pulmonary toilet and close observation for any signs of respiratory insufficiency or associated major injuries
- Active mechanical ventilatory support of respiration if needed

DI ICU (usually)

Hemothorax

KY A massive hemothorax is defined as a blood loss of > 1500 ml into the thoracic cavity.

HX Penetrating injuries (most commonly)

PX Absence of breath sounds and dullness to percussion on the ipsilateral side; signs and symptoms of hypovolemic shock

TX • **Simultaneous decompression of chest cavity** with a chest tube and **restoration of volume deficit** (may use autotransfused blood); placement of two large-bore IVs or a central venous line
 • **Cardiothoracic surgery consult** ASAP
 • **Chest tube insertion** (see Table 19.1) at the level of the fifth or sixth intercostal space, along the midaxillary line, ipsilateral to the hemothorax; the chest tube should not be inserted on the injury site but rather in a location away from the injury
 • **Cleansing and closure of the penetrating wound** to reduce the likelihood of tension pneumothorax
 • **Consideration of thoracotomy** based on the rate of blood loss (i.e., > 200 ml/hr for 2–3 consecutive hours) rather than on the initial volume of blood loss or the color of the draining blood
   A site of wound penetration medial to the nipple anteriorly or medial to the scapula posteriorly represents a higher probability for injury to the heart and the great vessels
   If the great vessels or myocardium have been injured, shock may persist despite aggressive fluid resuscitation
 • **Consideration of tetanus prophylaxis and empirical antibiotic coverage** in cases of penetrating injuries

DI ICU (usually)

Myocardial contusion

HX Blunt trauma to chest, especially with fractures or contusion of sternum or anterior ribs

PX Chest wall tenderness, bruising, and palpable rib fractures

LB Serial cardiac enzymes

IM • EKG changes (myocardial injury, dysrhythmia, BBB)
 • Two-dimensional echocardiogram (focal or regional wall motion abnormalities)

TX • **Cardiac monitoring;** aggressive management of emerging dysrhythmias

- **Observation with supportive measures** ensuring adequate oxygenation; correction of electrolyte abnormalities

DI ICU or monitored bed

Pericardial tamponade

HX Most common secondary to penetrating injuries

PX Beck's triad: JVD, hypotension, and muffled heart sounds

DD
- Rule out other causes of cardiac tamponade (pericarditis; penetration of a central line through the vena cava, atrium, or ventricle; infection)
- Consider other causes of hemodynamic instability that may mimic the signs and symptoms of cardiac tamponade (tension pneumothorax, massive pulmonary embolism, shock secondary to massive hemothorax), especially if the patient is unresponsive to pericardiocentesis

LB CBC, SMA-7, T&C, PT

IM
- Bedside US if available
- CXR (enlarged cardiac silhouette)
- EKG [total electrical alternans, electromechanical dissociation (PEA), decreased voltage]

TX
- Pericardiocentesis (Table 19.3) is indicated if:
  Acute cardiac tamponade with hemodynamic instability is suspected and pneumothorax and hemothorax have been ruled out
  Patient is unresponsive to the usual resuscitation measures for hypovolemic shock or
  The likelihood of injury to the myocardium or one of the great vessels is high (the pericardium can be opened at thoracotomy)
- All patients with a positive pericardiocentesis (recovery of nonclotting blood) due to trauma require open thoracotomy with inspection of the myocardium and the great vessels
- Immediate cardiothoracic surgery and cardiology consult

DI ICU or OR

Pneumothorax

KY This condition, which is rarely spontaneous, commonly results from blunt or penetrating trauma (see Chest Trauma, Tension Pneumothorax).

HX Dyspnea and pleuritic chest pain

PX Tympanitic to percussion, decreased breath sounds, and subcutaneous emphysema

Table 19.3   Guidelines for Pericardiocentesis

General instructions: Protect the airway, administer O$_2$, and have intubation and cardiopulmonary resuscitation equipment available. If the patient can be stabilized, pericardiocentesis should be performed by a specialist in the OR or catheter laboratory.*

1. Use the paraxiphoid approach for pericardiocentesis in most situations. Place the patient in the supine position, and cleanse and drape paraxiphoid area.

2. Infiltrate the skin and deep tissues with lidocaine 1% with or without epinephrine (if time permits).

3. Attach a long (12–18-cm), large-bore (16–18-gauge), short-bevel cardiac needle to a 50-ml syringe with a three-way stop cock. Use an alligator clip to attach a V-lead of the EKG to the metal of the needle.

4. Paraxiphoid approach: place the needle just below the costal margin, immediately to the left and inferior to the xiphoid process. Apply suction to the syringe while advancing the needle slowly at a 30°–45° angle to horizontal toward the midpoint of the left clavicle. As the needle penetrates the pericardium, resistance will be felt, and a characteristic "popping" sensation may be noted.

5. Monitor the EKG for ST segment elevation (indicating ventricular heart muscle contact) or PR segment elevation (indicating atrial epicardial contact). After the needle comes in contact with the epicardium, withdraw the needle slightly. Ectopic ventricular beats are associated with cardiac penetration.

6. Aspirate as much blood as possible. Blood from the pericardial space usually will not clot, unlike blood that is inadvertently drawn from inside the ventricles or atrium. If fluid is not obtained, redirect the needle toward the head.

7. Stabilize the needle by attaching a hemostat or Kelly clamp.

8. Consider emergency thoracotomy to determine the cause of hemopericardium (especially with active bleeding).

*Infusion of LR, crystalloid, colloid, or blood is a temporizing measure.

DD Tension pneumothorax, hemothorax

LB CBC, SMA-7, T&C, PT

IM CXR (upright and expiratory is more sensitive)

TX • **General measures; tube thoracostomy** (see Table 19.1)

   A 36F–40F thoracostomy tube is generally used with a traumatic pneumothorax

   A smaller tube may be used with a spontaneous pneumothorax

 • **Small primary spontaneous pneumothorax** (< 10%–15%) (not associated with any known underlying pulmonary disease; no dyspnea):

   Observe for 4–8 hours and repeat the CXR

   If the pneumothorax does not increase in size and the patient remains asymptomatic, consider discharge home with instructions for rest and curtailment of all strenuous activities

Instruct patient to return to the ED if dyspnea increases or chest pain recurs

- **Secondary spontaneous pneumothorax** (associated with known underlying pulmonary pathology, most commonly emphysema), **primary spontaneous pneumothorax** (> 15%), or **presence of symptoms:**

  Give high-flow oxygen

  Consider needle aspiration of the pneumothorax using a 16-gauge needle with an internal polyethylene catheter; insert in the anterior, second intercostal space in the midclavicular line

  Otherwise, insert a chest tube (see Table 19.1)

  Anesthetize and prepare the area before inserting the needle. Attach a 60-ml syringe via a three-way stopcock, and aspirate until no more air is aspirated.

  When no additional air can be aspirated and the volume is < 4 L, occlude the catheter and observe for 4 hours. If symptoms abate and the CXR does not show recurrence of the pneumothorax, the catheter can be removed, and the patient can be discharged home with instructions for rest and curtailment of all strenuous activities.

  If the volume is > 4 L and additional air is aspirated without resistance, this suggests an active bronchopleural fistula with continued air leak

  Admission is required for insertion of a chest tube and evaluation (see Table 19.1)

- **Traumatic pneumothorax** associated with penetrating or blunt thoracic injury, hemothorax, mechanical ventilation, and tension pneumothorax

  Give high-flow oxygen and insert a chest tube (see Table 19.1); do not delay the management of the tension pneumothorax until radiographic confirmation is obtained

  Perform aggressive hemodynamic and respiratory resuscitation as indicated

DI - Admission to trauma surgery service for trauma patients; obtain surgical consult for others

- Home with a unidirectional valve device (e.g., Heimlich) for some patients with spontaneous pneumothorax

Pulmonary contusion

KY Diagnosis is usually delayed because respiratory failure develops over time. Severe forms of this injury may be indistinguishable from ARDS.

HX Chest trauma

PX Chest wall tenderness, bruises, and palpable fractures

LB ABG

IM CXR (localized alveolar and or interstitial infiltrate, usually underlying the site of blunt injury or within the trajectory of the penetrating injury)

TX • Intubation is required whenever respiratory failure is severe or associated medical conditions [e.g., preexisting chronic pulmonary disease, renal failure, abdominal injury, head trauma with secondary depressed level of consciousness, prolonged immobilization (primarily secondary to skeletal injuries)] predispose to early intubation

DI ICU; conservative management in a critical care unit, with close observation, may be considered

Tension pneumothorax

HX Blunt or penetrating chest trauma

PX • Severe hemodynamic or respiratory compromise
• Specific signs: contralateral deviated trachea; decreased or absent breath sounds and hyperresonance to percussion on the affected side; JVD; asymmetrical chest wall motion with respiration; flattening or inversion of the ipsilateral hemidiaphragm; contralateral shifting of the mediastinum; flattening of the cardiomediastinal contour, and spreading of the ribs on the ipsilateral side

DD Pericardial tamponade

LB CBC, SMA-7, PT, PTT, T&C, toxicology screen

IM CXR

TX • Insert chest tube immediately (see Table 19.1); consider temporary ipsilateral placement of a large-bore IV catheter into the pleural space at the level of the second intercostal space at the midclavicular line until the chest tube is placed
• Insert two large-bore IV lines
• Consider CVP monitoring and arterial line
• Consider intubation if indicated

DI Trauma surgery service or OR, if indicated; arrange for cardiothoracic exploration with penetrating chest injury, persistent air leak, severe or persistent hemodynamic instability despite aggressive fluid resuscitation, or persistent active blood loss from the chest tube

Tracheobronchial injury

HX • Penetrating or blunt injuries to the upper torso, especially deceleration injuries
• Hoarseness, hemoptysis

PX Subcutaneous emphysema, palpable fracture, and crepitus

DD Associated injuries to the esophagus, carotid arteries, or jugular veins; tension pneumothorax (especially with large air leak through chest tube); abnormal breathing suggestive of airway obstruction

IM CXR (may show pneumomediastinum), chest CT, arteriogram

TX • Secure airway and ventilation
• Relieve tension pneumothorax
• Obtain early surgical correction of large vessel injury or esophageal disruption

DI OR or ICU

FACIAL TRAUMA

Dental trauma

KY Dental trauma may result in several tooth-related problems, including subluxation, which is the abnormal loosening of a tooth; displacement, which is partial to total tooth avulsion; and fracture, which may involve enamel, dentin, or pulp. Permanent teeth should be replaced as quickly as possible. For each minute the tooth is absent from the oral cavity, tooth survival decreases 1%.

HX **Important information:** knowledge about how, when, and where the trauma occurred, as well as the resulting treatment; past dental history
  Symptoms: pain, sensitivity to touch or temperature

PX Perform digital examination; check jaw/TMJ function, occlusion, fracture, tooth coloration, and soft tissue trauma

IM Radiographs: consider Panorex, soft tissue, or peripheral views

TX • Table 19.4 presents treatment guidelines for the specific types of dental trauma
• Transport teeth in mouth, milk, isotonic saline, or specialized solution

DI See Table 19.4

Eye trauma

HX Mechanism, environment, preexisting ocular disease, corrective lens or contact lens use, pain, photophobia, and vision loss

Table 19.4   Treatment Guidelines in Dental Trauma

Type of Trauma	Primary Teeth	Permanent Teeth
Subluxation	No stabilization; soft diet; dental follow-up	No stabilization; soft diet; dental follow-up
Displacement	Extraction if: • exfoliation will occur within 6 months or tooth is intruded and close to a permanent tooth • extruded tooth is allowed to reerupt	Nonmobile: no treatment; referral to dentist Mobile: repositioning; temporary stabilization
Avulsion	No reimplantation	Cleansing of tooth and socket (*no scrubbing*); reimplantation ASAP
Fracture (crown)	Hemostasis; pain control; removal of tooth fragment to prevent aspiration; referral to dentist	Same as for primary teeth
Root	Apical and middle one-third: repositioning; stabilization; referral to dentist Coronal one-third: crown removal; protection; stabilization; referral to dentist	Same as for primary teeth
Dentoalveolar	Repositioning; stabilization; removal of bone fragments; referral to dentist	Same as for primary teeth

PX • **Visual acuity:** ideally, check with Snellen chart; otherwise, check ability to read (record distance), count fingers, or differentiate light from dark
   • **Ocular anatomy:** eyelids; globe (fracture or penetration); orbit (step-off deformity and crepitus); pupil (size and shape); cornea (opacity, ulceration, and foreign bodies); conjunctiva (chemosis, subconjunctival emphysema, hemorrhage, and foreign bodies); anterior chamber (hyphema); iris (regular shape or reactive); lens (check displacement); vitreous (transparent unless hemorrhage); and retina (hemorrhage, tears, and detachment)

LB Visual field, slit-lamp, and funduscopic examination

IM CT of orbital soft tissues may be helpful

TX Management of injuries at various sites:

- **Lid:** ophthalmologic consult for wounds involving the medial canthus, injury to lacrimal sac or duct, horizontal lacerations of the upper lid that may involve the levator, and lacerations of the lid margins; superficial lid lacerations may be closed
- **Cornea:**
  For superficial abrasions: pain medication, antibiotic ointment (sulfacetamide, neomycin, bacitracin, polymyxin, and gentamicin), short-acting cycloplegic, and close follow-up
  Foreign bodies: removal with irrigation or extraction using slit-lamp biomicroscopy
  For anterior chamber hyphema: patching, hospitalization, upright bed rest, analgesics, and ophthalmologic referral
- **Lens displacement:** immediate ophthalmologic consult
- **Vitreous hemorrhage:** bed rest with patching and ophthalmologic referral
- **Retinal hemorrhage** (white, cloudy discoloration): ophthalmologic referral
- **Globe penetration:** immediate ophthalmologic referral
- **Chemical injury:** immediate irrigation with copious and continuous saline until pH = 7.4; immediate ophthalmologic referral
- **Orbital fracture:** careful examination for evidence of entrapment; ophthalmologic referral
- **Retrobulbar hematoma:** immediate lateral canthotomy or ophthalmologic referral if immediately available

Le Fort's fractures

KY Le Fort's fractures, which are fractures along characteristic midfacial fracture lines, result from blunt trauma. In all Le Fort's fractures, the jaw is free-floating.

PX Le Fort's fracture types:

- **Type I fracture** (horizontal maxillary fracture)
  Grasping the alveolar process between the index finger and thumb causes anterior–posterior motion
  Movement of the premaxilla signifies at least a type I fracture
- **Type II fracture** (pyramidal fracture)
  Inspection may reveal significant midfacial swelling, bilateral subconjunctival hemorrhages, periorbital ecchymosis, epistaxis, or CSF rhinorrhea (a result of a cribriform plate fracture)
  The diagnosis can be confirmed by gently holding the upper dental arch while palpating the base of the nose

- **Type III fracture** (craniofacial dysjunction, with a fracture line extending from the frontozygomatic sutures, across the orbits, and through the base of the nose and the ethmoid bones)

    Patient may have periorbital ecchymosis, with "dishface" features

    The diagnosis can be confirmed if there is movement of the zygomas and midfacial area

LB If CSF rhinorrhea, analysis of CSF fluid for glucose

IM Radiographs with Water's projections or CT of face required for all three types of Le Fort's fractures; CT of the orbits to help confirm the diagnosis of fracture types II and III

TX
- Any patient with suspected CSF leakage requires a neurosurgical consult prior to a maxillofacial surgery consult
- Tetanus and antibiotic prophylaxis should be administered

DI Admission versus outpatient treatment depends on ENT, ophthalmology, or neurosurgery consults

Mandibular fractures

KY The mandible is a "ring"-type bony structure, and thus examiners should look for two fractures. The most common area of fracture involves the angle of the mandible. Mandibular fractures are classified according to location: alveolar, condylar, angle, and body. Alveolar fractures are the most common type.

PX
- **Signs and symptoms:** malocclusion, bony crepitus, pain, deformity and deviation, and limited ROM
- **Extraoral examination:** possible swelling, ecchymosis, bony crepitus or step-off deformity, and point tenderness; test for anesthesia of the lower lip
- **Intraoral examination:** possible blood, malalignment or deformity of the dental arches or teeth; check for breaks in the mucosa and hematomas, especially of the sublingual area, and test for complete ROM

LB CBC, SMA-7, T&C

IM Radiographs: panoramic view of the maxilla and the mandible or otherwise, the standard three views (posterior–anterior view of the face and skull plus left and right lateral oblique views)

TX
- **General principles:**
    Restoration of form
    Restoration of function
- **Specific measures:**
    NPO; preserve all teeth and orthodontic devices

Tetanus prophylaxis
Antibiotic treatment (penicillin, cephalosporin, or clindamycin)
- **Definitive treatment** per oral surgeon:
Internal fixation
Alveolar fractures require stabilization via arch bars or wires

DI Per oral surgical consult

Midfacial fractures

KY Definitive treatment occurs within several days; ED treatment is supportive. Avulsed teeth should be reimplanted ASAP, however.

PX • **Zygomatic arch fracture:** depression of bone; patient may not be able to open or close mouth
- **Zygomatic–maxillary complex:** swelling/ecchymosis of the cheek or periorbital area, facial depression, unilateral epistaxis, anesthesia of the infraorbital nerve (cheek, upper lip, and teeth), diplopia, lateral subconjunctival hemorrhage, restriction of mandibular movements, and tissue crepitus; possible marked tissue edema
  Test for visual acuity and EOM
  Perform slit-lamp and funduscopic examination prn
- **Orbital floor fractures:** diplopia and inferior displacement of the globe, restriction of ocular movements secondary to tissue entrapment in the maxillary sinus
  Check lids for foreign bodies, orbital rims for edema/hemorrhage, corneas for abrasions, and sclera for tears
  Inspect anterior chamber for hyphema and the iris, lens, posterior chamber and retina for trauma

IM Radiographs:
- **Zygomatic arch:** basal skull view (jug-handle view and submental–occipital view)
- **Zygomatic–maxillary complex:** Water's projection and basal skull view; confirmation and further evaluation of the orbital and maxillary fractures may require tomograms
- **Orbital floor fractures:** Water's view and tomograms

TX • **Zygomatic arch fracture:** delayed surgical intervention for cosmetic defect or mandibular dysmobility
- **Zygomatic–maxillary complex:** open reduction and wire fixation or antral packing
- **Orbital floor fractures:** surgical reconstruction of the orbital floor

DI Per surgical consult

HEAD TRAUMA

KY Blunt trauma to the head is much more common than penetrating trauma. Brain injury from blunt trauma may result from axonal sheer; cerebral contusion; secondary edema; and subdural, epidural, or subarachnoid hemorrhage.

- **Increased ICP** may lead to herniation of the uncus adjacent to the edge of the tentorium, thus compressing the adjacent third cranial nerve and causing dilation of the ipsilateral pupil. As the ICP continues to rise, dilation of the contralateral pupil occurs with cessation of spontaneous respiration because of bilateral interruption of the pathways in the cerebral peduncles.
- **Subdural hematomas,** which are more common in elderly individuals, have a gradual onset of symptoms. Torn cortical vessels from contusions or cortical lacerations usually cause acute subdural hematomas. Tearing of bridging veins is associated with chronic subdural hematoma.
- **Epidural hematomas** are typically associated with a brief LOC, a "lucid interval," and then neurologic deterioration. Rapid accumulation of hematoma due to meningeal artery tearing results in rapid rise of ICP, ipsilateral uncal herniation, and compression of the peduncle and third cranial nerve. Survival depends on immediate surgical decompression.

HX Mechanism of injury, presence and duration of LOC, presence of a "lucid interval", PMH, and drug intake

PX
- Assume a cervical spine injury in all patients with multisystem trauma, especially those with injuries involving the head; *a normal neurologic examination does not rule out a cervical spine injury*
- Perform a mini-neurologic examination ASAP, and repeat frequently

    Use the GCS to determine level of consciousness (see Table 11.1) [score: < 8, severe head injury; 9–12, moderate head injury; 13–15, minor head injury]

    Evaluate lateralizing extremity weakness or changes in sensation and pupillary function

    Examine the skull for skull fracture

    Check for hemotympanum, ecchymosis over the mastoid process (Battle's sign), periorbital ecchymosis ("raccoon's eyes), and CSF rhinorrhea or otorrhea (signs associated with basilar skull fracture)

LB CBC, PT, PTT, Chem-7, T&C, toxicology screen

IM CT of brain; indications include:

- Transient or persistent unconsciousness with evidence of head injury or coma
- Skull fractures, including depressed and basilar fractures

TX • **General management:**

Airway, IV fluids, supplemental O_2, cardiac monitoring

Keep patient NPO

Treat shock aggressively with volume resuscitation, and search for underlying causes (head injuries do not usually cause shock except in terminal stages)

IV solutions for resuscitation should be isotonic (LR or NS)

Except for shock management, consider restricting fluid intake to maintenance levels or as indicated by hemodynamic monitoring

Emergency intubation may be indicated, usually with RSI (particular concern for ICP) for airway control with or without hyperventilation (see Table 16.1)

The intubation should be performed with in-line immobilization; cricothyrotomy prn

- **Other considerations:**

Consider hyperosmolar therapy [e.g., mannitol (1 g/kg IV push)] or hyperventilation (maintain P_{CO_2} at 30 mm Hg)

If seizures occur, treat with lorazepam (4–8 mg IV push); repeated until seizures are controlled; follow with phenytoin (17 mg/kg IV loading dose) at 50 mg/min

Analgesia and sedation as necessary

Clean and repair open head wounds

Give tetanus prophylaxis

DI Patients with minor concussions may be eligible for discharge home with head injury instructions, provided adequate support is available and return is possible

All other patients should be admitted for observation and ICU or OR per neurosurgical consult

SPINAL CORD TRAUMA

KY Assume the occurrence of spinal cord trauma until proven otherwise. Maintain spine immobilization until radiographs have ruled out fractures or dislocations; in selected patients, it may be possible to "clear" the cervical spine clinically.

HX Mechanism of injury, motor and sensory complaints, and pain

PX Avoid moving the patient; palpate for tenderness and deformity, and perform a complete motor and sensory examination

- **Tract dysfunction:**
    Corticospinal tract injuries: characterized by motor deficit on the
        same side of the body; test by voluntary muscle contractions or
        involuntary response to pain
    Spinothalamic tract injuries: characterized by decreased pain and
        temperature sensation contralateral to the injury; test by pin
        prick or pinch
    Posterior column injuries: characterized by proprioceptive deficit
        on the ipsilateral side; test by position sense of fingers and toes
        or tuning fork vibration
    Cervical cord injuries: findings may include flaccid areflexia,
        especially rectal sphincter; diaphragmatic breathing; priapism;
        hypotension with bradycardia; ability to flex but not extend the
        elbow; and pain above but not below the clavicle
- **Neurogenic shock** (particularly associated with cervical or high
    thoracic injury): loss of neurologic function and autonomic tone
    results in vasodilation; hypotension and bradycardia may occur
    Flaccidity and loss of reflexes are present initially
    Spinal shock may gradually disappear over days to weeks, and
        spasticity may replace the flaccid state
- **Spinal fractures** (Table 19.5)
- **LB** CBC, SMA-7, PT, T&C, toxicology screen
- **IM** • **Radiographs:** films should be examined for the AP diameter of the
    spinal canal; the contour and alignment of the vertebrae; and the
    presence of bone fragments, fractures, and soft tissue swelling
    Cervical spine: AP, oblique cervical, open-mouth (odontoid),
        cross-table lateral views (a swimmer's view may be required
        for the lower cervical vertebrae); all seven cervical vertebrae
        must be identified

Table 19.5   Spinal Fractures

Type of Fracture	Description	Mechanism
C1 (atlas)	Unstable (Jefferson fracture)	Axial load, "blowout" of ring
C2 (axis)	Stable or unstable (hangman's fracture)	Extension or compression
C3–C7	Stable or unstable	Flexion, extension, axial loading
T2–T10	Stable or unstable	Usually hyperflexion
Thoracolumbar	Stable or unstable	Usually hyperflexion and rotation
Lumbar	Stable or unstable	Usually hyperflexion

    Thoracic region: AP, lateral views
    Lumbar region: AP, lateral, oblique views
- CT scan may be necessary for definitive evaluation of suspected injuries

TX
- Immobilization on firm surface
- Treat shock with IV crystalloid
- Neurogenic shock:
    Pressors may be required
    Place patient in Trendelenburg's position
- Neurosurgery consult
- Steroids are indicated for penetrating spinal cord trauma and may be considered for blunt injury: methylpredisolone (30 mg/kg/hr for the next 23 hours)
- Placement of halo vest by orthopedic specialist or neurosurgeon for spinal stabilization
- Placement of Gardner-Wells tongs by neurosurgeon for cervical traction resulting from cervical dislocation

DI ICU

CHAPTER 20

Urogenital Emergencies

ACUTE URINARY RETENTION

KY Urinary retention is the inability to urinate. This problem primarily affects adult men.

- **Common causes:** BPH (most frequent); prostatic carcinoma, bladder carcinoma, urethral stricture, spinal cord disease or trauma, and blood clots
- **Uncommon causes:** phimosis, paraphimosis, urethritis, urethral calculus, foreign body, or medications (primarily anticholinergics but also narcotics, phenothiazines, sympathomimetics, cyclic antidepressants, antihistamines, antihypertensives, and muscle relaxants)

HX
- Low abdominal pain and inability to void
- Possible history of medication, neurologic disease or trauma, and occurrence of previous episodes

PX
- Abdominal examination: palpate for tenderness and distention of suprapubic region
- Rectal examination: check prostate size and consistency
- Pelvic examination: check for masses and tenderness
- Neurologic status: check for presence of abnormalities (e.g., saddle anesthesia, loss of rectal tone)

LB UA, C&S, CBC, SMA-7

TX
- Pass 16F Foley catheter (larger with many blood clots)
- Pass three-way catheter and perform bladder lavage with Murphy drip for gross hematuria
- If unable to pass Foley catheter, then try a 16F catheter coudé
- If still unable to pass this, try another size, obtain urologic consult, or perform suprapubic catheterization (treat UTI as indicated; see Chapter 9, Infectious Disease Emergencies, Cystitis and Pyelonephritis)

DI
- Consider admission to urology service for acute retention
- Possible discharge home with catheter and leg drainage bag for chronic conditions

DIALYSIS-RELATED EMERGENCIES

KY Patients with chronic renal failure may have a surgically created arteriovenous fistula or artificial vascular graft placed in the arm, and dialysis is performed for several hours several times per week. These patients are at increased risk for cardiac disease, including noninfectious pericarditis. *The involved arm should not be used for BP measurements, IV access, or blood drawing.*

HX Common complaints: faintness and dizziness, particularly after dialysis; shortness of breath, chest pain, bleeding, pain and swelling at the access site, and constipation

PX • **BP:**

Hypotension generally occurs during and immediately after dialysis

Hypertension is usually the result of volume overload, indicating the need for dialysis

• **Chest:** cardiac rhythm and heart sounds; friction rub; dyspnea, which may signify volume overload; and rales, which may indicate pneumonia or CHF

• **Access site:**

Bruising and bleeding from the site may be the result of thrombocytopenia

Loss of a thrill indicates possible thrombosis

Infection is common; signs are a warm red arm and fever

LB CBC, SMA-7, blood culture (if fever and infection are suspected)

IM EKG (peaked T waves and/or widened QRS suggest hyperkalemia; diffuse upward concave ST elevations indicate pericarditis), CXR

TX Airway, IV fluids, supplemental O_2, monitoring

Hypotension usually responds to infusion of NS; vasopressors are seldom necessary

Hypertension and dyspnea

O_2: 4 L/min by nasal cannula (6 L by mask)

NTG (to reduce preload and afterload): 0.4 mg SL q30min prn

Sodium nitroprusside (for severe hypertension): 0.5 µg/kg/min, titrated to DBP > 100 mm Hg

Dialysis may be indicated

• Cardiac arrhythmias, pulmonary edema, and bleeding abnormalities are treated in the standard fashion (see Chapter 1, Cardiovascular Emergencies, Arrhythmias; Chapter 8, Hematologic/Oncologic Emergencies; and Chapter 16, Pulmonary Emergencies)

• Pericarditis usually does not result in cardiac tamponade, and pericardiocentesis is rarely necessary

- Infection of access site: vancomycin (1 g IV) loading dose; thrombosis of access site: immediate surgical consult
- Severe hyperkalemia (EKG manifestations, chest pain, and/or K^+ level > 7.5 mEq/L): calcium gluconate 10% solution (10 ml over 5 minutes), followed by 50% glucose (50 ml) plus regular insulin (20 U) and $NaHCO_3$ (50 mEq IV); definitive treatment is dialysis
- Constipation usually responds to docusate sodium: 200 mg PO daily

DI Admission to medical service and emergency dialysis for volume overload and/or pulmonary edema

EPIDIDYMITIS

KY Epididymitis, the infection and/or inflammation of epididymis from retrograde spread of organisms up the vas deferens, is the most common cause of acute scrotal mass in adult men. Etiologic factors are STDs, chronic prostatitis, and urethral instrumentation. In men < 35 years of age, the causal organisms are *Chlamydia trachomatis and Neisseria gonorrhoeae;* in men > 35 years of age, the causal organisms are *Escherichia coli,* enterococci, *Pseudomonas,* and *Proteus.*

HX
- Acute onset of scrotal pain and swelling on one side over several hours; severe pain in the posterior testicle that is relieved by elevation
- Sometimes earlier history of STD and/or penile discharge; intercourse with new sexual partners

PX
- Check for fever
- Palpate for abdominal tenderness and auscultate for bowel sounds
- Observe for penile discharge, genital lesions, hernia, and lymphadenopathy
- Gently palpate both testes with the patient lying and standing; the affected testis is low-riding, with posterior induration and point tenderness over the area of the epididymis

DD Testicular torsion, orchitis, torsion of appendix testis, tumor, hernia

LB UA (usually shows pyuria or bacteriuria), urine C&S, CBC, blood culture (if sepsis suspected)

IM Scrotal US may confirm the diagnosis and rule out torsion

TX
- Ceftriaxone: 250 mg IM once plus
  Doxycycline: 100 mg bid ×10 days
- Antibiotics appropriate for UTI for those age > 35

DI
- Admission to medical or urologic service for febrile, toxic-appearing patients

- Outpatient management for other patients, with urologic consultation in several days

HEMATURIA

KY Hematuria is defined as > 5 RBCs per HPF in a 10-ml urine sediment. (Urine dipstick detects < 5 RBCs.) Most cases of hematuria result from UTIs, but sudden, severe back pain suggests ureteral stones.

- Most common causes: < 20 years of age, UTI and GN; > 20 years, UTI and ureteral stones; > 50 years, UTI, stones, BPH, bladder and kidney cancer
- Renal causes: IgA nephropathy (Berger's disease); GN (from streptococcal infection, SLE, Goodpasture's syndrome, vasculitis); pyelonephritis; trauma; tumors (renal epithelial or vascular); SBE
- Lower urinary tract causes: calculus, tumor, infection, prostatitis
- Hematologic causes: coagulopathy, sickle cell disease
- Other causes: rupture of AAA or renal artery aneurysm cyclophosphamide; foreign bodies; Henoch-Schönlein purpura; blood clots, which can cause secondary obstruction

HX
- Fever, dysuria, frequency, urgency, and retention, which suggest hemorrhagic cystitis and pyelonephritis
- Renal colic pain, which indicates calculus or mimicking of AAA
- History of sickle cell disease and coagulopathy or anticoagulant use, which suggests a hematologic etiology
- Lack of significant history, which may indicate neoplasm
- Streptococcal pharyngitis within the past few weeks, which suggests GN

PX
- Fever, tachycardia, and ill appearance, which suggest an infectious cause; consider malignancy if age > 40 years
- Mass or bruit on abdominal examination, which suggests renal artery aneurysm or AAA
- Prostate tenderness, which suggests prostatitis

DD Pigmenturia caused by porphyria, myoglobin, free Hgb, beets, rhubarb, and some medications

LB
- CBC, SMA-7, UA
  - RBC casts (suggest GN, SLE, SBE)
  - WBCs (suggest infection); WBC casts (suggest pyelonephritis)
  - Proteinuria (suggests pyelonephritis, GN, nephrotic syndrome); if GN is suspected, especially in children, check for the other components of nephritis syndrome (e.g., edema, hypertension, renal insufficiency)

IM IVP (appropriate in the ED to evaluate hematuria after trauma or for suspected renal stones) or CT (for suspected renal stone or aneurysm)

TX Treatment according to etiology; place a three-way catheter and perform bladder irrigation with Murphy drip for gross hematuria or hematuria with urinary retention

DI • Admission for cases complicated by severe illness, dehydration, renal insufficiency or failure, diabetes, or obstruction, and new GN; possible cancer or ongoing bleeding may also require inpatient evaluation and intervention
   • Outpatient management for further evaluation for other cases

PROSTATITIS

KY Prostatitis, an inflammation of the prostate gland, may be acute or chronic. Most cases are caused by bacterial infection with the same organisms that cause UTIs: *E. coli* (most common), *Pseudomonas,* and enterococci. Chronic prostatitis is the most common cause of recurrent UTI in men; in some chronic cases, however, cultures are negative. Younger men are more apt to have acute prostatitis, whereas older men are more likely to have chronic prostatitis with exacerbations.

HX • **Acute prostatitis:** fever, chills, dysuria, frequency, and urgency; recent onset of low back or groin pain
   • **Chronic prostatitis** (exacerbations): low-grade fever, chronic low back pain, frequency, and dysuria
   • **Useful information:** inquire about penile discharge, genital lesions, sexual partners, previous episodes and recent urinary catheterization

PX • Check for fever
   • Palpate abdomen, flanks, lumbar region for tenderness (suprapubic or CVA tenderness)
   • Examine genitalia for urethral discharge, lesions, and inguinal adenopathy; palpate testes for swelling, tenderness, or masses
   • Perform rectal examination to check prostate (tender and soft in acute prostatitis; slightly tender with normal consistency in chronic prostatitis); *do not massage the prostate gland,* because bacteremia may occur

DD Epididymitis, orchitis, renal colic, UTI

LB CBC, UA, urine C&S, blood culture (if applicable)

TX • **Acute prostatitis:** gentamicin (1–2 mg/kg IV load) plus ampicillin (2 g IV); ciprofloxacin or ofloxacin (200 mg IV) may be used

- **Chronic prostatitis:** ciprofloxacin (250 mg PO tid × 4 weeks) or ofloxacin (200 mg bid × 4 weeks)

DI • Admission (usually) to medical floor for acute prostatitis
- Outpatient therapy with urology consult for chronic prostatitis

RENAL COLIC

KY Renal colic is severe pain from obstruction of urinary outflow tract by one or more calculi. A large majority (80%) of these stones are calcium salts that are commonly associated with dehydration.

HX • **Symptoms:** abrupt onset of severe abdominal or flank pain, usually at night or early morning; the pain, which is usually intermittent, is sometimes accompanied by nausea and vomiting
- **Useful information:** inquire about a family history of stones

PX • Appearance: patient writhing in pain; unable to find comfortable position; may prefer standing position, leaning on gurney (a patient with peritonitis lies curled up and motionless, because any movement aggravates pain)
- Vital sign–related conditions: tachypnea, tachycardia, and hypertension related to discomfort
- Abdomen:
  Moderate abdominal or flank tenderness over the site of obstruction; no point tenderness or rebound; sometimes decreased bowel sounds
  Search carefully for bruits and pulsatile mass (see differential diagnosis)

DD • **Most common:** pancreatitis, biliary colic, pyelonephritis, bowel obstruction, appendicitis
- **Less common:** perforated peptic ulcer or diverticulum, ruptured abdominal aorta (in elderly patients, renal colic must be differentiated from a leaking or ruptured abdominal aortic aneurysm, which is a lethal condition), mesenteric artery occlusion, cervical cancer, endometriosis

LB UA (almost always contains a large amount of blood), CBC, SMA-7

IM KUB (many calcium stones evident on plain film), IVP (shows delayed filling and dilatation on involved side), spiral stone CT, renal US prn

TX • IV fluids, supplemental O_2, monitoring prn
- Pain control
  Meperidine: 25–50 mg IV q10min or 50–100 mg IM q3–6hr
  Alternatively, consider ketorolac: 30 mg IM or 10 mg IV or morphine 3–5 mg IV and titrate
- Hydration with IV NS

DI • Admission for infection and/or fever, high-grade obstruction, and intractable pain, with urologic consult for stones > 6 mm
   • Discharge home with acetaminophen with codeine or NSAIDs; increase fluids and strain all urine; follow-up in 2 days

RENAL FAILURE

KY In renal failure, the kidneys no longer adequately filter nitrogenous wastes, leading to azotemia with accumulation of urea and creatinine in the bloodstream.

HX Few specific symptoms:
   • Acute abdominal pain with nausea and vomiting, which may suggest a prerenal cause
   • Acute onset of oliguria [decreased urine output (< 500 ml/day)], high BP, and shortness of breath, which may represent nephritis
   • Oliguria plus suprapubic pain, which may indicate a postrenal cause

PX • Appearance: note skin turgor, color, and edema
   • Vital signs: check for hypotension or hypertension; cardiac and respiratory signs [e.g., rub (uremia), rales (CHF and volume overload)]
   • Abdomen: abdominal and flank tenderness, which may suggest a postrenal cause; listen for bruit, suggesting vascular etiology
   • Prostate and pelvis: evaluate for masses

DD • **Prerenal causes:** reduction in cardiac output (CHF, cirrhosis), hypovolemia (fluid loss)
   • **Renal causes:** ATN secondary to shock, hemorrhage, and some antibiotics; acute interstitial nephritis from drugs, including some antibiotics, and NSAIDs
   • **Postrenal causes:** obstruction of collecting system, urethra, bladder, and ureters

LB CBC, SMA-7, Ca, phosphate, BUN, UA, urine sediment (measurement of urinary and serum Na primarily helpful outside of ED)

IM EKG, CXR

TX • **Supportive measures:** airway, IV fluids, supplemental O_2, monitoring prn
   • **Prerenal causes:** NS or LR (rapid infusion) for hypovolemia
   • **Renal causes:** dialysis; low-dose dopamine (may increase renal blood flow in ATN): 2 µg/kg/min
   • **Postrenal causes:** Foley catheter (may relieve bladder outlet obstruction)

DI Admission to medical floor

TESTICULAR TORSION

KY Testicular torsion is twisting of the spermatic cord and testis, thus occluding the venous system and decreasing arterial flow. This condition commonly occurs in puberty (average age, 17 years). The cause relates to an abnormally developed tunica vaginalis. *To salvage a testis, detorsion must occur in < 6 hours.*

TX
- Sudden onset of pain in the scrotum, which may radiate to the abdomen; sometimes nausea and vomiting
- Possible history of previous milder attacks

PX
- Palpate the abdomen for tenderness; auscultate for bowel sounds
- Observe for penile discharge, genital lesions, hernia and lymphadenopathy
- Gently palpate both testes with the patient lying and standing; the affected testis is tender, high-riding, slightly swollen, and sometimes lies horizontally or is malrotated anteriorly
- Feel posteriorly for an enlarged tender spermatic cord (epididymitis) or other masses

Transilluminate for hydrocele

DD Epididymitis, orchitis, torsion of appendix testis, tumor, hernia, hydrocele, hematocele

LB UA (negative), CBC (one-third of patients have leukocytosis); lab preparation for surgery

IM Radionuclide scanning is the diagnostic test of choice, but no test-associated delays should interfere with treatment. Scrotal ultrasound may also be used to identify torsion.

TX Brief attempt at manual detorsion in the emergency department; urologic consult; preparation for immediate surgical detorsion

DI OR

CHAPTER 21

Wounds

GENERAL EVALUATION AND TREATMENT

HX Important factors are:

- Mechanism of injury: simple laceration, crushing injury, CFI, bite wound, puncture
- Age of the wound (golden period for closure: < 6–12 hours depending on location)
- Environment: clean or contaminated
- Patient factors:

  Age (infection is increased if < 2 or > 50 years)

  Preexisting health problems (i.e., diabetes, alcoholism, or immunosuppression)

  Nutritional status, smoking status (smoking delays distal extremity healing)

  Use of medications (i.e., steroids), allergies, and tetanus immunization

PX • Location of the wound (degree of vascularity, stress on the wound, or skin area with high bacteria count) and presence of underlying structures (e.g., nerves, tendons, vascular structures, bones or joints)

- Sensory–motor function (two-point discrimination, ROM, and strength) and circulation (distal pulses, capillary refill time, and color and temperature)

DD Simple laceration, stellate laceration, avulsion, puncture, crush wound, bite, CFI

IM Consider radiograph to check for foreign body or underlying fracture

TX • **Skin preparation** (disinfection of the skin is necessary before any procedure)

  All of the available various soaps and disinfectants should be used only on the skin, not in the wound; disinfectants are known to be toxic to wound tissue, and they may slow healing while increasing the infection rate

  Povidone–iodine and chlorhexidine are two common, excellent skin disinfectants

  Hair may be cut but should not be shaved (never shave the eyebrows)

Table 21.1 Anesthetic Agents Used in Wound Care

Amides:* lidocaine, mepivacaine, bupivacaine
Esters:* procaine, tetracaine, chloroprocaine, benzocaine, cocaine (not for injection)
Antihistamines: diphenhydramine hydrochloride (an amide antihistamine)†
Epinephrine: increases the time of anesthesia and decreases bleeding; because of some resultant increase in the infection rate, this agent should be avoided in infection-prone wounds. *It should also be avoided in areas of distal vascularity (fingers, toes, penis, tip of the nose, and ears).*
Topical agents: TAC (TEC), a mixture of tetracaine, adrenaline (epinephrine), and cocaine is a good local anesthetic. Because of concern about increased infection rates and severe reactions with exposure of TAC to mucous membranes, *TAC should not be allowed to come in contact with mucous membranes.*

*An agent from the amide group may be used in patients who are allergic to the ester group of local anesthetics, and vice versa.
†May be used in patients who are allergic to esters.

- **Wound anesthesia:** direct infiltration (through the wound edge), parallel margin infiltration (field block), or regional blocks (digital blocks are the most common)
    Anesthetic agents (Table 21.1)
    Pain associated with anesthetic administration: buffering anesthetics with $NaHCO_3$ (1 ml $NaHCO_3$ per 10 ml 1% anesthetic) raises the pH to near neutral and decreases the pain of injection); warmed anesthetics also reduce pain
- **Inspection and irrigation:** *the two most important aspects of wound care*
- **Wound inspection** (*this should occur in a bloodless field*):
    Check for foreign bodies and involvement of deep structures (tendons, bones, joints, nerves, vascular structures, and organs)
    Culture all infected wounds but not uninfected (fresh) wounds
    Débride all devitalized tissue and remove all foreign bodies
- **Wound irrigation:** Large volumes (250–2000 ml) of irrigating solution (usually sterile NS) at high pressures are necessary for nearly all wounds; povidone–iodine, other soaps, and hydrogen peroxide should not be used inside wounds. Adequate pressure may be obtained using a 19-gauge Angiocath with a 35-ml syringe.
- **Débridement:** débride necrotic or devitalized tissue using forceps and a scalpel or scissors
- **Wound closure:** most wounds can be closed with nylon sutures through the skin (Table 21.2)
    Suture instructions are beyond the scope of this book; refer to larger texts or ask for demonstrations of suture placement

Table 21.2   Guide to Suture Size and Removal

Location	Suture or Staple Size	Days Until Removal
Scalp*	3–0 or 4–0	7–10
Face*	6–0	3–5
Eyelid*	6–0 or 7–0	3
Ear*	4–0 or 5–0	7–10
Inside mouth†	4–0 or 5–0	7–10
Trunk*	4–0 or 5–0	7–10
Arm*	4–0 or 5–0	10–12
Leg	3–0 or 4–0	12–14
Foot (top)*	4–0 or 5–0	10–12
Foot (bottom)*	3–0 or 4–0	10–12
Other joints	4–0 or 5–0	14
		Days to Dissolve
Subcutaneous tissue or fascia	3–0 or 4–0	7–14 (plain gut)
		20–40 (chromic gut)
		60–90 (Vicryl)
		100–120 (Dexon)

*A monofilament, nonabsorbable suture material (nylon or polypropylene) is preferred.
†Use silk or absorbable sutures (Dexon, Vicryl, or gut).

> In wounds involving deep tissue, subcutaneous sutures may be needed to bring the tissues together; these sutures may increase the rate of infection

- **Wound care:**
  > Antibiotic ointment helps keep the skin soft and promotes healing
  >
  > Dressings absorb fluids from the wound and protect it from contamination
  >
  > Immobilization of a joint with a splint may be necessary (prevents the wound from opening)

DI Immediate referral to the appropriate surgical specialty for large or deep wounds that involve underlying structures; otherwise, patients can be discharged home with care instructions. Pain medication (e.g., acetaminophen with codeine or hydrocodone, NSAIDs) should be prescribed; when the local anesthesia wears off, pain can be expected. Patient instructions include:

- Watch for signs of infection (redness, swelling, pain, and drainage); about 2%–5% of all wounds become infected
- *Keep the wound clean and dry for 1 day and clean thereafter;* the bandage should be changed every day (at this time, the wound may be gently cleaned, and new antibiotic ointment may be applied).
- Have the sutures removed as instructed (see Table 21.2).

BITE WOUNDS

KY Characteristically, 80%–90% of bite wounds are dog bites, 5%–10% are cat bites, 2%–3% are human bites, and 2%–3% are from other animals (e.g., rats, hamsters). Cat bites rank first in terms of infection rate, human bites are second, and dog bites are third.

- All bite wounds should receive proper wound inspection, débridement, and irrigation. Radiographs should be considered for evaluation of deep structures and retained foreign bodies.
- Closure of bite wounds is controversial; if closure is considered, it may be accomplished in a delayed manner in 2–4 days. Wounds to the face can generally be closed primarily, whereas wounds to the hands should generally not be closed primarily.
- Antibiotics (penicillin and a cephalosporin) should be prescribed for most bite wounds; erythromycin and tetracycline should be considered for penicillin-allergic patients
- Frequent follow-up visits to watch for infection are essential

Cat bites

KY Cat bites tend to result in puncture wounds with infection rates approaching 50%. The animals' long, narrow teeth often produce wounds that have a high risk for development of tenosynovitis. Typical causal organisms include *Staphylococcus aureus, Streptococcus* spp., *Klebsiella, Enterobacter* spp., anaerobes, and *Pasteurella multocida.*

HX
- Headache, fever, malaise, and tender regional lymphadenopathy are apparent about 1 week after a cat scratch or bite; a transient macular or vesicular rash may be present
- The immunization and health status of the cat should be determined

PX
- Lymphadenopathy, possible rash, and suppurative lymph nodes
- Local extremity wounds may be red, swollen, and digit partially flexed with tenderness on passive extension

DD Plague, syphilis, lymphogranuloma venereum, sporotrichosis, anthrax, fungal infection, mononucleosis, lymphoma, bacterial adenitis

TX
- Copious irrigation and débridement of devitalized tissue
- Tetanus prophylaxis
- Closure: normal hosts with relatively clean lacerations, especially of the face, can safely be sutured primarily if seen within a few hours of injury; delayed primary closure and healing by secondary intention are less apt to result in infection
- Antibiotic agents: amoxicillin–clavulanate (250 mg tid × 7 days) or penicillin (500 mg tid × 7 days) [first choice]; doxycycline

(100 mg bid × 7 days) or tetracycline (500 mg qid × 7 days) for penicillin-allergic patients (second choices)
- Cat-scratch disease resolves spontaneously in 1–2 months; antibiotics have not been shown to be effective

DI Admission for IV antibiotics for those patients who are septic, immunocompromised, or show infectious signs of CNS, head, joint, or deep structure involvement; all patients who do not require admission should be rechecked in 24–48 hours

Dog bites

KY Dog bites are usually crush-type lacerations with devitalized adjacent tissue. About 10% of all dog bite wounds become infected, with much higher rates in full-thickness bites. The causal organisms are the same as for cat bites (see Bite Wounds, Cat Bites).

HX Circumstances surrounding the bite (time, immunization and health status of the offending animal, and whether it has been captured) and the nature of attack (provoked versus unprovoked) should be obtained

PX Check for wound infection, septic arthritis, and osteomyelitis; if wound infection occurs within 24 hours of the bite, assume that *P. multocida* is the causative agent

IM Consider radiography to check for associated fracture

TX • Irrigation and débridement of devitalized tissue; hand wounds should be explored; wounds should be cultured only if infected
- Tetanus prophylaxis
- Closure:
  Small puncture wounds and lacerations can be cleansed and left open
  Most lacerations, except those of the hand with potential for joint or tendon involvement, should be closed primarily
- Antibiotics: penicillin V (500 mg qid × 7 days) or ampicillin (500 mg qid × 7 days) (first choices); amoxicillin–clavulanate and doxycycline (alternatives)

DI Home (usually); admission if signs of severe infection are present

Human bites

KY Human bites may represent dangerous wounds, especially when distal extremities are involved. Both aerobic and anaerobic bacteria from the mouth may become embedded in the wound, potentially leading to tenosynovitis, septic arthritis, or osteomyelitis if untreated. The infection rate is about 20%.

HX Wounds over the knuckles, ears, nose, tongue, nipples, fingertips, or penis should lead to a suspicion of a human bite

PX • Erythema, swelling, warmth, and purulence, with more pain than would normally be expected
 • Lymphangitis and adenopathy suggest proximal spread of infection and increased risk for sepsis

LB If the patient is immunocompromised, obtain a CBC and SMA-7; consider blood culture if infection is apparent

IM Radiographs of all significant hand wounds and wounds that overlie bones and joints

TX • Copious irrigation and débridement of devitalized tissue
 • Tetanus prophylaxis
 • Closure: facial wounds can be closed if they are free of infection; wounds of the hands and wounds with tendon injury or joint space involvement should be referred to a surgeon
 • Treat fractures as open fractures
 • Antibiotics (to cover *Staphylococcus, Streptococcus, Eikenella corrodens,* and other Gram-negative organisms); if the patient is sent home, treat with:
   Amoxicillin–clavulanate (prophylaxis): 250–500 mg PO tid × 5–7 days [erythromycin (500 mg PO qid) in penicillin-allergic patients]; theoretically, amoxicillin–clavulanate is a good combination drug
   Penicillin (500 mg PO qid) with dicloxacillin (500 mg PO qid) [alternative]

DI • Home (see treatment); wounds should be rechecked in 24 hours
 • Admission, after receipt of IV antibiotics in the ED, for patients with signs of soft tissue infection, including lymphangitis, adenopathy, or symptoms of systemic infection (e.g., fever, chills, rigors)
 • Admission for immunocompromised patients

CLOSED-FIST INJURIES (CFIS)

KY CFIs frequently occur while individuals are intoxicated, and patients often present to the ED many hours after their injury has taken place.

 • Radiographs of CFIs should be obtained in all cases.
 • Inspection, débridement, and irrigation should be performed.
 • CFIs have a high rate of infection, so patients with these wounds should receive IV antibiotics. Splinting is important to prevent infection. Patients may require admission to a hand surgery service for close follow-up and continued antibiotics.

PUNCTURE WOUNDS

KY Most puncture wounds occur to the feet. In punctures through tennis shoes, *Pseudomonas aeruginosa* infections are a possibility.

- Soaking puncture wounds is not adequate. The wound should be opened, inspected, débrided, irrigated, and left open.
- Prophylactic antibiotics are usually not required. Frequent follow-up visits on days 1, 3, 5, and 7 to watch for infection are recommended.

TETANUS IMMUNIZATION

KY All patients should be evaluated regarding their tetanus immunization status. Proper wound management (débridement and irrigation) is the most significant component of the prevention of tetanus. Table 21.3 provides guidelines for tetanus immunization.

Table 21.3   Guidelines for Tetanus Immunization*

History	Non–tetanus-prone Wounds	Tetanus-prone Wounds[†]
Unknown or less than three injections	Td	Td plus tetanus immune globulin
At least three injections (last injection: 0–5 years)	None	None
At least three injections (last injection: 5–10 years)	None	Td
At least three injections (last injection: 10+ years)	Td	Td

*Tetanus immunizations are safe in pregnancy.
[†]Tetanus-prone wounds are characterized by one or more of the following: > 6 hours old; contaminated, infected, or nonviable tissue; puncture, crush, or missile wound; burn or frostbite.

Advanced Cardiac Life Support (ACLS) Algorithms

VENTRICULAR FIBRILLATION/PULSELESS VENTRICULAR TACHYCARDIA (VF/VT) ALGORITHM

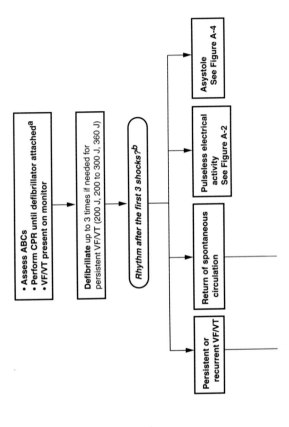

- Assess ABCs
- Perform CPR until defibrillator attached[a]
- VF/VT present on monitor

Defibrillate up to 3 times if needed for persistent VF/VT (200 J, 200 to 300 J, 360 J)

Rhythm after the first 3 shocks?[b]

Persistent or recurrent VF/VT

Return of spontaneous circulation

Pulseless electrical activity
See Figure A-2

Asystole
See Figure A-4

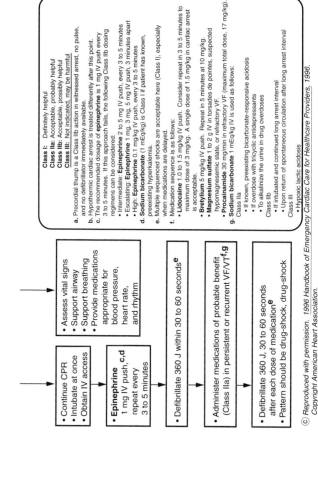

Class I: Definitely helpful
Class IIa: Acceptable, probably helpful
Class IIb: Acceptable, possibly helpful
Class III: Not indicated, may be harmful

- Continue CPR
- Intubate at once
- Obtain IV access

- **Epinephrine**
  1 mg IV push,^c,d
  repeat every
  3 to 5 minutes

- Assess vital signs
- Support airway
- Support breathing
- Provide medications appropriate for blood pressure, heart rate, and rhythm

- Defibrillate 360 J within 30 to 60 seconds^e

- Administer medications of probable benefit (Class IIa) in persistent or recurrent VF/VT^f,g

- Defibrillate 360 J, 30 to 60 seconds after each dose of medication^e
- Pattern should be drug-shock, drug-shock

a. Precordial thump is a Class IIb action in witnessed arrest, no pulse, and no defibrillator immediately available.
b. Hypothermic cardiac arrest is treated differently after this point.
c. The recommended dosage of **epinephrine** is 1 mg IV push every 3 to 5 minutes. If this approach fails, the following Class IIb dosing regimens can be considered:
   - Intermediate: **Epinephrine** 2 to 5 mg IV push, every 3 to 5 minutes
   - Escalating: **Epinephrine** 1 mg, 3 mg, 5 mg IV push, 3 minutes apart
   - High: **Epinephrine** 0.1 mg/kg IV push, every 3 to 5 minutes
d. **Sodium bicarbonate** (1 mEq/kg) is Class I if patient has known, preexisting hyperkalemia.
e. Multiple sequenced shocks are acceptable here (Class I), especially when medications are delayed.
f. Medication sequence is as follows:
   - **Lidocaine** 1.0 to 1.5 mg/kg IV push. Consider repeat in 3 to 5 minutes to maximum dose of 3 mg/kg. A single dose of 1.5 mg/kg in cardiac arrest is acceptable.
   - **Bretylium** 5 mg/kg IV push. Repeat in 5 minutes at 10 mg/kg.
   - **Magnesium sulfate** 1 to 2 g IV in torsades de pointes, suspected hypomagnesemic state, or refractory VF.
   - **Procainamide** 30 mg/min in refractory VF (maximum total dose, 17 mg/kg).
g. **Sodium bicarbonate** 1 mEq/kg IV is used as follows:
   Class IIa
   - If known, preexisting bicarbonate-responsive acidosis
   - If overdose with tricyclic antidepressants
   - To alkalinize the urine in drug overdoses
   Class IIb
   - If intubated and continued long arrest interval
   - Upon return of spontaneous circulation after long arrest interval
   Class III
   - Hypoxic lactic acidosis

PULSELESS ELECTRICAL ACTIVITY (PEA) ALGORITHM

PEA includes the following:
- Electromechanical dissociation (EMD)
- Pseudo-EMD
- Idioventricular rhythms
- Ventricular escape rhythms
- Bradyasystolic rhythms
- Postdefibrillation idioventricular rhythms

- Continue CPR
- Intubate at once
- Obtain IV access

- Assess blood flow using Doppler ultrasound, end-tidal CO_2, echocardiography, or arterial line

Consider possible causes
(Possible therapies are given in parentheses.)

- Hypovolemia (volume infusion)
- Hypoxia (ventilation)
- Cardiac tamponade (pericardiocentesis)
- Tension pneumothorax (needle decompression)
- Hypothermia
- Massive pulmonary embolism (surgery, **thrombolytics**)

- Drug overdoses, such as tricyclics, digitalis, beta-blockers, calcium channel blockers
- Hyperkalemia[a]
- Acidosis[b]
- Massive acute myocardial infarction

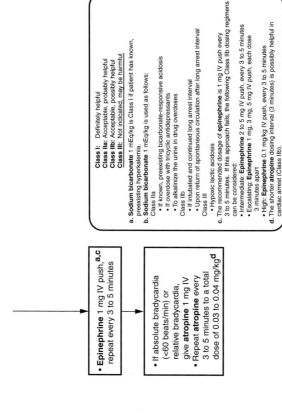

- **Epinephrine** 1 mg IV push,[a,c] repeat every 3 to 5 minutes

- If absolute bradycardia (<60 beats/min) or relative bradycardia, give **atropine** 1 mg IV
- Repeat **atropine** every 3 to 5 minutes to a total dose of 0.03 to 0.04 mg/kg[d]

Class I: Definitely helpful
Class IIa: Acceptable, probably helpful
Class IIb: Acceptable, possibly helpful
Class III: Not indicated, may be harmful

a. **Sodium bicarbonate** 1 mEq/kg is Class I if patient has known, preexisting hyperkalemia.

b. **Sodium bicarbonate** 1 mEq/kg is used as follows:

Class IIa
 • If known, preexisting bicarbonate-responsive acidosis
 • If overdose with tricyclic antidepressants
 • To alkalinize the urine in drug overdoses

Class IIb
 • If intubated and continued long arrest interval
 • Upon return of spontaneous circulation after long arrest interval

Class III
 • Hypoxic lactic acidosis

c. The recommended dosage of **epinephrine** is 1 mg IV push every 3 to 5 minutes. If this approach fails, the following Class IIb dosing regimens can be considered:

 • Intermediate: **Epinephrine** 2 to 5 mg IV push, every 3 to 5 minutes
 • Escalating: **Epinephrine** 1 mg, 3 mg, 5 mg IV push, each dose 3 minutes apart
 • High: **Epinephrine** 0.1 mg/kg IV push, every 3 to 5 minutes

d. The shorter **atropine** dosing interval (3 minutes) is possibly helpful in cardiac arrest (Class IIb).

© Reproduced with permission. 1996 Handbook of Emergency Cardiac Care for Healthcare Providers, 1996. Copyright American Heart Association.

263

TACHYCARDIA ALGORITHM

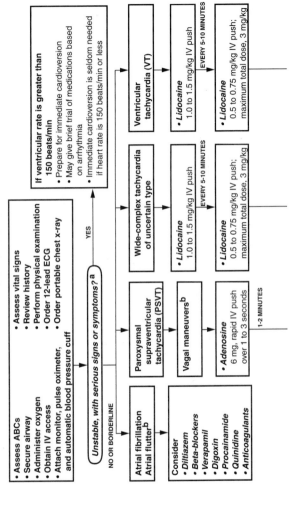

- Assess ABCs
- Secure airway
- Administer oxygen
- Obtain IV access
- Attach monitor, pulse oximeter, and automatic blood pressure cuff

- Assess vital signs
- Review history
- Perform physical examination
- Order 12-lead ECG
- Order portable chest x-ray

Unstable, with serious signs or symptoms?[a]

If ventricular rate is greater than 150 beats/min
- Prepare for immediate cardioversion
- May give brief trial of medications based on arrhythmia
- Immediate cardioversion is seldom needed if heart rate is 150 beats/min or less

YES

NO OR BORDERLINE

Atrial fibrillation
Atrial flutter[b]

Consider
- *Diltiazem*
- *Beta-blockers*
- *Verapamil*
- *Digoxin*
- *Procainamide*
- *Quinidine*
- *Anticoagulants*

Paroxysmal supraventricular tachycardia (PSVT)

Vagal maneuvers[b]

- *Adenosine*
  6 mg, rapid IV push over 1 to 3 seconds

1-2 MINUTES

Wide-complex tachycardia of uncertain type

- *Lidocaine*
  1.0 to 1.5 mg/kg IV push

EVERY 5-10 MINUTES

- *Lidocaine*
  0.5 to 0.75 mg/kg IV push; maximum total dose, 3 mg/kg

Ventricular tachycardia (VT)

- *Lidocaine*
  1.0 to 1.5 mg/kg IV push

EVERY 5-10 MINUTES

- *Lidocaine*
  0.5 to 0.75 mg/kg IV push; maximum total dose, 3 mg/kg

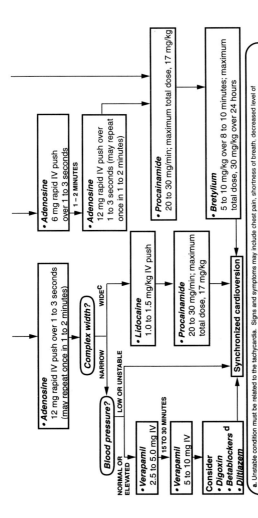

- **Adenosine**
6 mg rapid IV push over 1 to 3 seconds
1 - 2 MINUTES

- **Adenosine**
12 mg rapid IV push over 1 to 3 seconds (may repeat once in 1 to 2 minutes)

- **Procainamide**
20 to 30 mg/min; maximum total dose, 17 mg/kg

- **Bretylium**
5 to 10 mg/kg over 8 to 10 minutes; maximum total dose, 30 mg/kg over 24 hours

- **Adenosine**
12 mg rapid IV push over 1 to 3 seconds (may repeat once in 1 to 2 minutes)

Complex width?

NARROW · WIDE[c]

Blood pressure?

LOW OR UNSTABLE

NORMAL OR ELEVATED

- **Verapamil**
2.5 to 5.0 mg IV
15 TO 30 MINUTES

- **Verapamil**
5 to 10 mg IV

Consider
- **Digoxin**
- **Betablockers** [d]
- **Diltiazem**

- **Lidocaine**
1.0 to 1.5 mg/kg IV push

- **Procainamide**
20 to 30 mg/min; maximum total dose, 17 mg/kg

Synchronized cardioversion

a. Unstable condition must be related to the tachycardia. Signs and symptoms may include chest pain, shortness of breath, decreased level of consciousness, low blood pressure, shock, pulmonary congestion, congestive heart failure, AMI.

b. Carotid sinus pressure is contraindicated in patients with carotid bruits; avoid ice-water immersion in patients with ischemic heart disease.

c. If the wide-complex tachycardia is known with certainty to be PSVT and blood pressure is normal or elevated, sequence can include **verapamil**.

d. IV **beta-blockers** combined with IV **verapamil** may cause severe hypotension.

© *Reproduced with permission. 1996 Handbook of Emergency Cardiac Care for Healthcare Providers, 1996. Copyright American Heart Association.*

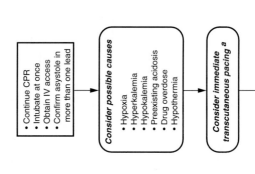

- Continue CPR
- Intubate at once
- Obtain IV access
- Confirm asystole in more than one lead

Consider possible causes

- Hypoxia
- Hyperkalemia
- Hypokalemia
- Preexisting acidosis
- Drug overdose
- Hypothermia

Consider immediate transcutaneous pacing [a]

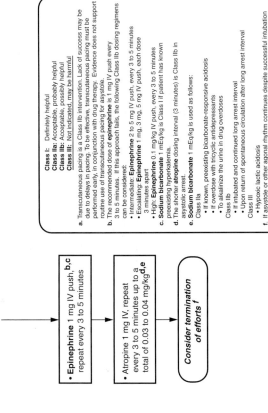

- **Epinephrine** 1 mg IV push, repeat every 3 to 5 minutes [b,c]

- Atropine 1 mg IV, repeat every 3 to 5 minutes up to a total of 0.03 to 0.04 mg/kg [d,e]

Consider termination of efforts [f]

Class I: Definitely helpful
Class IIa: Acceptable, probably helpful
Class IIb: Acceptable, possibly helpful
Class III: Not indicated, may be harmful

a. Transcutaneous pacing is a Class IIb intervention. Lack of success may be due to delays in pacing. To be effective, transcutaneous pacing must be performed early, in conjunction with drug therapy. Evidence does not support routine use of transcutaneous pacing for asystole.

b. The recommended dose of **epinephrine** is 1 mg IV push every 3 to 5 minutes. If this approach fails, the following Class IIb dosing regimens can be considered:
  • Intermediate: **Epinephrine** 2 to 5 mg IV push, every 3 to 5 minutes
  • Escalating: **Epinephrine** 1 mg, 3 mg, 5 mg IV push, each dose 3 minutes apart
  • High: **Epinephrine** 0.1 mg/kg IV push, every 3 to 5 minutes

c. **Sodium bicarbonate** 1 mEq/kg is Class I if patient has known preexisting hyperkalemia.

d. The shorter **atropine** dosing interval (3 minutes) is Class IIb in asystolic arrest.

e. **Sodium bicarbonate** 1 mEq/kg is used as follows:
  Class IIa
    • If known, preexisting bicarbonate-responsive acidosis
    • If overdose with tricyclic antidepressants
    • To alkalinize the urine in drug overdoses
  Class IIb
    • If intubated and continued long arrest interval
    • Upon return of spontaneous circulation after long arrest interval
  Class III
    • Hypoxic lactic acidosis

f. If asystole or other agonal rhythm continues despite successful intubation and initial medications and no reversible causes are identified, a physician may consider termination of resuscitative efforts. Consider duration of arrest.

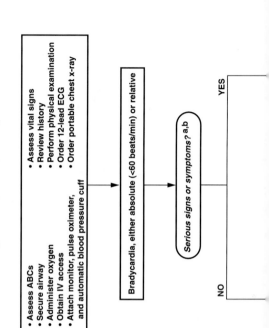

BRADYCARDIA ALGORITHM
(patient is not in cardiac arrest)

- Assess ABCs
- Secure airway
- Administer oxygen
- Obtain IV access
- Attach monitor, pulse oximeter, and automatic blood pressure cuff
- Assess vital signs
- Review history
- Perform physical examination
- Order 12-lead ECG
- Order portable chest x-ray

Bradycardia, either absolute (<60 beats/min) or relative

Serious signs or symptoms? [a,b]

NO   YES

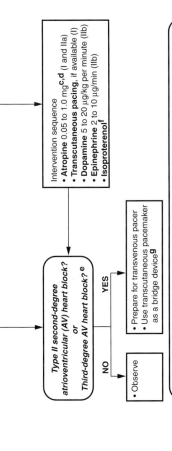

Type II second-degree atrioventricular (AV) heart block?
or
Third-degree AV heart block?[e]

NO
- Observe

YES
- Prepare for transvenous pacer
- Use transcutaneous pacemaker as a bridge device[g]

Intervention sequence
- **Atropine** 0.05 to 1.0 mg[c,d] (I and IIa)
- **Transcutaneous pacing**, if available (I)
- **Dopamine** 5 to 20 µg/kg per minute (IIb)
- **Epinephrine** 2 to 10 µg/min (IIb)
- **Isoproterenol**[f]

a. Serious signs or symptoms must be related to the slow rate. Clinical manifestations include the following:
  - Symptoms (chest pain, shortness of breath, decreased level of consciousness)
  - Signs (low blood pressure, shock, pulmonary congestion, congestive heart failure, AMI)

b. If patient is symptomatic, do not delay transcutaneous pacing while awaiting IV access or for **atropine** to take effect.

c. Denervated transplanted hearts will not respond to **atropine**. Go at once to pacing, **catecholamine** infusion, or both.

d. **Atropine** should be given in repeat doses every 3 to 5 minutes up to a total of 0.03 to 0.04 mg/kg. Use the shorter dosing interval (3 minutes) in severe clinical conditions. It has been suggested that **atropine** should be used with caution in AV block at the His-Purkinje level (type II AV block and new third-degree block with wide QRS complexes) (Class IIb).

e. Never treat third-degree heart block plus ventricular escape beats with **lidocaine**.

f. **Isoproterenol** should be used, if at all, with extreme caution. At low doses it is Class IIb (possibly helpful); at higher doses it is Class III (harmful).

g. Verify patient tolerance and mechanical capture. Use analgesia and sedation as needed.

APPENDIX B

Radiographic Evaluation of Common Interventions

Placement of central IV line

KY A central venous catheter should be located in the superior vena cava, well above the right atrium, and a pulmonary artery catheter centrally and posteriorly, not more than 3–5 cm from the midline. Rule out a pneumothorax by checking that the lung markings extend completely to the ribs on both sides. An upright, end-expiratory CXR may be helpful. Examine the hydropericardium for a "water bottle" sign or mediastinal widening.

Insertion of ET tube

KY Using a CXR, verify that the tube is located 3 cm below the vocal cords, 2–4 cm above the carina, and that its tip is level with the aortic arch.

Tracheostomy

KY Verify by CXR that the tube is located one-half the distance from the stoma to the carina. The tube should be parallel to the long axis of the trachea, and it should be approximately two-thirds the width of the trachea. The cuff should not cause bulging of the trachea walls. Check for subcutaneous air in the neck tissue and for mediastinal widening secondary to air leakage.

Insertion of NG tube

KY Verify that the tube is located in the stomach and not coiled in the esophagus or in trachea using a CXR. The tip of the tube should not be near the gastroesophageal junction.

Insertion of chest tube

KY The tip of a chest tube for drainage of a pneumothorax should be directed posteriorly and superiorly, near the level of the third intercostal space, pointing toward the apex. The tube should be located inferoposteriorly, at or about the level of the eighth intercostal space, to drain a free-flowing pulmonary effusion. Verify that the proximal side port of the tube is within the chest cavity using a CXR.

Use of mechanical ventilator

🄺 After initiation, obtain a CXR to rule out pneumothorax, subcutaneous emphysema, pneumomediastinum, or subpleural air cysts. Infiltrates may diminish or disappear as a result of increased aeration and expansion of the affected lung lobe.

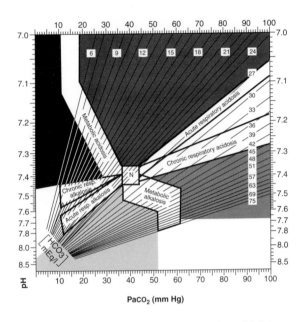

The significance bands for the various simple disorders are labeled on the map. Probable interpretations for points falling in the cross-hatched areas between are:

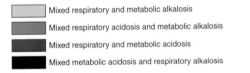

Mixed respiratory and metabolic alkalosis

Mixed respiratory acidosis and metabolic alkalosis

Mixed respiratory and metabolic acidosis

Mixed metabolic acidosis and respiratory alkalosis

Redrawn with permission from Goldberg M: Computer-based instruction and diagnosis of acid-base disorders. *JAMA* 223: 269, 1973.

Goldberg Acid-Base Map

The Goldberg acid-base map can be used to determine the type of acid-base disturbance, as well as to predict the serum bicarbonate value.

Determining the type of acid-base disturbance

1. Obtain the arterial pH and the arterial carbon dioxide ($PaCO_2$) values from an arterial blood gas (ABG) determination, and plot their intersection on the Goldberg acid-base map.
2. If the **point is within a labeled band** (e.g., "metabolic acidosis"), the patient may have a simple acid-base disturbance with its appropriate, physiologic compensation. The patient may also have a mixed acid-base disturbance. The patient's clinical situation can help the physician to determine whether the patient is suffering from a simple or a mixed acid-base disturbance.

   Example: A patient with diabetes but no known respiratory problems has an arterial pH of 7.20 and a $PaCO_2$ of 20 mm Hg. These values intersect within the metabolic acidosis band, suggesting that the patient has a metabolic acidosis with the appropriate compensatory respiratory alkalosis.

   Example: An elderly man with a barrel chest, wheezing, rhonchi, rales, and very mild respiratory distress has an arterial pH of 7.35 and a $PaCO_2$ of 60 mm Hg. A chest radiograph reveals a flattened diaphragm. Plotting the $PaCO_2$ and the pH on the Goldberg acid-base map reveals that the patient most likely has chronic respiratory acidosis with its appropriate compensatory metabolic acidosis, a diagnosis supported by the clinical evidence.

   Example: A previously healthy teenager with a 3-day history of vomiting suffers from aspiration and acute respiratory distress. Like the elderly gentleman in the previous example, the teenager's arterial pH is 7.35 and his $PaCO_2$ is 60 mm Hg, which translates to chronic respiratory alkalosis on the Goldberg acid-base map. However, the clinical situation would suggest that the patient has a mixed acid-base disturbance characterized by a metabolic alkalosis (owing to the protracted vomiting) and an acute respiratory acidosis (owing to the aspiration pneumonia).
3. If the point is outside any of the labeled bands, the patient has at least two primary acid-base disturbances (within 95% probability used to construct the *in vivo* confidence bands).

Example: A patient has an arterial pH of 7.30 and a $Paco_2$ of 20 mm Hg. These values intersect in the area below the metabolic acidosis band and above the two respiratory alkalosis bands, suggesting that the patient has a mixed acid-base disturbance consisting of a metabolic acidosis and a primary (not a compensatory) respiratory alkalosis. The clinical situation can help the physician determine whether the respiratory alkalosis is chronic or acute.

Predicting the serum bicarbonate value

The point where the arterial pH and $Paco_2$ values intersect on the Goldberg acid-base map can be used to predict the serum bicarbonate value. The *bicarbonate lines* run from the lower left to the top and right side of the map. The *bicarbonate values* are shown on the top and right side of the map and are calculated using the Henderson-Hasselbalch equation.

APPENDIX D

Common Medications

Generic Name	Trade Name	Therapeutic Range*
Acetaminophen	Tylenol	< 150 µg/ml (at 4 hr)
Amitriptyline	Elavil	100–250 ng/ml
Aspirin (ASA)	. . .	15–25 mg/dl
Carbamazepine	Tegratol	4–10 µg/ml
Chloramphenicol	Chloromycetin	10–15 µg/ml (peak); < 5 µg/ml (trough)
Digitoxin	. . .	10–30 ng/ml
Digoxin	Lanoxin	0.8–2.0 ng/ml
Disopyramide	Norpace	2–5 µg/ml
Ethosuximide	Zarotin	40–100 µg/ml
Flecainide	Tambocor	0.2–1.0 µg/ml
Gentamicin	Garamycin	6.0–8.0 µg/ml (peak); < 2.0 µg/ml (trough)
Imipramine	Tofranil	150–300 ng/ml
Lidocaine	Xylocaine	2–5 µg/ml
Lithium	Eskalith	0.5–1.4 mEq/L
Nortriptyline	Pamelor	50–150 ng/ml
Phenobarbital	Luminal	10–30 mEq/L
Phenytoin[†]	Dilantin	8–20 µg/ml
Procainamide	Pronestyl	4.0–8.0 µg/ml
Quinidine	Quinaglute	2.5–5.0 µg/ml
Theophylline	Theo-Dur	8–20 µg/ml
Valproic acid	Depakene	50–100 µg/ml
Vancomycin	Vancocin	30–40 µg/ml (peak); < 10 µg/ml (trough)

*Values may vary depending on the laboratory used.
[†]The therapeutic level of phenytoin is 4–10 µg/ml in cases of significant azotemia and/or hypoalbuminemia.

Dermatomes

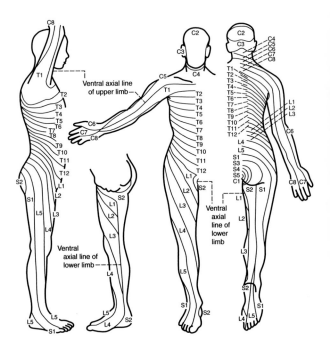

INDEX

*Page numbers in *italics* denote figures; those followed by a *t* denote tables.

Abdominal aortic aneurysm, 1
Abdominal pain
  acute, 49–50
  somatic, 49
  visceral, 49
Abdominal trauma, 221–224
Abortions, types of, 151
Abruptio placentae, 153
Abscess
  anorectal, 16
  cutaneous, 16
  peritonsillar, 76–77
  retropharyngeal, 179–180
Acetaminophen toxicity, 199, *200*
Acid-base disorders
  metabolic acidosis, 127, *127*
  metabolic alkalosis, 128
  respiratory acidosis, 128–129
  respiratory alkalosis, 129
Acid-base disturbance, 272–273
Acidosis
  anion gap metabolic, 202–203, 203*t*
  metabolic, 127, *127*
  respiratory, 128–129
Acquired immunodeficiency syndrome (AIDS), 93–94
Activated charcoal, 198
Acute abdominal pain, 49–50
Acute aortic dissection, 1–2
Acute aspirin poisoning, 215
Acute hemolytic transfusion reaction, 91
Acute myocardial infarction (AMI), 2–3, 4*t*
Acute urinary retention, 243
Adrenal crisis, 32
Advanced Cardiac Life Support (ACLS), *260–269*

Airway management, 220
  and intubation, 186, 187*t,* 188*t*
Albuterol for asthma, 188
Alcohol poisoning, 201–202
Alcoholic ketoacidosis, 32–33
Alkalis, 207
Alkalosis
  metabolic, 128
  respiratory, 129
Allergic emergencies. (*See* Rheumatologic/allergic emergencies)
Allergic rhinitis, 193
Altered mental status (AMS), 52
  causes of, *134*
  and coma, 133, 133*t*
  physical findings and causes in, 134*t*
Amenorrhea, 155–156
Amides in wound care, 252*t*
Amoxicillin for chlamydial disease, 119
Ampicillin
  for epiglottitis, 100
  for meningitis, 107
Amputation, *164*
Amyotrophic lateral sclerosis, 135
Analgesia/sedation, 171, 172*t*
Anaphylaxis, 194–195
Anemia, 85–87
  chronic, 85
  hemorrhagic, 85, 86
Anesthetic agents for wound care, 252*t*
Aneurysm, abdominal aortic, 1
Angina, Ludwig's, 74, 75
Angioedema, 194
Anion gap, 202
  elevated, 127
  metabolic acidosis, 202–203, 203*t*
  normal, 127

Anorectal abscess, 16
Anorexia nervosa, 181
Ant stings, 42–43
Anterior uveitis, 77, 78, 80
Antibiotic-associated colitis, 95
Antibiotics for chronic obstructive pulmonary disease (COPD), 190
Anticholinergic toxicity, 203–204
Anticoagulation therapy for atrial fibrillation, 6
Antiemetics for conjunctivitis, 80
Antihistamines in wound care, 252t
Antipsychotic toxicity, 204–205
Antiretroviral therapy for human immunodeficiency virus (HIV) infection, 94
Anxiolytic for acute myocardial infarction (AMI), 4
Aortic disruption, 227
Aortic dissection, acute, 1–2
Aplastic crisis, 90
Apley compression test, 165
Apnea, 172–173
Apparent life-threatening episode (ALTE), 173
Appendicitis, 50–51
Arrhythmias, asystole, 4–5
Arteritis, 140
Arthritis
  crystal-induced, 197
  hemorrhagic, 197
  infectious, 197
  monarticular, 195, 195t, 196t, 197
  septic, 117–118
Aspirin poisoning, acute, 215
Asthma, 186, 188–189
Asystole, 4–5
Athlete's foot, 21, 22
Atrial fibrillation, 6
  flutter, 6–7
  paroxysmal supraventricular tachycardia, 7–8
    premature ventricular contractions, 8
    pulseless electrical activity, 8–9
    ventricular, 9
    ventricular tachycardia, 9–10
Atrial flutter, 6–7
Atropine
  for pediatric resuscitation, 170t
  in rapid-sequence induction, 187t
Auditory canal, foreign bodies in, 72
Azithromycin for gonorrheal infection, 120

β-Blockers
  for acute myocardial infarction (AMI), 3
  for atrial fibrillation, 6
  for atrial flutter, 7
  for conjunctivitis, 80
  overdose of, 205
Bacterial skin infections
  cutaneous abscess, 16
  impetigo, 16–17
  meningococcemia, 17
  Rocky Mountain spotted fever, 17–18
  scarlet fever, 18
Bee stings, 42–43
Benzodiazepines
  for panic disorder, 185
  toxicity of, 217
Bite wounds, 254–256
Black widow spiders, bites of, 43–44
Bleeding, gastrointestinal (GI) tract, 55–56
Blepharitis, marginal, 103
Blood destruction disorders, 86
Blood production disorders, 85
Bloody show, 149

Blunt trauma, 222
Boutonnière deformity, *164*
Bradycardia, 168, 170
Bretylium for pediatric
    resuscitation, 170*t*
Bronchiolitis, 173–174
Bronchodilators
    for chronic obstructive pulmonary
        disease (COPD), 190
    for congestive heart failure
        (CHF), 12
Brown-recluse spider bites, 44–45
Brudzinski's sign, 98
Bulimia nervosa, 181–182
Burns, 224–225, *226, 227*

Calcium channel blocker
        overdose, 205
Calcium channel blockers
    for atrial flutter, 7
    overdose of, 205
Candida albicans, 20
Candida cystitis, 97
Candidiasis, 20–21
    vulvovaginal, 69
Carbon monoxide poisoning, 206
Carbonic anhydrase inhibitors for
        conjunctivitis, 80
Carbuncle, 16
Cardiac dysrhythmias, 168
Cardiovascular emergencies
    abdominal aortic aneurysm
        (AAA), 1
    acute aortic dissection, 1–2
    acute myocardial infarction
        (AMI), 2–3, 4*t*
    arrhythmias, 4–5
        asystole, 4–5
    atrial fibrillation, 6
        flutter, 6–7
        paroxysmal supraventricular
            tachycardia, 7–8

pulseless electrical activity,
    8–9
ventricular contractions, 8
ventricular fibrillation, 9
ventricular tachycardia, 9–10
    chest pain, 10, 11*t, 12t*
    congestive heart failure, 10–12
    hypertensive, 13–14, 13*t*
    pulmonary embolism, 14–15
    syncope, 15
Cardioversion
    for atrial fibrillation, 6
    for atrial flutter, 7
Carpal tunnel syndrome, 157
Cat bites, 254–255
Caustic ingestions, 207
Cefaclor for impetigo, 17
Cefamandole for
        meningococcemia, 17
Cefotaxime
    for epiglottitis, 100
    for meningitis, 107
    for meningococcemia, 17
Cefoxitin for pelvic inflammatory
        disease (PID), 64–65
Ceftizoxime for
        meningococcemia, 17
Ceftriaxone
    for epiglottitis, 100
    for gonorrheal infection, 120
    for meningitis, 107
    for meningococcemia, 17
    for pelvic inflammatory disease
        (PID), 64–65
Cefuroxime
    for epiglottitis, 100
    for meningococcemia, 17
Cellulitis, 16, 124–125, 173–174
    facial, 75
    of odontogenic origin, 74
Central IV line, placement of, 270
Central nervous system (CNS)
        toxoplasmosis, 94
Central vertigo, 82

Cerebellar hemorrhage, 137*t*

Cerebrovascular accident (CVA), 135–137

signs and symptoms of, 137*t*

Cervical spondylosis, *134,* 135

Charcoal, activated, 198

Chemical injury, 236

Chemical restraints for management of difficult patients, 184

Chest pain, 10, 11*t,* 12*t*

Chest trauma
aortic disruption, 227
esophageal injury, 228
flail, 228
hemothorax, 229
myocardial contusion, 229–230
pneumothorax, 230–232
pulmonary contusion, 232–233
tension pneumothorax, 233
tracheobronchial injury, 234

Chest tube, insertion of, 219*t,* 229, 270–271

Chickenpox, 29

Child molestation, 65

Chin lift, 220

Chlamydial disease, 119

Chloramphenicol
for epiglottitis, 100
for meningococcemia, 17
for Rocky Mountain spotted fever, 18

Cholecystitis, 51

Cholinergic crises, 144

Chronic anemia, 85

Chronic aspirin poisoning, 215

Chronic obstructive pulmonary disease (COPD), 189–191

Ciprofloxacin for gonorrheal infection (GC), 120

Cirrhosis, 52–53

Clindamycin for pelvic inflammatory disease (PID), 64–65

Closed fractures, 160

Closed-fist injuries (CFIS), 256

Clostridium toxins, 53

Cloxacillin for impetigo, 17

Cluster headache, 138, 140

Cocaine toxicity, 208

Cold-induced tissue injuries, 38

Cold-related conditions
cold-induced tissue injuries, 38
hypothermia, 39

Colitis
antibiotic-associated and pseudomembranous, 95
ulcerative, 57

Coma
causes of, *134*
physical findings and causes in, 134*t*

Compartment syndrome, 157–158

Conception, retained products of, 156

Congestive heart failure (CHF), 10–12

Conjunctivitis, 77, 78, 79–80

Contact dermatitis, 19

Continuous ambulatory peritoneal dialysis (CAPD), 95–96

Contrast enemas, 222

Contrast gastroduodenography, 222

Conversion disorders, 182–183

Corneal abrasion, 77, 79

Corneal laceration, 77, 78

Corneal ulceration, 77

Coronary artery bypass graft for acute myocardial infarction (AMI), 4

Cortocosteroids for conjunctivitis, 80

Cricothyrotomy, 221

Crohn's disease, 57

Cryptococcal meningitis, 94

Crystal-induced arthritis, 197

Cutaneous abscess, 16

Cyclic antidepressant overdose, 208–210
Cyst, ovarian, 63
Cystitis, 96–97
Cytomegalovirus (CMV), 94

De Quervain's tenosynovitis, *164*
Debridement, 252
Deep venous thrombosis (DVT), 87–88
Dehydration, 175, 175*t*
Delivery, 150
  emergency, 149–151
Dental emergencies, 70
Dental trauma, 234, 235*t*
Depression and suicide, 183
Dermatitides, 19
  contact dermatitis, 19
  Rhus (toxicodendron) dermatitis, 19
  seborrheic dermatitis, 19–20
Dermatitis
  contact, 19
  Rhus (Toxicodendron), 19
  seborrheic, 19–20
Dermatologic emergencies
  bacterial skin infections
    cutaneous abscess, 16
    impetigo, 16–17
    meningococcemia, 17
    Rocky Mountain spotted fever, 17–18
    scarlet fever, 18
  dermatitides
    contact dermatitis, 19
    Rhus (toxicodendron) dermatitis, 19
    seborrheic dermatitis, 19–20
  erythema nodosum, 20
  fungal infections
    candidiasis, 20–21
    tinea, 21–22

life-threatening dermatoses
  erythema multiforme/Stevens-Johnson syndrome, 22–23
  staphylococcal scalded skin syndrome (SSSS), 23
  toxic epidermal necrolysis (TEN), 23–24
  toxic shock syndrome, 24
papulosquamous eruptions
  pityriasis rosea, 24–25
  psoriasis, 25
  urticaria, 25–26
purpuric lesions
  Henoch-Schönlein, 26
  idiopathic thrombocytopenic purpura (ITP), 26–27
  thrombotic thrombocytopenic purpura, 27
vesicular lesions (herpetic)
  herpes simplex, 27–28
  herpes zoster (shingles), 28–29
  varicella (chickenpox), 29
viral exanthems
  roseola, 29–30
  rubella (German measles), 30
  rubeola (measles), 30–31
Dermatomes, *276*
Dexamethasone for meningitis, 107
Diabetic ketoacidosis (DKA), 33–34
Dialysis-related emergencies, 244–245
Diarrhea, 53
Diazepam for pediatric resuscitation, 170*t*
Digoxin
  for atrial fibrillation, 6
  for congestive heart failure (CHF), 12
  toxicity of, 210–211
Disk herniation, 166
Dislocations, 158–159

Disseminated intravascular coagulation (DIC), 88–89
Diverticular disease, 54
Dobutamine for congestive heart failure (CHF), 12
Dog bites, 255
Dopamine for pediatric resuscitation, 170*t*
"Double-blind" edrophonium test, 145
Doxycycline
  for chlamydial disease, 119
  for gonorrheal infection, 120
Dysfunctional uterine bleeding, 61
Dysmenorrhea, 61–62

Eating disorders
  anorexia nervosa, 181
  bulimia nervosa, 181–182
Eaton-Lambert syndrome, 145
Eclampsia, 153
Ectopic pregnancy, 148–149
Edrophonium, 145
Electrical injuries, 39–40
Elevated anion gap, 127
Emergency delivery, 149–151
Emergent angioplasty for acute myocardial infarction, 3
Encephalitis, 97–98
Endocarditis, 98–99
Endocrinologic emergencies
  adrenal crisis, 32
  alcoholic ketoacidosis, 32–33
  diabetic ketoacidosis, 33–34
  hypoglycemia, 34
  nonketotic hyperosmolar coma, 34–35
  thyroid disorders
    hypothyroidism and myxedema coma, 35–36
    thyroid storm, 36
  Wernicke-Korsakoff syndrome, 37

Endometriosis, 62–63
Enemas, contrast, 222
Enterobiasis, 110, 111
Environmental emergencies
  cold-related conditions
    cold-induced tissue injuries, 38
    hypothermia, 39
  electrical injuries, 39–40
  heat-related conditions, 40–41
  high-pressure injection injuries, 41–42
  insect and spider bites and stings
    bee, wasp, and ant stings, 42–43
    black widow spiders, 43–44
    brown-recluse spider bites, 44–45
    mosquito and fly bites, 45
  smoke inhalation, 45–46
  snakebite, 46–47
  submersion injuries, 47–48
Epididymitis, 245–246
Epidural hematomas, 239
Epiglottitis, 99–100
Epinephrine
  for asthma, 188
  for pediatric resuscitation, 170*t*
  in wound care, 252*t*
Epistaxis, 71–72
Erysipelas, 125–126
Erythema multiforme/Stevens-Johnson syndrome, 22–23
Erythema nodosum, 20
Erythromycin
  for chlamydial disease, 119
  for gonorrheal infection, 120
  for impetigo, 17
  for scarlet fever, 18
Esophageal injury, 228
Esters in wound care, 252*t*
ET intubation, 220
ET tube, insertion of, 270

Ethylene glycol toxicity, 201
Euvolemic hyponatremia, 132
Extensor tendon injury, *164*
Eye
 foreign bodies in, 77, 78, 79
 trauma to, 234–236

Facial cellulitis, 75
Facial trauma
 dental, 234, 235*t*
 eye, 234–236
 Le Fort's fractures, 236–237
 mandibular, 237–238
 midfacial fractures, 238
Febrile seizure, 145–146
Febrile transfusion reaction, 91
Fentanyl in rapid-sequence
  induction, 187*t*
Fetal distress, 150
Fever, 175–176, 177*t*
First-degree burn, 224
First-trimester hemorrhage, 151
Fistula test, 82
Flail chest, 228
Fleas, 103–104
Flexor tendon injury, *164*
Fly bites, 45
Focal seizure, 145
Folliculitis, 16
Foreign bodies, 72–74
 in airway, 74, 168
 in auditory canal, 72
 in eye, 77, 78, 79
 in nasal passages, 73–74
 in upper airway, 74
Fractures, 159–161
 closed, 160
 complications of, 159*t*
 Le Fort's, 236–237
 mandibular, 237–238
 midfacial, 238
 nondisplaced, 160

 open, 160
 pelvic, 166–167
 Salter-Harris classification of
   physeal, *161*
 spinal, 241*t*
 terms used to describe, 160
 types of, 160
Frostbite, 38
Fungal infections
 candidiasis, 20–21
 tinea, 21–22
Furosemide for congestive heart
  failure, 12
Furuncle, 16

Ganglion cyst, *164*
Gangrene, gas, 126
Gas gangrene, 126
Gastric lavage, 198
Gastroduodenography, contrast,
  222
Gastrointestinal emergencies
 acute abdominal pain, 49–50
 appendicitis, 50–51
 bleeding, 55–56
 cholecystitis, 51
 cirrhosis, 52–53
 diarrhea, 53
 diverticular disease, 54
 inflammatory bowel disease,
   56–57, 56*t*
 intestinal obstruction, 57–58
 pancreatitis, 58–59
 peptic ulcer disease, 59–60
Gastrointestinal tract
 bleeding in, 55–56
 candidiasis in, 94
Generalized seizure, 145
German measles, 30
Gestational hypertension,
  153–154
Giardiasis, 110, 111

Glasgow Coma Scale, 133t
Glaucoma, 77, 78, 84
Globe penetration, 236
Goldberg acid-base map, *272,*
    273–274
Gonorrheal infection, 119–121
Grand mal seizure, 145
Gynecologic emergencies
    dysfunctional uterine bleeding, 61
    dysmenorrhea, 61–62
    endometriosis, 62
    Mittelschmerz, 63
    ovarian cyst, 63
    ovarian torsion, 64
    pelvic inflammatory disease,
        64–65
    sexual assault, 65–67
    uterine leiomyoma, 67
    vaginal infections
        vaginitis, 67–68
        vaginosis (bacterial), 68–69
        vulvovaginal candidiasis, 69

Hall-Pike maneuver, 82–83
Hallucinogen use, 211–212
Hand
    infections in, 161–162
    injuries to, 162, 163, 164t
Head and neck emergencies
    dental, 70
    epistaxis, 71–72
    foreign bodies, 72–74
    infection of mouth and salivary
        glands, 74–75
    neck mass, 75–76
    peritonsillar abscess, 76–77
    red eye, 77–80, 79t
    temporomandibular joint (TMJ)
        problems, 80–81
    tonsillitis, 81–82
    vertigo, 82–84, 83t
    vision loss (sudden), 84

Head trauma, 239–240
Headache, 138, 140–141
    cluster, 138, 140
    migraine, 138
    types of, 139–140t
Heat exhaustion, 41
Heat-related conditions, 40–41
Hematologic/oncologic
        emergencies, 85, 86t
    anemia, 85–87
    deep venous thrombosis, 87–88
    disseminated intravascular
        coagulation, 88–89
    heparin overdose, 89–90
    sickle-cell crisis, 90–91
    transfusion reaction, 91–92
    warfarin overdose, 92
Hematomas
    epidural, 239
    subdural, 239
Hematuria, 246–247
Hemolytic crisis, 90
Hemolytic transfusion reaction,
        acute, 91
Hemoptysis, 191
Hemorrhage
    cerebellar, 137t
    first-trimester, 151
    intracranial, 141–142
    pontine, 137t
    postpartum, 152
    putamen, 137t
    third-trimester, 152–153
Hemorrhagic anemia, 85, 86
Hemorrhagic arthritis, 197
Hemorrhagic shock, 221
Hemothorax, 229
Henoch-Schönlein purpura, 26
Heparin
    for acute myocardial infarction
        (AMI), 4
    overdose of, 89–90
    for pulmonary embolism, 14
Hepatic encephalopathy, 53

Hepatitis, 101–102
Herpes simplex, 27–28
Herpes simplex virus (HSV), 94,
    102–103
Herpes zoster, 28–29, 94
High-pressure injection injuries,
    41–42
Hip fractures and dislocations, 162
Human bites, 255–256
Human immunodeficiency virus
    (HIV), 93
Human papillomavirus (HPV),
    121
Hydralazine for hypertensive
    emergencies, 13
Hyperemesis gravidarum,
    154–155
Hyperkalemia, 129–130
Hypernatremia, 130–131
Hyperosmotic agents for
    conjunctivitis, 80
Hypertension, gestational,
    153–154
Hypertensive emergencies,
    13–14, 13*t*
Hypervolemic hyponatremia, 132
Hypoglycemia, 34
Hypokalemia, 131
Hyponasal voice, 179
Hyponatremia, 132
Hypothermia, 39
Hypothyroidism and myxedema
    coma, 35–36
Hypovolemic hyponatremia, 132
Hypoxia, 168

Idiopathic thrombocytopenic
    purpura (ITP), 26–27
Immersion foot, 38
Immunization, 176, 178*t*
    tetanus, 257, 257*t*
Impetigo, 16–17
Infantile spasm, 146

Infections
    bacterial skin, 16–18
    fungal, 20–22
    gonorrheal, 120
    of mouth and salivary glands,
        74–75
    opportunistic, 94
    parasitic, 110–111
    soft tissue, 124–126
Infectious arthritis, 197
Infectious disease emergencies
    acquired immunodeficiency
        syndrome (AIDS), 93–94
    antibiotic-associated and
        pseudomembranous colitis, 95
    continuous ambulatory peritoneal
        dialysis (CAPD), 95–96
    cystitis, 96–97
    encephalitis, 97–98
    endocarditis, 98–99
    epiglottitis, 99–100
    hepatitis, 101–102
    herpes simplex virus (HSV),
        102–103
    infestations (mites, lice, and
        fleas), 103–104
    Lyme disease, 104–106
    meningitis, 106–108
    osteomyelitis, 108–109,
        109*t*, 110*t*
    parasitic, 110–111
    pharyngitis, 111–112
    pneumonia, 112–113, 114–115*t*
    pyelonephritis, 96–97
    scarlet fever, 113, 116
    sepsis, 116–117
    septic arthritis, 117–118
    sexually transmitted disease
        (STD)
        chlamydial, 119
        gonorrheal, 119–121
        human papillomavirus
            (HPV), 121
        syphilis, 121–123

sinusitis, 123–124
soft tissue infections
cellulitis, 124–125
erysipelas, 125–126
myonecrosis (gas gangrene),
126
Infestations (mites, lice, and
fleas), 103–104
Inflammatory bowel disease,
56–57, 56t
Insect bites and stings
bee, wasp, and ant stings, 42–43
mosquito and fly bites, 45
Intestinal obstruction, 57–58
Intracranial hemorrhage, 141–142
Intubation
nasotracheal, 186, 188t
orotracheal, 186, 187t
Iron (Fe) toxicity, 212–213
Isopropyl alcohol, 202
ingestion of, 201
Isoproterenol for pediatric
resuscitation, 170t
Isovolemic hyponatremia, 132

Jaundice, 52
Jaw thrust, 220
Jet insufflation, 221

Kernig's sign, 98
Ketoacidosis, alcoholic, 32–33
Kleihauer-Betke test, 224
Knee soft tissue injuries, 162

Labetalol for hypertensive
emergencies, 13
Landry-Guillain Barré syndrome,
142–143

Laryngotracheobronchitis (croup),
178–179
Le Fort's fractures, 236–237
Lens displacement, 236
Lice, 103, 104
Lidocaine
for pediatric resuscitation, 170t
in rapid-sequence induction, 187t
Life-threatening dermatoses
erythema multiforme/Stevens-
Johnson syndrome, 22–23
staphylococcal scalded skin
syndrome (SSSS), 23
toxic epidermal necrolysis
(TEN), 23–24
toxic shock syndrome, 24
Low back complaints, 165–166
Ludwig's angina, 74, 75
Lyme disease, 98, 104–106

Magnesium sulfate for acute
myocardial infarction
(AMI), 4
Malaria, 111
Mallet finger, 164
Mandibular fractures, 237–238
Marginal blepharitis, 103
Maxillofacial trauma, 219
Measles, 30–31
Mechanical ventilator, use of, 271
Medications, common, 274t
Meningitis, 106–108
Meningococcemia, 17
Metabolic acidosis, 127, 127
Metabolic alkalosis, 128
Metabolic emergencies
acid-base disorders, metabolic
acidosis, 127, 127
hyperkalemia, 129–130
hypernatremia, 130–131
hypokalemia, 131
hyponatremia, 132

Metaproterenol for asthma, 188

Methanol toxicity, 201

Midazolam in rapid-sequence induction, 187*t*

Midfacial fractures, 238

Migraine headache, 138

Miotics for conjunctivitis, 80

Mites, 103, 104

Mittelschmerz, 63

Monarticular arthritis (hot joint), 195, 195*t*, 196*t*, 197

Morphine sulfate for congestive heart failure (CHF), 12

Mosquito bites, 45

Multiple sclerosis (MS), 143–144

Myasthenia gravis, *144*, 144–145

Myasthenic crises, 144

Mycoplasma pneumoniae, 173

Myocardial contusion, 229–230

Myocardial infarction, acute, 2–3, 4*t*

Myonecrosis, 126

NaCl-responsive conditions, 128

NaCl-unresponsive conditions, 128

Nafcillin for staphylococcal scalded skin syndrome (SSSS), 23

NaHCO₃ for pediatric resuscitation, 170*t*

Naloxone for pediatric resuscitation, 170*t*

Narcotic overdose, 213

Nasal passages, foreign bodies in, 73–74

Nasogastric tube, insertion of, 270

Nasopharyngeal airway, 220

Nasotracheal intubation, 186, 188*t*

Neck emergencies. (See Head and neck emergencies)

Neck mass, 75–76

Needle cricothyrotomy, 221

Neoplasia, 166

Neurogenic shock, 241

Neuroleptic drugs for management of difficult patients, 184

Neurologic emergencies
altered mental status and coma, 133, 133*t*
amyotrophic lateral sclerosis, 135
cerebrovascular accident, 135–137
headache, 138, 140–141
types of, 139–140*t*
intracranial hemorrhage, 141–142
Landry-Guillain Barré syndrome, 142–143
multiple sclerosis, 143–144
myasthenia gravis, *144,* 144–145
seizures, 145–147

Newborn resuscitation, 168–169, 169*t*, 170*t*

Nitroglycerin
for acute myocardial infarction (AMI), 4
for congestive heart failure (CHF), 12
for hypertensive emergencies, 13

Nitroprusside
for acute aortic dissection, 2
for congestive heart failure (CHF), 12
for hypertensive emergencies, 13

Nonallergic rhinitis, 193

Nondisplaced fractures, 160

Nonketotic hyperosmolar coma, 34–35

Norfloxacin for gonorrheal infection, 120

Normal anion gap, 127

Obstetric emergencies
  delivery, 149–151
  ectopic, 148–149
  gestational hypertension,
    153–154
  hemorrhaging
    first-trimester, 151
    postpartum, 152
    third-trimester, 152–153
  hyperemesis gravidarum,
    154–155
  postabortion sepsis, 155
  pregnancy, 155–156
  retained products of conception,
    156
Ocular anatomy, 235
Ocular headache, 141
Ofloxacin for pelvic inflammatory
    disease (PID), 64–65
Oncologic emergencies. (*See*
    Hematologic/oncologic
    emergencies)
Open fractures, 160
Opportunistic infections, 94
Orbital cellulite, 174
Orbital floor fractures, 238
Orbital fracture, 236
Oropharyngeal airway, 220
Orotracheal intubation, 186, 187*t*
Orthopedic emergencies
  carpal tunnel syndrome, 157
  compartment syndrome, 157–158
  dislocations, 158–159
  fractures, 159–161
    complications of, 159*t*
  hand infections, 161–162
  hand injuries, 162, *163*, 164*t*
  hip fractures and dislocations, 162
  knee soft tissue injuries, 162
  low back complaints, 165–166
  pelvic fractures, 166–167
  sprains, 167
  strains, 167
Osmolar gap, 203

Osteomyelitis, 108–109, 109*t*,
    110*t*, 166
Ovarian cyst, 63
Ovarian torsion, 64

Pain management, use of
    medications for, 171, 172*t*
Pancreatitis, 58–59
Panic disorder, 184–185
Papulosquamous eruptions
  pityriasis rosea, 24–25
  psoriasis, 25
  urticaria, 25–26
Parasitic infections, 110–111
Paroxysmal supraventricular
    tachycardia (PSVT), 7–8, 168
Patients, management of difficult,
    183–184
PEA, 170
Pediatric emergencies
  analgesia/sedation, 171, 172*t*
  apnea, 172–173
  bronchiolitis, 173–174
  cellulitis (orbital and
    periorbital), 173–174
  dehydration, 175, 175*t*
  fever, 175–176, 177*t*
  immunization, 176, 178*t*
  laryngotracheobronchitis
    (croup), 178–179
  resuscitation, 168–171, 169*t*, 170*t*
  retropharyngeal abscess, 179–180
Pelvic fractures, 166–167
Pelvic inflammatory disease
    (PID), 64–65
Penetrating trauma, 222
Penicillin G
  for meningococcemia, 17
  for scarlet fever, 18
Penicillin VK for scarlet fever, 18
Pentamidine for phencyclidine
    (PCP), 94

Peptic ulcer disease, 59–60
Pericardial tamponade, 230, 231*t*
Pericardiocentesis, 230, 231*t*
Peripheral vertigo, 82
Peritonsillar abscess, 76–77
Petit mal seizure, 145
Petroleum distillates, 214
Pharyngitis, 111–112, 179
Phenazopyridine
  for cystitis, 96
  for pyelonephritis, 96
Phencyclidine (PCP), 94
Phenobarbital for pediatric
    resuscitation, 170*t*
Phenobarbital poisoning, 217
Phentolamine for hypertensive
    emergencies, 13
Phenytoin pearls, 147
Phenytoin toxicity, 214–215
  symptoms of, 147*t*
Pityriasis rosea, 24–25
Placenta previa, 152–153
Pleural effusion, 191–192
Pneumonia, 112–113, 114–115*t*
  causes of, in patients by age
    group, 112*t*
  types of, 114–115*t*
Pneumothorax, 230–232
Poisoning. (*See* Toxicologic
    emergencies)
Pontine hemorrhage, 137*t*
Postabortion sepsis, 155
Postpartum hemorrhage, 152
Prednisone for phencyclidine
    (PCP), 94
Preeclampsia, 153
Pregnancy, 155–156
  ectopic, 148–149
  trauma in, 223–224
  vaginosis in, 69
Premature ventricular
    contractions (PVCs), 8
Prolapse, 150
Prostatitis, 247–248

Pseudomembranous colitis, 95
Psoriasis, 25
Psychiatric emergencies
  anorexia nervosa, 181
  bulimia nervosa, 181–182
  conversion disorders, 182–183
  depression and suicide, 183
  management of difficult
    patients, 183–184
  panic disorder, 184–185
Pulmonary contusion, 232–233
Pulmonary embolism, 14–15
Pulmonary emergencies
  airway management
    and intubation, 186,
    187*t*, 188*t*
  asthma, 186, 188–189
  chronic obstructive pulmonary
    disease (COPD), 189–191
  hemoptysis, 191
  pleural effusion, 191–192
  respiratory failure and ventilator
    management, 192
  rhinitis, 193
Pulseless electrical activity
    (PEA), 8–9
Puncture wounds, 257
Purpura, Henoch-Schönlein, 26
Purpuric lesions
  Henoch-Schönlein, 26
  idiopathic thrombocytopenic
    purpura (ITP), 26–27
  thrombotic thrombocytopenic
    purpura, 27
Putamen hemorrhage, 137*t*
Pyelonephritis, 96–97

Radiographic evaluation of
    common interventions,
    270–271
Rape, 65
  counseling for, 66

Red blood cells (RBC)
  excessive destruction of, 85
  insufficient production of, 85
Red eye, 77–80, 79*t*
Renal colic, 248–249
Renal failure, 249
Rescue angioplasty for acute
    myocardial infarction
    (AMI), 4
Respiratory acidosis, 128–129
Respiratory alkalosis, 129
Respiratory failure and ventilator
    management, 192
Respiratory syncytial virus
    (RSV), 173
Resuscitation, 168–171,
    169*t*, 170*t*
Retained products of conception,
    156
Retinal artery occlusion, 84
Retinal hemorrhage, 236
Retrobulbar hematoma, 236
Retropharyngeal abscess, 179–180
Rheumatologic/allergic
    emergencies
  anaphylaxis, 194–195
  monarticular arthritis (hot joint),
    195, 195*t*, 196*t*, 197
Rhinitis, 193
Rhus (Toxicodendron) dermatitis,
    19
Rickettsia rickettsii, 17–18
Rocky Mountain spotted fever,
    17–18, 98
Roseola, 29–30
Roth's spots, 99
Rubella, 30
Rubeola, 30–31

Salicylate/nonsteroidal anti-
    inflammatory drug (NSAID)
    toxicity, 215–216

Salter-Harris classification of
    physeal fractures, *161*
Scarlet fever, 18, 113, 116
Seborrheic dermatitis, 19–20
Second-degree burn, 224
Sedation, 171, 172*t*
Sedative-hypnotic overdose, 217
Seizures, 145–147
  types of, 145
Sepsis, 116–117
  postabortion, 155
Septic arthritis, 117–118
Sequestration crisis, 90
Serum bicarbonate value,
    predicting, 274
Sexual assault, 65–67
Sexually transmitted disease
    (STD)
  chlamydial, 119
  gonorrheal, 119–121
  human papillomavirus (HPV),
    121
  syphilis, 121–123
Shingles, 28–29, 94
Shock
  hemorrhagic, 221
  neurogenic, 241
Sickle cell crisis, 90–91
Sinusitis, 123–124
Smoke inhalation, 45–46
Snakebite, 46–47
Soft tissue infections
  cellulitis, 124–125
  erysipelas, 125–126
  myonecrosis (gas gangrene), 126
Somatic abdominal pain, 49
Spectinomycin
  for gonorrheal infection, 120
  for pelvic inflammatory disease
    (PID), 64–65
Spider bites
  black widow, 43–44
  brown recluse, 44–45
Spinal cord trauma, 240–242, 241*t*

Spinal fractures, 241*t*

Spleen and liver injury, 221

Sprains, 167

Stab wounds, 223

Staphylococcal scalded skin syndrome (SSSS), 23

Staphylococcus toxins, 53

Steeple sign, 178

Steroids
  for asthma, 188
  for chronic obstructive pulmonary disease (COPD), 190

Strains, 167

Subarachnoid hemorrhage (SAH), 141

Subdural hematomas, 239

Submersion injuries, 47–48

Subungual hematoma, *164*

Succinylcholine in rapid-sequence induction, 187*t*

Suction, 220

Sudden infant death syndrome (SIDS), 172–173

Supraventricular VT, 171

Suture size and removal, 253*t*

Syncope for pulmonary embolism, 15

Synovial fluid characteristics, 196*t*

Syphilis, 121–123
  stages of, 122*t*

Temporal arteritis, 84

Temporal lobe seizure, 145

Temporomandibular joint (TMJ) problems, 80–81

Tenosynovitis, 254

Tension headache, 141

Tension pneumothorax, 233

Terbutaline for asthma, 188

Testicular torsion, 250

Tetanus immunization, 257, 257*t*

Tetracycline
  for chlamydial disease, 119
  for Rocky Mountain spotted fever, 18

Thiopental in rapid-sequence induction, 187*t*

Third-degree burn, 225

Third-trimester hemorrhage, 152–153

Thrombolytic therapy
  for acute myocardial infarction (AMI), 3, 3*t*, 4*t*
  for pulmonary embolism, 15

Thrombotic thrombocytopenic purpura, 27

Thumb sign, 178

Thyroid disorders
  hypothyroidism and myxedema coma, 35–36
  thyroid storm, 36

Thyroid storm, 36

Tinea, 21–22

Tinea capitis, 21, 22

Tinea corporis, 21, 22

Tinea cruris, 21

Tinea pedis, 21, 22

Tinea unguium, 21, 22

Tinea versicolor, 22

Todd's paralysis, 146

Tonsillitis, 81–82

Tooth avulsion, 70

Tooth fracture, 70

Topical agents in wound care, 252*t*

Toxic epidermal necrolysis (TENS), 23–24

Toxic shock syndrome (TSS), 24

Toxicologic emergencies
  acetaminophen toxicity, 199, *200*
  alcohol poisoning, 201–202
  anion gap metabolic acidosis, 202–203, 203*t*

anticholinergic toxicity,
203–204
antipsychotic toxicity, 204–205
β-Blockers/calcium channel
blocker overdose, 205
carbon monoxide poisoning, 206
caustic ingestions, 207
cocaine toxicity, 208
cyclic antidepressant overdose,
208–210
digoxin toxicity, 210–211
general evaluation and
treatment, 198–199
hallucinogen use, 211–212
iron (Fe) toxicity, 212–213
narcotic overdose, 213
petroleum distillates, 214
phenytoin toxicity, 214–215
salicylate/nonsteroidal anti-
inflammatory drug,
215–216
sedative-hypnotic overdose, 217
Tracheobronchial injury, 234
Tracheostomy, 270
Transfusion reaction, 91–92
Trauma
abdominal, 221–224
burns, 224–225, 226, 227
chest
aortic disruption, 227
esophageal injury, 228
flail, 228
hemothorax, 229
myocardial contusion,
229–230
pneumothorax, 230–232
pulmonary contusion,
232–233
tension pneumothorax, 233
tracheobronchial injury, 234
facial
dental, 234, 235t
eye, 234–236
Le Fort's fractures, 236–237

mandibular, 237–238
midfacial fractures, 238
general evaluation
primary survey, 218, 219t
secondary survey, 218–221
head, 239–240
spinal cord, 240–242, 241t
Trichomoniasis, 67–68
Tuberculosis (TB), 94

Ulcerative colitis, 57
Upper airway, foreign bodies in,
74, 168
Urinary retention, acute, 243
Urogenital emergencies
acute urinary retention, 243
dialysis-related, 244–245
epididymitis, 245–246
hematuria, 246–247
prostatitis, 247–248
renal colic, 248–249
renal failure, 249
testicular torsion, 250
Urticaria, 25–26, 194
Uterine leiomyoma, 67
Uveitis, anterior, 78, 80

Vaginal infections
vaginitis (trichomoniasis),
67–68
vaginosis (bacterial), 68–69
vulvovaginal candidiasis, 69
Vaginosis (bacterial), 68–69
Varicella, 29
Vaso-occlusive crisis, 90
Ventricular fibrillation, 9, 168
Ventricular tachycardia (VT),
9–10, 168, 171
Vercuronium in rapid-sequence
induction, 187t

Versicolor, 22
Vertigo, 82–84, 83*t*
Vesicular lesions (herpetic)
　herpes simplex, 27–28
　herpes zoster, 28–29
　varicella, 29
VF/pulseless VT, 171
Viral exanthems
　roseola, 29–30
　rubella, 30
　rubeola, 30–31
Visceral abdominal pain, 49
Vision loss, 84
Vitreous hemorrhage, 236
Vulvovaginal candidiasis, 69

Warfarin overdose, 92
Wasp stings, 42–43
Wernicke-Korsakoff syndrome,
　37

Wolff-Parkinson-White syndrome,
　168
Wounds
　bite, 256
　care of, 253
　closed-fist injuries, 256
　closure of, 252–253, 253*t*
　general evaluation and
　　treatment, 251–253,
　　252*t*, 253*t*
　inspection of, 252
　irrigation of, 252
　puncture wounds, 257
　tetanus immunization, 257, 257*t*

Zygomatic arch fracture, 238
Zygomatic-maxillary complex,
　238